The Bloomsbury Companion to
Contemporary Philosophy of Medicine

Bloomsbury Companions

The *Bloomsbury Companions* series is a major series of single volume companions to key research fields in the humanities aimed at postgraduate students, scholars and libraries. Each companion offers a comprehensive reference resource giving an overview of key topics, research areas, new directions and a manageable guide to beginning or developing research in the field. A distinctive feature of the series is that each companion provides practical guidance on advanced study and research in the field, including research methods and subject-specific resources.

Titles currently available in the series

Aesthetics, edited by Anna Christina Ribeiro

Aristotle, edited by Claudia Baracchi

Continental Philosophy, edited by John Mullarkey and Beth Lord

Epistemology, edited by Andrew Cullison

Ethics, edited by Christian Miller

Existentialism, edited by Jack Reynolds, Felicity Joseph and Ashley Woodward

Hegel, edited by Allegra de Laurentiis and Jeffrey Edwards

Heidegger, edited by Francois Raffoul and Eric S. Nelson

Hobbes, edited by S. A. Lloyd

Hume, edited by Alan Bailey and Dan O'Brien

Kant, edited by Gary Banham, Dennis Schulting and Nigel Hems

Leibniz, edited by Brendan Look

Locke, edited by S.-J. Savonious-Wroth, Paul Schuurman and Jonathan Walmsley

Metaphysics, edited by Robert W. Barnard and Neil A. Manson

Philosophical Logic, edited by Leon Horston and Richard Pettigrew

Philosophy of Language, edited by Manuel Garcia-Carpintero and Max Kolbel

Philosophy of Mind, edited by James Garvey

Philosophy of Science, edited by Steven French and Juha Saatsi

Plato, edited by Gerald A. Press

Political Philosophy, edited by Andrew Fiala

Pragmatism, edited by Sami Pihlström

Socrates, edited by John Bussanich and Nicholas D. Smith

Spinoza, edited by Wiep van Bunge

The Bloomsbury Companion to Contemporary Philosophy of Medicine

Edited by
James A. Marcum

Bloomsbury Academic
An imprint of Bloomsbury Publishing Plc

B L O O M S B U R Y
LONDON · OXFORD · NEW YORK · NEW DELHI · SYDNEY

Bloomsbury Academic

An imprint of Bloomsbury Publishing Plc

50 Bedford Square	1385 Broadway
London	New York
WC1B 3DP	NY 10018
UK	USA

www.bloomsbury.com

BLOOMSBURY and the Diana logo are trademarks of Bloomsbury Publishing Plc

First published 2017

British Library Cataloguing-in-Publication Data
A catalogue record for this book is available from the British Library.

ISBN: HB: 978-1-4742-3300-2
ePDF: 978-1-4742-3302-6
ePub: 978-1-4742-3301-9

Library of Congress Cataloging-in-Publication Data
A catalog record for this book is available from the Library of Congress.

Series: Bloomsbury Companions

Typeset by Newgen Knowledge Works (P) Ltd., Chennai, India
Printed and bound in Great Britain

Contents

Contents

Notes on Contributors

Robyn Bluhm is an associate professor at Michigan State University with a joint appointment in the Department of Philosophy and Lyman Briggs College. Her research examines philosophical issues in neuroscience and in medicine, with particular focus on the relationship between ethical and epistemological questions in these areas. She has written extensively on evidence-based medicine and on sex/gender difference research in neuroscience. She is a coeditor of *Neurofeminism: Issues at the Intersection of Feminist Theory and Cognitive Science* and of the *International Journal of Feminist Approaches to Bioethics* (IJFAB).

Marianne Boenink is an assistant professor at the Department of Philosophy, University of Twente in the Netherlands. She has a background in health sciences and philosophy. Her research focuses on the conceptual, hermeneutical, and normative analysis of visions of the future of biomedicine and healthcare, and on how these visions shape actual practices of biomedical innovation and vice versa. She is particularly interested in science and technologies pursuing "personalized and predictive medicine." From 2009 to 2015 she was project leader of the research project "Responsible early diagnostics for Alzheimer's disease," funded by the Netherlands Organisation for Scientific Research (NWO). Currently, she leads a project on the early ethical and social assessment of new technologies to prognosticate patients in coma (also funded by NWO) and a project on the effects of involving patients and caregivers in dementia biomarkers research (funded by the Netherlands Organisation for Health Research and Development).

Hillel D. Braude studied medicine at the University of Cape Town Medical School (1988–1993) and obtained a PhD in philosophy cum laude with The University of Chicago's Committee for the History of Culture (1998–2006). He completed a Fellowship at the MacLean Center for Clinical Medical Ethics (2001–2003), and has worked as a clinical medical ethicist in Paris and Montreal. Dr. Braude also completed postdoctoral fellowships in neuroethics with McGill University's Biomedical Ethics Unit and Religious Studies Faculty (2008–2011). He is the author of *Intuition in Medicine: A Philosophical Defense of Clinical Reasoning* (University of Chicago Press, 2012). His multidisciplinary research interests include neuroethics, phenomenology, cognition, and clinical reasoning. He is currently director of research at the Mifne Center in the North of Israel for the treatment of infants with autism and their whole families.

Alex Broadbent is professor of philosophy and executive dean of the Faculty of Humanities at the University of Johannesburg (UJ). Previously he held various research, teaching, and visiting positions at Cambridge, Vienna, Athens, and Harvard, before joining the UJ in 2011. Alex is a philosopher of science with particular interests in philosophy of epidemiology, philosophy of medicine, and philosophy of law, connected by the philosophical themes of causation, explanation, and prediction. He is committed to finding philosophical problems in practical contexts, and to contributing something useful concerning them. He holds a P-rating from the National Research Foundation of South Africa (2013–2018) and is a member of the South African Young Academy of Sciences. He has published a number of articles in top-ranked international journals across three disciplines (philosophy, epidemiology, law). His first book, *Philosophy of Epidemiology*, was published by Palgrave Macmillan in 2013, and has been translated into Korean. His second book, *Philosophy for Graduate Students: Metaphysics and Epistemology*, was published by Routledge in February 2016. He is currently working on his third book, *Philosophy of Medicine*, under contract with Oxford University Press.

Brendan Clarke is lecturer in history and philosophy of medicine at the Department of Science and Technology Studies, University College London. After qualifying in medicine in 2007, he moved into philosophy of medicine via PhD research on causality in medicine (UCL, 2011). His current research concerns contemporary questions in medical practice. He is coinvestigator on the Evaluating Evidence in Medicine project, funded by the UK Arts and Humanities Research Council, which investigates the role of evidence in science and health policy. He is particularly interested in investigating the intersection between traditional epistemology and the social and political functions of health policy.

Rachel Cooper is a senior lecturer in philosophy at Lancaster University, United Kingdom. Her publications include *Diagnosing the Diagnostic and Statistical Manual of Mental Disorders* (Karnac, 2014), *Psychiatry and the Philosophy of Science* (Routledge, 2007), and *Classifying Madness* (Springer, 2005).

Lydie Fialová studied medicine, philosophy, and history at Charles University in Prague. Initially trained in child psychiatry with a focus on the genetics of autism, she then pursued doctoral studies in anthropology at the University of Edinburgh, conducting her fieldwork in psychiatric hospitals in the Czech Republic. She was a postdoctoral fellow at the Center for Philosophy and History of Science at Boston University and is currently a fellow in medical ethics at the University of Edinburgh. Among her publications is *Medicine in the Context of Western Thought* (in Czech), which explores the philosophical, historical, and sociocultural dimensions of medicine. She has also published articles in the areas of psychiatry and anthropology. Her research explores the inter-relatedness of the epistemological, ethical, and cultural dimensions of contemporary medicine and life sciences.

Tania Gergel, after completing her doctorate on Plato's *Phaedo*, joined the Classics Department at King's College London as a lecturer specializing in ancient philosophy, and has also taught at Birkbeck College, the Open University, and Cambridge. Following an extended career break, she returned to King's in 2011 and developed an interest in the philosophy of medicine as a visiting research fellow with the Wellcome Funded Centre for Humanities and Health, publishing on medicine and phenomenology. As well as continuing interests in ancient philosophy, she is now a visiting research fellow in philosophy and psychiatry at the Institute of Psychiatry, Psychology and Neuroscience and a member of the Mental Health, Ethics and Law Research Group, with research focusing on stigma, coercion, identity, and advance directives in psychiatry.

Mona Gupta is a consultation-liaison psychiatrist at the Centre Hospitalier de l'Université de Montréal (CHUM) and a researcher at the CRCHUM (Centre de Recherche du CHUM) in Montreal. She is also associate professor in the Department of Psychiatry at the University of Montreal. Her areas of academic interest are in bioethics and the philosophy of psychiatry. Dr. Gupta is the author of several articles and books chapters on ethics in psychiatry, particularly on the subject of ethics and evidence-based medicine in psychiatry. Her research monograph on this topic was published in the International Perspectives on Philosophy and Psychiatry series by Oxford University Press in 2014 and nominated for a BMA Medical Book of the Year award in 2015.

Jeremy Howick investigates questions that require input from philosophy and clinical epidemiology. These include: the ontology, effects, and ethics of placebo treatments in clinical trials and clinical practice; the benefits and harms of informed consent; and the problem with too much medicine, which has an economic dimension due to rising healthcare costs and resource wasting. With over 60 academic publications (including two books), he has been funded by the Medical Research Council and the National Institutes of Health Research, and his research has been used to shape policy. He is also a dedicated teacher and science communicator who is writing a popular science book about the placebo effect.

Saana Jukola completed her PhD in philosophy in 2015 (University of Jyväskylä, Finland) and is currently a postdoctoral researcher at the DFG Research Training Group Integrating Ethics and Epistemology of Scientific Research (Bielefeld University, Germany). She is also a member of the Academy of Finland Centre of Excellence in the Philosophy of Social Sciences (*TINT*) and a research associate at the University of Johannesburg. Jukola's research interest is the objectivity of socially relevant research, particularly medicine. Her post-doctoral project focuses on the interplay between evidence and nonepistemic factors in nutrition research.

Ashley Graham Kennedy holds degrees in astrophysics, humanities, and philosophy and is currently assistant professor of philosophy and assistant professor of clinical biomedical science at Florida Atlantic University, where she teaches philosophy of medicine, biomedical ethics, and symbolic logic to undergraduate students. Her main area of research concerns evidential and ethical issues that arise in medical diagnostic practice. Some of her recent work has appeared in *Studies in History and Philosophy of Science, British Medical Journal, Journal of Medicine and Philosophy*, and *Journal of Evaluation in Clinical Practice*.

Michael Loughlin is the professor of applied philosophy at Manchester Metropolitan University. He has written extensively on the relationship between knowledge, science, and value in clinical practice, applying arguments developed in his PhD (on the relationship between epistemology and ethics) and early publications in philosophy to analyses of the nature and role of rationality, evidence, judgment, and intuition in medicine and healthcare. His early work (including a 2002 book *Ethics, Management and Mythology*) raised methodological questions about quality measures, bioethics, and the use of evidence in health policy, criticized the role of management theory in undermining professional autonomy, and defended a conception of professional judgment with reference to a "virtues" approach to practical wisdom. He has written many articles in academic journals and popular media, and addressed international audiences of practitioners and policy makers on evidence-based medicine. He has coauthored policy documents and advised professional groups on the philosophical education of practitioners. As associate editor of the *Journal of Evaluation in Clinical Practice*, he has edited several special issues on philosophical aspects of healthcare. He is the editor of *Debates in Values-based Practice: Arguments for and Against* (CUP, 2014) and currently chairs the Special Interest Group in Health Philosophy for the European Society for Person Centred Healthcare.

James A. Marcum is professor of philosophy and a member of the Institute for Biomedical Studies at Baylor University in Texas. He earned doctorates in philosophy from Boston College and in physiology from the University of Cincinnati Medical College. He was a faculty member at Harvard Medical School as a molecular biologist for over a decade before joining Baylor's philosophy department. His research interests include the philosophy and history of science and medicine, and examples of his publications appear in such journals as *Synthese, Perspectives on Science, History and Philosophy of the Life Sciences, Perspectives in Biology and Medicine*, and *Theoretical Medicine and Bioethics*. His book publications include *An Introductory Philosophy of Medicine: Humanizing*

Modern Medicine (Springer, 2008) and *The Virtuous Physician: The Role of Virtue in Medicine* (Springer, 2012).

Michael Ruse is Lucyle T. Werkmeister Professor of Philosophy and director of the Program in the History and Philosophy of Science at Florida State University. He is particularly interested in philosophical and historical questions about evolutionary theory and has written extensively on the topic from the viewpoint of science, from the viewpoint of philosophy, from the viewpoint of history, and increasingly recently from the viewpoint of religion. He is the sometime recipient of a Guggenheim fellowship, a former Gifford lecturer, and holder of several honorary degrees. His next book is *Darwinism as Religion: What Literature Tells Us about Evolution.*

Federica Russo is assistant professor in philosophy of science at the University of Amsterdam. She is interested in causality and evidence in the social, biomedical, and policy sciences, as well as in the relation between science and technology. Among her recent publications are *Causality: Philosophical Theory Meets Scientific Practice* (coauthored with Phyllis Illari, Oxford University Press, 2014) and *Causality and Causal Modelling in the Social Sciences: Measuring Variations* (Springer, 2009). Federica also authored several articles in international journals and spanning various themes, such as causation and causal modeling, explanation, evidence, and technology. She edited the volume *Causality in the Sciences* with Phyllis Illari and Jon Williamson (Oxford University Press, 2011). Federica sits in the steering committee of the "Causality in the Sciences" Conference Series and is activity leader of the Society for the Philosophy of Information.

Jacob Stegenga is assistant professor in the Department of Philosophy at the University of Victoria. His research focuses on philosophy of science, including methodological problems of medical research, conceptual questions in evolutionary biology, and fundamental topics in reasoning and rationality. Stegenga's present work is culminating in a book tentatively titled *Medical Nihilism*, in which he argues that if we attend to the extent of bias in medical research, the thin theoretical basis of many interventions, the malleability of empirical methods in medicine, and if we employ our best inductive framework, then our confidence in medical interventions ought to be low. His research employs empirical findings, analysis, and formal methods to establish normative conclusions about science.

Fredrik Svenaeus is professor at the Centre for Studies in Practical Knowledge, Södertörn University, Sweden. His main research areas are philosophy of medicine, bioethics, medical humanities, and philosophical anthropology. Current research projects focus on the concept of suffering in bioethics and on psychiatric diagnosis and the concept of medicalization. Recent publication include: "The Phenomenology of Suffering in Medicine and Bioethics," *Theoretical Medicine* *and Bioethics* (2014); "Organ Transplantation Ethics from the Persepctive of Embodied Selfhood," in *The Routledge Companion to Bioethics* (2015); and "The Relationship between Empathy and Sympathy in Good Health Care," *Medicine, Health Care and Philosophy* (2015).

Alfred I. Tauber, professor of philosophy, emeritus, and Zoltan Kohn Professor of Medicine, emeritus, at Boston University, served as chief of the Hematology-Oncology Division, Boston City Hospital (1982–1991) and as director of the Center for Philosophy and History of Science (1993–2010). As a hematologist and biochemist, Dr. Tauber's laboratory interests focused on phagocyte cell biology and the inflammatory reaction, which eventually oriented his later studies in the philosophy and history of science. He has published extensively in ethics and science studies with an emphasis on the critical examination of immunology's theory and historical development, most recently *Immunity: The Evolution of an Idea* (Oxford, 2017). He is the author of two medical ethics monographs: *Confessions of a Medicine Man* (MIT Press, 1999) and *Patient Autonomy and the Ethics of Responsibility* (MIT Press, 2005). These philosophical texts explore contemporary issues of the doctor–patient relationship.

Şerife Tekin is an assistant professor of philosophy at Daemen College, New York, and an associate fellow of the Center for Philosophy of Science at the University of Pittsburgh, Pennsylvania. She works in philosophy of mind, philosophy of science, and medical ethics. Her work has appeared in journals such as *Philosophy, Psychiatry and Psychology*, *Public Affairs Quarterly*, *Journal of Medical Ethics*, *Philosophical Psychology*, *The American Journal of Bioethics*; in books such as *Classifying Psychopathology: Mental Kinds and Natural Kinds* (MIT Press, 2014); *The Psychiatric Babel: Assessing the DSM-5* (Springer, 2015); *Anthology on Pharmaceuticals* (Springer, 2015); and in encyclopedias such as *Encyclopedia of Clinical Psychology* (Wiley-Blackwell Press, 2015) and *The Encyclopedia of Bioethics* (Macmillan Reference, 2013). Her coedited book, *Extraordinary Science: Responding to the Current Crisis in Psychiatric Research* (with Jeffrey Poland) is scheduled to be published in July 2016 with the MIT University Press.

Part I

Introduction: Philosophy of
Medicine, Research Problems,
and Methods

1 Introduction: Contemporary Philosophy of Medicine

James A. Marcum

Introduction

Modern medicine is pluralistic in terms of its nature and practice, and *The Bloomsbury Companion to Contemporary Philosophy of Medicine* (*The Companion*) reflects that pluralism. Traditionally, the notion of medical pluralism refers to "employment of more than one medical system or the use of both conventional and complementary and alternative medicine (CAM) for health and illness" (Wade et al., 2008, p. 829).[1] In *The Companion*, the notion is restricted to contemporary Western medicine and its practice, particularly what Arthur Kleinman (1980) calls the "professional sector." Basically, modern medicine is fragmented in that approaches to its nature range from logico-rational explanations to humanistic accounts, while approaches to its practice range from evidence-based medicine (EBM) to patient-centered care (Hsu, 2008).[2] These approaches often involve different philosophical perspectives, such as analytical, empirical, phenomenological, or personalist views. *The Companion* aims to provide a practical and extensive guide to assist the reader in exploring the ontological, epistemological, and methodological (and to a limited extent, ethical) issues — vis-à-vis modern medicine's pluralism — challenging contemporary philosophers of medicine.

Structurally, *The Companion* begins with this general introductory chapter, which provides not only a background for contemporary philosophy of medicine but also a framework and narrative to integrate the individual chapters. The next chapter introduces various research problems in contemporary philosophy of medicine and methodological approaches to them. The main section, "Current Research and Future Directions," is composed of eleven chapters, which can be divided into three subsections. The first, chapters 3–6, pertains chiefly to medicine qua science, beginning with the individual in terms of molecular and genomic medicine (traditional pathophysiology accounts of disease) and the population with respect to epidemiology (global healthcare) and then proceeding to EBM and finally to evolutionary medicine. The next subsection, chapters 7–10, focuses mainly on medicine qua art—commencing with medical humanism and then focusing on embodiment, gender, and personhood. Chapters 11–13 constitute the final subsection in which special topics in contemporary philosophy of medicine are explored, particularly disease, health, medical causation, and clinical reasoning (CR) and decision-making. Also included in *The Companion* is a final chapter on new directions in the philosophy of medicine, especially in terms of an "epistemological turn." Moreover, a series of scholarly tools for conducting research in contemporary philosophy of medicine is included in *The Companion*, specifically a glossary of key terms, a guide to research sources, and an annotated bibliography.

Since medical pluralism is even more extensive than covered in *The Companion*, a section of this chapter is devoted to briefly discussing these additional types of or approaches to medicine and its practice—including logic of medicine, translational medicine, integrative medicine, systems medicine, biopsychosocial (BPS) medicine, narrative medicine, and virtue-based medicine—that space within *The Companion* eventually could not permit. Finally, this chapter concludes with a discussion of a "metaphysical turn" with respect to ontology and presuppositions in contemporary philosophy of medicine.

Background

Although contemporary philosophy of medicine—particularly in the Western tradition—is an emerging discipline in modern philosophy, with its own journals, introductory texts, specialized monographs, professional societies, conferences, and so on, it is an ancient discipline historically, with its origins in classical Greece and Rome. An important aspect of its history is a major shift in traditional Greek medicine from the physician as priest to the physician as philosopher. Along with this shift was an emphasis on the rational rather than on the mystical basis of disease etiology. The Hippocratic corpus clearly illustrates this in terms of the sacred disease, epilepsy: "It is not, in my opinion, any more divine or more sacred than any other diseases, but has a natural cause" (Jones, 1923, p. 139). Thus, disease in general could be studied not only rationally—having a natural cause—but also empirically—having a material cause—and thereby treated intelligibly and physically. As the rational–empirical approach became the tradition in medicine, another shift transpired beginning with the scientific revolution in the sixteenth and seventeenth centuries and culminating in the early twentieth century, the physician as scientist.

Besides the rational–empirical tradition, another tradition runs deep in medicine—humanism. Historically, medical rationalism–empiricism has been at odds with medical humanism—especially during the early part of the twentieth century when the science of medicine eclipsed its art. For example, William Welch (1908) advocated securing the practice of medicine exclusively in scientific rationality. But, medical scientism need not preclude the art of medicine; and several early twentieth-century physicians promoted the integration of medicine's science and art. Francis Peabody (1927), for instance, advocated an integrative approach in his well-known lecture, "The care of the patient." According to Peabody, science is not just technical inquiry but also includes nontechnical information that makes up the patient as an "impressionistic painting." Finally, for medical humanism, the goal is not simply an accurate diagnosis, although that is important in delivering quality patient care, but the relief of human suffering and the restoration of human dignity.

For contemporary medicine and its philosophy, the science versus art controversy of the early twentieth century morphed into the evidence-based versus person-centered medicine debate of the late twentieth and early twenty-first centuries. Besides these two approaches to the nature of medicine and its practice, other approaches emerged during the twentieth century, including molecular and genomic medicine, epidemiology, and evolutionary medicine. To add to medicine's pluralism, medical humanism—in response to medicine's addiction to science and its technology—championed the patient qua person, phenomenological embodiment, and recently genderness. Another shift in the conception of the physician is under way today—the physician qua person. The outcome with respect to modern medicine's pluralism at the end of the twentieth century is a plethora of new problems and issues, which contemporary philosophers of medicine are now pursuing.

Framework

In chapter 2—"Research Problems ad Methods in the Philosophy of Medicine"—Michael Loughlin, Robyn Bluhm, and Mona Gupta explore the ontological and epistemological research problems and issues that have emerged with medicine's pluralism, and the methods philosophers of medicine use to address them. Besides introducing the reader to the contemporary philosophy of medicine, their chapter serves to frame the remaining chapters within the "Current Research and Future Directions" section. Just as the approaches to medicine and its practice range from the molecular and genomic to the person and evolving populations, so the philosophical methods used to investigate and ultimately to make sense of medicine's pluralism range from the logico-analytical and positivistic to the humanistic and phenomenological.[3] To that end, the metaphysical presuppositions and ontological commitments that contemporary philosophers of medicine employ methodologically are analyzed in the chapter.

One of the more critical ontological issues that surfaces in several chapters within *The Companion* is the nature of personhood, especially of the patient in terms of the illness experience.[4] What drives this ontological issue is often the reduction of the patient to laboratory results or epidemiological evidence, which also has important ethical and moral implications for what Loughlin and coauthors call "usual" clinical practice. They also explore the epistemological issues associated with foundationalism and empiricism, that is, whether empirical evidence constitutes the only—or even an adequate—empirical base for medical practice. Finally, the reliance on metaphors like "base" and "center" are compared collectively to determine whether they share any conceptual similarities. For the authors, the goal of contemporary philosophy of medicine is whether it can contribute intelligibly and productively to the ongoing discussion over medical pluralism. Equipped with these different methodologies to the problems and issues challenging contemporary philosophers of medicine, the reader is able to appreciate and engage the issues raised in the remaining chapters.

The Science of Medicine

As noted earlier, the "Current Research and Future Directions" section can be divided into three subsections. The first (chapters 3–6) pertains to the impact the natural sciences have had on the nature and practice of medicine. The common thread that connects these chapters is an increasing complexity, along with uncertainty, which emerges when spanning a spectrum with molecular and genomic medicine (chapter 3) on one end and evolutionary medicine (chapter 6) on the other. Along that spectrum is epidemiology (chapter 4) in which disease prevalence and patterns within specific populations provide the basis for examining the distribution of health and disease in human populations, along with EBM (chapter 5) in which therapeutic modalities are tested clinically on populations made up of well-defined patient and control groups. The challenge facing contemporary philosophy of medicine involves not only the unique problems and issues emerging within each of these approaches to medicine and its practice but also ascertaining the relationship among them to provide a suitable notion of modern medicine and its "usual" clinical practice. For example, the role of mechanistic thinking in developing therapies based on an understanding of pathological mechanisms is a source of contention between advocates of molecular and genomic medicine and those of epidemiology and EBM.

In chapter 3—"Disease in the Era of Genomic and Molecular Medicine"— Marianne Boenink examines not only the ontological and epistemological issues emerging from the development of genomics and molecular biology—the foundations of current biomedical research and practice—but also their ethical and political implications. Boenink begins with the nascence of medical genetics and the drive to sequence the human genome, based on the underlying assumption of "one gene-one disease" hypothesis and biomedicine's ontological conception of disease. According to her, disease and even medicine itself has become technologically mediated, that is, technology defines the possibilities of what constitutes health and disease.[5] With the completion of the Human Genome Project, however, the genetic etiology of disease has broadened to include multiple genes and molecular pathways— what is called the cascade model of disease based on various biomarkers. The model represents a physiological conceptualization of disease in terms of complex temporal processes and interactions among the cascade's components. The problem with the model, for Boenink, is that the notion of biomarker used to identify and monitor a cascade's components is ambiguous and requires clarification.

Associated with the geneticization and molecularization of medicine has been the rise of P3 medicine, which is predictive, preventive, and personalized.[6] Boenink explores the reductionist and mechanistic assumptions underlying P3 medicine, which she claims leads to fragmentation of the patient. To counter this deterministic approach to medicine, she employs epigenetics and systems biology approaches to rethink the complex interactions among genome, lifestyle choices, and environmental contexts for explicating health and disease. She then substitutes an entanglement model of health and disease, in terms of multiple variables and factors, for the cascade model. She argues that current developments in nanotechnology, including information and communications technology—which permits monitoring the body, lifestyle, and environmental context—may lead to a genuinely personalized medicine. However, she concludes that these developments can obfuscate the boundaries between normal and abnormal, and between medical research and standard or "usual" clinical care.

In chapter 4—"Philosophy of Epidemiology"—Alex Broadbent examines the philosophical issues surrounding epidemiology, especially the notion of causation. He begins with identifying the salient feature for defining epidemiology, "the distribution and determinants of disease." Epidemiology's goal, then, is to understand the patterns of those distributions and determinants, in order to improve human health—especially in terms of populations. Although epidemiology only emerged in the second half of the twentieth century, after the pioneering work of John Snow and Ignaaz Semmelweis in the first-half of the nineteenth century, diseases such as bubonic plague have scrounged humanity for centuries. But what Broadbent finds intriguing philosophically about epidemiology is its "outside-the-box" thinking vis-à-vis conventional theorizing and experimenting.

Broadbent focuses on three important philosophical issues concerning the determinants or causes of disease in populations. The first issue is multifactorialism in which disease causation is the outcome of various factors and elements. He examines two chief metaphors for representing multifactorialism—web of causation and causal pie—and discusses the challenges facing a nuanced classification of diseases based on them. The next issue is the causal interpretation problem, which pertains to the correct construal of measures of association for determining disease causation, and he proposes a novel solution to the problem. The final issue is the causal inference problem, which involves the criteria for justifying causal inferences. He first discusses Bradford Hill's viewpoints and notes their similarity to "inference to the best explanation." He then comments on the shift to the current counterfactual view of causation and claims that the issue of causation is one of the more pressing issues for philosophy of epidemiology. Finally, he briefly discusses several topics—ethical and methodological issues, risk relativism, epidemiology and the law, and social determinants of health—which he claims are fertile ground for philosophical toiling.

In chapter 5—"Justification of Evidence-Based Medicine Epistemology"— Jeremy Howick first explores the roots of EBM, especially with respect to the failure of mechanistic reasoning and clinical experience to support "usual" clinical practice. He goes on to define EBM according to the Evidence Based Medicine Working Group and to clarify EBM's relationship to clinical experience, pathophysiological or mechanistic reasoning, and clinical research. He next turns to the question of what the philosophy of EBM is. For Howick, that philosophy consists chiefly of an analysis of hierarchies of evidence in order to address EBM's critics. These critics claim that much of what can be called "usual" clinical practice does not require randomized controlled trials (RCTs) to warrant their use in treating patients. Moreover, they claim that there is scant evidence for the superiority of EBM over other methods for clinical practice.

Howick also introduces a number of philosophical controversies surrounding EBM, such as diagnostic reasoning, clinical expertise, prognostic markers, and so on, but limits his comments to two controversies. The first is the epistemological priority between observational studies and RCTs for supplying the best evidence for clinical practice. Although observational studies, such as case and cohort studies, do furnish useful information and evidence for clinical practice, they are prone to allocation, performance, and self-selection biases. He then enlists RCTs to the rescue in terms of providing two features generally not employed in observational studies: double masking and placebo controls. The second controversy concerns the necessity of mechanistic or pathophysiological reasoning in clinical research and practice, especially with respect to the Russo–Williamson thesis (see chapter 12). Howick argues that the role of mechanistic reasoning is overemphasized and that empirical trial and error is often sufficient for generating the best evidence for clinical practice. He then concludes that RCTs do deliver the best evidence for clinical practice, compared with either clinical expertise or mechanistic reasoning.

In chapter 6—"Evolutionary Medicine: Philosophical Aspects"—Michael Ruse begins with the question of why it took so long for evolutionary medicine to appear on the medical scene, with the publication in 1994 of Randolph Nesse and George Williams's book on Darwinian medicine. Part of the reason, according to Ruse, was the inability of Darwinian evolutionists, as exemplified by Thomas Huxley's response to Father Hahn, to envision how evolutionary theory could assist in treating patients practically. Ruse next turns to Peter Gluckman and coauthors' *Principles of Evolutionary Medicine* to address how an evolutionary perspective assists in clinical practice and in understanding notions such as health and disease. He then considers the philosophical issues surrounding the role of natural selection, especially multilevel selection, for examining diseases such as preeclampsia and bacterial infection.

Ruse concludes the chapter with a discussion of the nature of health and disease, as well as related concepts, particularly in terms of the debate surrounding the naturalist or objectivist and normativist or constructivist conceptions of health and disease. For Ruse, objective or natural causes of health and disease are necessary but insufficient from an evolutionary perspective since we are interested in why we get sick—as Nesse and Williams entitled their book. He also invokes Hans-Georg Gadamer's notion of health to argue that biology and evolution do play a role in medicine. In the end, Ruse raises an alarming philosophical question about medicine for an aging population—why should we treat people past their reproductive prime?

In sum, there is a plurality of approaches to the science of medicine and its practice, ranging from the genomic and molecular to the organismic and evolving populations. Certainly science is critical for "usual" clinical practice; but what entails or defines precisely the scientific approach raises challenging philosophical problems and issues for molecular and genomic medicine, epidemiology and population medicine, EBM, and evolutionary medicine. These issues include, for example, the role of mechanistic thinking in analyzing and justifying causal relationships, the nature of evidence upon which to base the best possible clinical practice, or Ruse's alarming insight that evolution is not interested in the diseases of individuals past their reproductive prime and the even more alarming question of why we should then be concerned with treating them.

Moreover, the plurality of approaches to medicine divulges a deep ideological rift in the Western ontological conception of natural phenomena, as well as how to investigate them experimentally or empirically and to understand them theoretically or rationally. For example, from the sixteenth to eighteenth centuries rationalists and empiricists debated the best approach to medicine

(King, 1978). According to the seventeenth-century physician Giorgio Baglivi (1723, pp. 7–8),

> Those who oppose Reason to Experience, whether Empiricks or Rational Physicians, seem to be all Mad: For how can we make Reason to act all the Parts of Science, that, as all wise Men ought to acknowledge, is acquir'd by Tryal and Use Continu'd thro' a long progress of Time? And, on the other hand, why should Experience be only regarded, and Reason turn'd out of doors? . . . I understand that Queen Reason, that is plac'd above all the rest, by which a Physician looks into the Principles and Causes of Diseases, foretells their progress and event, and gathers Futurities from what's present.

Baglivi's comment is as relevant today as it was over three centuries ago. Philosophers of medicine can certainly contribute to the ongoing discussion concerning the metaphysical, epistemological, and methodological issues that challenge modern scientific medicine.

The Art of Medicine

The next subsection (chapter 7–10) addresses the problems and issues arising from clinical practice that restricts its delivery to simply the scientific and technical dimension of healthcare. Although medical humanism arose with a vengeance during the mid-part of the twentieth century to redress the abuses and neglect of the patient at the hands of overly technologized medicine, as discussed in the second part of chapter 7, its roots originated with the Enlightenment, as discussed in the first part. Medical humanism, as introduced in the chapter, represents the attempt to recover medicine's moral imperative to relieve human suffering and to restore human dignity, and it provides a context for the remaining chapters. In the next chapter on phenomenology and medicine, medical humanism is advanced with respect to the notion of embodiment, which is used to explore a patient's illness narrative—especially in terms of the meaning of illness. Chapter 9 incorporates gender medicine—a rapidly developing field of contemporary philosophy of medicine—into medical humanism, especially in terms of the notion of phenomenological embodiment. And in the last chapter of this subsection on patient- and person-centered medicine, the problems attendant to patient or person qua center holding clinical encounters together are discussed and healthcare personalism is introduced to address the problems.

In chapter 7—"Medical Humanism Part 1: Philosophical and Historical Underpinnings"—Alfred Tauber explores the roots of humanism beginning with the Enlightenment and follows its development to the end of the nineteenth century with the dawn of positivism. As Tauber notes, whereas the impetus for humanism was initially religious dogmatism, by the end of the nineteenth century it was scientific dogmatism or scientism. The impact of paradigmatic scientism, especially in terms of positivism, on medicine and its practice was inevitable—given scientism's epistemic hegemony. Indeed, as Tauber demonstrates, the paradigm governing medical practice over the past century or so has been a scientific or mechanistic approach to understanding and explaining pathophysiological processes—particularly in an effort to master and manipulate disease through rational therapeutic intervention. For Tauber, this paradigm has had a particular devastating impact on the moral dimension of the patient–physician relationship. What has been transgressed morally through medical scientism has been the dignity of the person, whether patient or physician. The proper humanistic response to this transgression, Tauber argues, should not be the rejection of the science of medicine but the morally inappropriate application of it to treating patients qua persons by physicians qua persons. In the end, for Tauber, scientism and humanism vis-à-vis medical practice is not oppositional or antithetical but rather complementary.

In chapter 7—"Medical Humanism Part 2: Inspirations of the Twentieth Century"—Lydie Fialová advances into the twentieth century the discussion of medical humanism begun by Tauber. To that end, she discusses not only the medicalization of human developmental stages, especially birth and death, but also the institutionalization of medicine as a "medico-industrial complex." Fialová begins with the "objects" of medicine—patients—and shows how the objectification of patients results is their fragmentation, with a loss of personhood. In order to rejoin the fragments of patients to recover their personhood, she turns to twentieth-century phenomenology. Fialová first introduces Husserl's "life-world" and Heidegger's "being-in-the-world"; then she discusses the attempts of twentieth-century phenomenologists, such as Lévinas, Arendt, Jaspers, among others, to forge a philosophical system to rejoin the fragmented person into a contiguous whole. She finally appropriates these phenomenological insights into contemporary medicine and its practice, especially in terms of relieving not only physical but also existential suffering. Fialová concludes that the animating virtue for medical humanism is compassion, as the physician cares about and for the patient.

In chapter 8—"Phenomenology and Medicine"—Fredrik Svenaeus advances the discussion of the role of phenomenology in medical humanism, introduced by Fialová. Specifically, Svenaeus begins with a brief history of the phenomenology of medicine, with its appearance as an academic discipline in the 1980s, and defines its goal as hermeneutics of the patient's illness experience—especially its existential features—in order to make sense of illness vis-à-vis the patient's life-world. Importantly, the goal of phenomenological medicine is the relief of suffering associated with illness and not necessarily with a physical cure, which is an important goal of medicine qua applied biology but not always attainable. Svenaeus then contrasts the goal of phenomenological medicine to the goal of the biomedical sciences, which is to address the physical features of the patient's diseased condition with respect to either cure or management. He articulates this contrast in the goals between phenomenological medicine and the biomedical sciences in terms of the "lived" body and the "living" body, respectively.

According to Svenaeus, the living body—as the domain of the biomedical sciences—is reduced to its various tissue, cellular, molecular, and genomic components. As he notes, it is a third-person perspective, which is objective and neutral. In other words, the biomedical physician's gaze is one of emotionally detached concern. And the contact between the physician and patient is often mediated through technology. On the other hand, as a lived body—the domain of phenomenological medicine—the patient qua whole is embedded or contextualized within a life-world. It represents a first-person perspective in terms of the patient's illness experience and a second-person experience as the physician responds empathically to the patient's illness and the suffering associated with it.

Svenaeus next articulates the existential anxiety associated with illness in terms of Heidegger's notion of "unhomelike being-in-the-world" and the alienation from not only the self and the body but also others and society. The physician's role is to assist the patient in navigating this alienation and in forging a meaningful life in the face of illness and even death. Svenaeus also employs Heidegger's notion of *Gestell* or "enframing" to discuss the judicious use of new medical technology rather than being used by it, especially in terms of the dying experience or the "final homecoming." In sum, phenomenological medicine enriches the truncated approach of the biomedical sciences by taking into account the patient's life-world with respect to living a flourishing and meaningful life.

In chapter 9—"Gender Medicine and Phenomenological Embodiment"—Tania Gergel explores the relationship of gender to medicine and its practice vis-à-vis medical humanism and phenomenology. She commences with the naissance of gender studies around the end of the twentieth century and then analyzes the distinction between the concepts of sex and gender. She argues that the notion of gender realism in which gender is equated to sex is too simplistic, since either concept can vary considerably within a given social or cultural context. This has important implications for the philosophy of medicine in terms of labeling concepts such as health or disease as either natural, with respect to sex, or normative, with respect to gender. Importantly, she next examines the problems with this facile taxonomy, especially in terms of gender stereotypes—particularly for diagnosis. For example, she discusses the impact these stereotypes have for women in terms of overdiagnosis for psychiatric diseases such as depression and underdiagnosis for physical diseases such as heart disease. Of course, gender stereotypes also have an impact on the delivery of healthcare to men, such as underdiagnosis of depression.

Gergel then takes up the philosophical issues surrounding the male-as-norm both in biomedical research and clinical practice. She explores the assumptions underlying the male-as-norm position, such as physiological processes are common to the sexes or protection of women of childbearing age from possible harm from experimental or clinical trials. Interestingly, while women are excluded from or underrepresented in clinical trials, yet their life-stages, such as pregnancy and menopause, have been overmedicalized. She concludes by proposing a phenomenological approach to address gender issues and the assumptions underlying them in medicine and its practice. Specifically, she suggests that the notion of embodiment can be used to construct a framework to resolve the artificial distinction between dichotomies, such as male and female, mind and body, or the self and environment, and the difficulties associated with gender bias in medicine.

In chapter 10—"Patient- and Person-Centered Medicine: Does the Center Hold?"—the problems associated with centering clinical encounters on the patient or even the person are examined. Although patient-centered medicine empowers patients, especially through respect for their autonomy, it risks the abandonment of patients in the sense that the healthcare system has become fragmented in its delivery of quality care. Thus, patients qua center cannot sustain clinical encounters, since they do not have the training to make sound clinical decisions. Person-centered medicine, with its shift from the patient to person, avoids this problem but unfortunately has been unable to provide a robust definition of personhood to maintain the centrality of either patients or physicians in clinical encounters. To address the problems associated with both patient- and person-centered medicine, healthcare personalism is then introduced. It is based on the philosophical movement of personalism and relies on an emergent notion of personhood in which dignity is the chief characteristic of the person. Moreover, it champions a network metaphor for clinical encounters. Finally, its goal is the delivery of quality healthcare in terms of ameliorating suffering and restoring human dignity.

In sum, just as there is a plurality of approaches to the science of medicine and its practice, so there is a plurality to the art of medicine and its practice—ranging from medical humanism to person-centered medicine. Traditionally, the science and the art of medicine have been viewed as antithetical or oppositional approaches, especially in terms of their presuppositions (Table 1.1). For example, medical scientism assumes objectivity while medical humanism subjectivity. However, as argued in this subsection, medical humanism provides the motivation, as well as the means, for addressing many of the issues

Table 1.1 Presuppositions for medical scientism and humanism

Medical scientism	Medical humanism
Objectivity	Subjectivity
Naturalism	Normativism
Reductionism	Holism
Absolutism	Relativism
Realism	Idealism
Analytical	Phenomenological
Positivism	Historicism

in medicine and its practice that arise with an overdependence on the natural sciences. Thus, medical humanism, especially in terms of phenomenological medicine and person-centered care, can legitimate the first-person experience of the patient as an important dimension for clinical encounters by including the second-person experience of the clinician. Moreover, as several of the authors of the chapters in this subsection argue, the relationship between medical scientism and humanism can be something other than antithetical—it can be complementary. For example, the fundamental presuppositions often used to distinguish between medical scientism and humanism—objectivity and subjectivity—need not be oppositional. Rather, they can complement or supplement one another, particularly in the sense articulated by Bernard Lonergan (1972, p. 292): "Genuine objectivity is the fruit of authentic subjectivity." In other words, a trustworthy person can function in a frankly neutral manner, without succumbing to personal bias or prejudice. Medical scientism and humanism, then, are not antithetical but are necessary for a comprehensive understanding of medicine and its practice.

Finally, medical humanism, especially in terms of the person-centered approach, helps to address the problem of treating persons for their illnesses past their reproductive prime—a problem that surfaced with an evolutionary approach to medicine. As seen in the subsection's chapters, persons are more than simply reproductive machines. As discussed in chapter 10, Christian Smith (2010) champions a notion of person based on critical realist personalism and has identified human dignity as the sine qua non of personhood. Since what defines a person is dignity and not reproductive capacity and since illness robs persons of their dignity, then a moral obligation exists to treat persons suffering from an illness—whether they are in their reproductive prime or not. Moreover, medicine through addressing the suffering associated with an illness—its chief goal according to Eric Cassell (1991)—reinstates that dignity and the opportunity of the person to live a flourishing and meaningful life.

Topics

In the final subsection (chapters 11–13) of "Current Research and Future Directions," specific perennial problems and issues in traditional philosophy of medicine are examined. The notions of health and disease are probably the most notable historical problems facing contemporary philosophy of medicine. They are examined in the first chapter of this subsection—particularly with respect to the concept of disorder, both physically and mentally, the notion of positive health, and the forms of disability. Medical causality is discussed in chapter 12, using a "causal mosaic" metaphor to capture its multifaceted nature. Last, in chapter 13, the nature of CR and decision-making are explicated not simply in terms of the mechanics of logical or formal reasoning but also, and more importantly, with respect to a practical reasoning or Aristotelian *phronesis* that includes the moral dimension of clinical decision-making. Such an approach to CR respects the patient's dignity and addresses the suffering associated with illness. Finally, this subsection exhibits a specific structure: it begins with what concerns medicine most, health and disease, and then moves to their underlying causes that are important for making sound clinical decisions that benefit—and do not harm—persons, whether patients or clinicians. Moreover, this raises moral issues concerning medical decisions made under complex and uncertain conditions (Hayward, 2006).

In chapter 11—"Health and Disease"—Rachel Cooper begins with the traditional debate over the nature of health and disease in terms of function and dysfunction as championed by Christopher Boorse, especially with respect to descriptive and normative accounts. A major issue in the debate is exactly what normal function is, compared with deviations from it. Moreover, she explores the debate as it centers on whether health and disease vis-à-vis function and dysfunction are value-free. She then turns to the question of whether dysfunction is sufficient and/or necessary for defining health and disease. Another critical issue for defining disease is whether it is bad. In other words, are diseases always harmful? She contrasts the Aristotelian position in which the harm associated with disease is objective in nature to the position in which harm reflects social norms. Next, Cooper discusses the issue of whether diseases must be unusual or unexpected with respect to statistical and modal approaches. Another issue she examines is whether diseases must be medically treatable. She then entertains briefly several issues concerning health and disease, including the compatibility of descriptive and normative accounts, Wittgensteinian versus Roschian conceptualizations, a multiple account notion of disorder, and finally simply doing without accounts of disorder.

Cooper also explores the issues surrounding mental versus physical health and disease or disorder. She begins with the antipsychiatry movement in the

1970s and proceeds to the biologically based approach of today, in terms of the neurosciences. She then discusses the appropriateness of splitting disorders along the binary plane of mental and physical, since many diseases exhibit both mental and physical dimensions. In conclusion, Cooper presents the reader with several emerging philosophical issues concerning health and disease. First, she discusses the first-person perspective of phenomenology and how best to integrate it with the third-person perspective of the biomedical sciences in order to understand health and disease more fully. Next, she examines the impact of medicalization and demedicalization on the changing nature of health and disease. Finally, she explores the issues facing a number of medical conditions, such as disabilities, aging, and artificial organs and organisms—which represent important areas for philosophical reflection.[7]

In chapter 12—"Causation in Medicine"—Brendan Clark and Federica Russo examine the philosophical issues pertaining to the notion of causation in the biomedical sciences and clinical practice. Their thesis is that no single understanding of medical causation captures its complexity entirely, whether in terms of making a diagnosis, evaluating a risk factor, or listening to a patient's illness narrative. They begin by noting the various understandings and uses of causation and utilize this plurality to champion a causal mosaic metaphor for an approach to medical causation. To that end, they invoke casuistry to operationalize their metaphor in terms of two episodes in medicine. The first is hypertension. They discuss what is problematic about causation in this medical episode with respect to a treatment's efficacy and effectiveness. Another critical issue is the reference class problem for which they offer several principles, such as the broadness of the reference class, to assist in addressing it. The next episode is actually a series of deficiency diseases, which they analyze vis-à-vis causation in terms of omission, evidence, and inference. Their examples include the Ottawa ankle rules, gender medicine, and asbestos-related deaths.

Clark and Russo argue that medical causation is multifactorial and then introduce a causal mosaic metaphor to capture the diversity of uses for causal thinking in medicine. They begin by identifying the two predominate causal theories in the philosophy of science, the counterfactual theory and mechanistic theory, and proceed to discuss the biological and epidemiological notions of causation. Next, they turn their attention to the question of the use of causal knowledge. From a survey of its uses, they conclude that the "one-theory of causality" is inadequate to capture the plurality of types and uses of causation in medicine. Their mosaic metaphor is an attempt to integrate the different philosophical notions of causation, whether metaphysical or epistemological, and scientific notions, whether inferential or predictive. Just as tiles positioned correctly within a mosaic allows a picture to emerge, so proper positioning of philosophical and scientific accounts allows the medical causal picture to emerge. Finally, Clark and Russo acknowledge the challenges facing them to provide a full mosaic for medical causation, and they invite both the philosophical and medical communities to join them in working toward that end.

In chapter 13—"Clinical Reasoning and Knowing'"—Hillel Braude conducts an analysis of CR in terms of current cognitive sciences. For Braude, however, CR involves not only a cognitive dimension but also a moral one, which he explores in terms of Aristotelian *phronesis*. He begins the cognitive analysis discussing Alvan Feinstein's *Clinical Judgment* and the physician's personal role in the art of clinical judging and knowing. This leads him to the nonanalytical or tacit dimension of reasoning, especially as espoused by Michael Polanyi, and to the paradox that this dimension is critical for explicit reasoning but is resistant to analysis via such reasoning. Braude next takes up the recent work on decision analysis, especially Daniel Kahneman and Amos Tversky's prospect theory based on heuristic rules or mental shortcuts as opposed to logical algorithmic rules involved in rational choice or expected utility theory. He goes on to discuss the relevance of this work in debiasing CR. Braude then considers the dual process theory of cognition with its intuitive system 1 processes and logical system 2 processes, as well as the role of metacognition—self-evaluative cognitive processes—to bridge the gap between the two systems, and the theory's application to CR.

Having furnished the background for examining CR in terms of contemporary cognitive science, Braude then turns to the Aristotelian notion of *phronesis* or practical reason to provide a comprehensive model for CR, which combines both the epistemic and moral dimensions of clinical knowing and decision-making. For Braude, *phronesis* represents the best method for CR since it incorporates the necessary epistemic virtues involved in clinical medicine, especially *episteme* (analytic reasoning), *techné* (technical reasoning), and *nous* (intuitive reasoning). In addition, *phronesis* also includes both *poiesis*—an act of crafting a product— and *praxis*—a practical act of achieving a good end. *Phronesis*, particularly for reliable CR, involves the competence not simply to deliver a diagnosis and to recommend a treatment but an accurate diagnosis and an efficacious treatment for a particular patient. According to Braude, *phronesis* represents the most effective way to make clinical decisions and judgments—particularly given the uncertainties and complexities associated with clinical practice. Indeed, he concludes that *phronesis* not only entails the cognitive dimension of CR but also stipulates its moral dimension for delivering the medical goods.

In sum, uncertainty and complexity are hallmarks of modern medicine, as illustrated not only in the topics of health, disease, medical causation, and clinical reasoning and knowing but also in the plurality of approaches to the nature of medicine per se and its practice. The problems arising because of the complexity involved in defining disease, health, and medical causation undergirds the gravity of uncertainty's impact on clinical decision-making and the need to embed it in a moral framework for delivering the medical goods and for not harming the patient unnecessarily (Hayward, 2006). As Braude discusses in his chapter, *phronesis* is undoubtedly a means for bridging the gap between medicine's technical and moral imperatives vis-à-vis clinical uncertainty and complexity. Virtue theory also provides an important avenue for philosophers of medicine to contribute to the issues raised over the uncertainties and complexities associated with clinical practice. For example, compassionate wisdom, as a compound virtue, has been proposed to address them (Marcum, 2012a). There are definitely many issues in contemporary medicine for philosophers of medicine to analyze and contribute to in the future—to which we now turn.

Philosophy of Medicine's Future

In the last chapter—"New Directions in Philosophy of Medicine"—Jacob Stegenga and coauthors explore the immediate future of contemporary philosophy of medicine with respect to its perennial problems, such as health and disease, and assess the directions it may take in addressing them. The specific problems they examine include RCTs and their meta-analysis, clinical diagnosis, philosophy and psychiatry, and objectivity and medical research. Although no permanent solutions to these problems are imminent, they contend that contemporary philosophy of medicine helps to bring clarity to issues challenging modern medicine and its practice, whether for a specific medical discipline like psychiatry or for a particular clinical skill like diagnosis. Contemporary philosophy of medicine's future is certainly an issue of concern for the discipline (Lemoine et al., 2014; Loughlin et al., 2014), and this chapter helps to address that concern and to provide a clear path on which to proceed.

Stegenga and coauthors embed their commentary on philosophy of medicine's future in terms of an "epistemological turn" in the recent literature. They identify two features of this turn. The first concerns the epistemic status of RCTs and their meta-analysis and systematic reviews, while the second pertains to the intersection among the methodological, social, and ethical dimensions of medical research. As for the first feature, they explore the philosophical issues arising from RCTs in terms of generalizability to clinical care and outcomes with respect to specific patient groups. For the second feature, they examine the relationship between objectivity and medical research, as well as the social context in which such research is conducted. Specifically, the authors examine the traditional view of objectivity as a virtue associated with neutral investigation and explanation, and discuss the issues arising with this view in terms of social constraints, particularly in terms of funding sources.

Stegenga and coauthors also examine the philosophical issues surrounding clinical diagnosis, especially whether there is a logic of diagnosis. And they explore the philosophical issues pertaining to the relationship between diagnostic accuracy and clinical outcomes and between diagnostics and predictive or prognostic value. The authors also discuss recent developments within psychiatry, especially with the publication of the DSM 5 and the neuroscientific approach to the etiology of psychiatric disorders. They specifically consider the concerns over whether the DSM-5 approach provides the best means for classifying and investigating psychiatric disorders. Finally, they conclude that contemporary philosophy of medicine with its "epistemological turn" introduces multiple directions for philosophical reflection to proceed.

Research Resources

The Companion is structured not only to reflect the pluralism within modern medicine and its practice but also to provide the reader with a dynamic framework for conducting scholarship in contemporary philosophy of medicine vis-à-vis modern medicine's pluralism and thereby to offer the reader guidance in accessing and utilizing the literature on the contemporary philosophy of medicine. To that end, it also contains a final section on research sources, including a glossary of key terms, a guide to these sources, and an annotated bibliography. In conclusion, *The Companion* strives to equip the reader with the knowledge and skills needed to participate in and to contribute to contemporary philosophy of medicine.

Additional Types of Medicine

Besides the types of medicine covered in *The Companion*'s chapters, there are other important types that also represent fertile ground for philosophical toiling. Space restrictions do not permit their inclusion, in any depth. In this section, a few of them are briefly discussed. For medical scientism, the types of medicine include the logic of medicine along with analytic medicine, translational medicine, integrative medicine, and systems medicine. For medical humanism, the types of medicine include BPS medicine, narrative medicine, and virtue-based medicine.

Logic of medicine, which includes analytic medicine, is an important type of or approach to medicine and its practice (Black, 1968; Murphy, 1997; Sadegh-Zadeh, 2015). One of the main goals of this approach is to reduce the incidence of clinical errors, especially in CR for both diagnosis and treatment selection. Another goal is to clarify and to bring precision to the conceptual, epistemological, methodological, and ontological foundations of medicine. In terms of reducing the incidence of error, the logic of medicine stresses intellectual rigor through some type of logical system, whether traditional logic, logico-statistical analysis, Bayesian logic, or fuzzy logic. With respect to clarifying the foundations of medicine, it employs linguistic analysis of epistemic statements, especially in terms of the definition and classification of disease, as well as critical analysis of the standards for discovering and justifying medical knowledge. Finally, the focus of the logic of medicine and analytic medicine is not simply on medical knowledge per se but on providing the best opportunity for a successful and an efficacious clinical encounter between patient and physician.

Translational medicine is aptly captured in the motto "bench-to-bedside" and is considered the gateway toward realizing personalized medicine (Luciano et al., 2011). Although defining translational medicine is challenging, it is generally delineated in terms of at least two basic stages (Woolf, 2008). The first, T1, is the translation or application of knowledge gained from biomedical research to clinical trials, while the second, T2, is the translation or utilization of knowledge obtained from clinical trials to treat patients at the bedside. There are epistemological issues with the use of the metaphor "translation" to represent the generation and application of medical knowledge (Greenhalgh and Wieringa, 2011; Solomon, 2015). First, the generation of biomedical or clinical knowledge is not as simple or straightforward as many scientists or clinicians assume. Rather, the process of discovering such knowledge and justifying it involves personal preferences and social values that problematize the process. Next, the transfer or application of medical knowledge is not simply a unidirectional flow from bench-to-bedside but also includes a retrograde flow from bedside-to-bench (Marincola, 2003). Finally, various stakeholders, especially policy makers, have a significant impact on how such knowledge is translated at the bedside.[8]

Integrative medicine comes in at least two types. The first is the integration of Western medical specialties and subspecialties to provide patients with seamless and contiguous healthcare (Rakel, 2012). A common complaint of patients with Western medicine is the fragmented nature of its healthcare delivery. In other words, patients may see various specialists with no overall guidance from a single healthcare professional. One means of achieving integration might include the incorporation of one of the humanistic approaches to medicine, such as patient-centered care (Maizes et al., 2009). The second type involves the integration of Western allopathic medicine with Eastern complementary and alternative medicine, especially Chinese traditional or Ayurveda medicine, or with homeopathic medicine (Baer, 2004; Kligler and Lee, 2004). Whereas the first type of integrative medicine addresses the fragmented care of Western medicine, the second focuses on the perceived ineffectualness of Western therapies either to cure or manage illness effectively or on the pernicious side effects of allopathic therapies. Finally, although both types differ in significant ways, they do share a common goal of integrating both the body and mind to provide holistic healthcare.

Systems medicine is a recent type of scientific medicine that represents an outgrowth of systems and big biology (Auffray et al., 2009).[9] With the initial completion of the Human Genome Project in the early 2000s, new technologies for the investigation and analysis of experimental data from genomics, proteomics, and metabolomics, for instance, began to transform the understanding of physiological and pathological processes in terms of linear mechanistic causal processes to network interactive causal processes (Barabási et al., 2011). Philosophically, this represents a shift from a reductionistic framework to a holistic one (Marcum, 2009a). In other words, a complex phenomenon is simply more than the summation of its individual components' properties. The challenge, however, has been the realization or operationalization of this shift both methodologically and conceptually. Besides translational medicine, systems medicine also champions a personalized medicine or P4 medicine: predictive, preventive, personalized, and participatory (Hood, 2013). However, criticism has been leveled against systems or P4 medicine in that it does not take into consideration the patient's illness experience (Pavelić et al., 2015). One potential means to address this criticism is to integrate systems-P4 medicine with Traditional Chinese Medicine (Guoan et al., 2011).

As for other types of humanistic medicine, George Engel (1977) introduced a BPS model for clinical practice in contrast to traditional scientific medicine or the biomedical model of healthcare. According to Engel, quality healthcare should include not only the biological and technical but also the psychological and social dimensions. Although the medical community, both nationally and internationally, embraced BPS medicine initially, the challenge facing it was empirical testing of its principles (Schwartz, 1982). Moreover, the philosophical assumptions grounding BPS medicine have been analyzed in terms of defending the necessity of incorporating the patient's illness experience into clinical practice (Borrell-Carrió et al., 2004). And, the BPS model has been revised to include the spiritual dimension of healthcare, based on a philosophical anthropology of personhood (Sulmasy, 2002). However, the operationalization of BPS medicine has been criticized, at least for psychiatry, as being an unprincipled eclectic approach, and a principled noneclectic alternative based on Karl Jaspers's methods-based approach has been proposed to replace it (Ghaemi, 2010).[10]

Besides BPS medicine, another response to the marginalization of patients due to technological intervention in clinical practice is narrative medicine. Certainly objective clinical observations and facts are critical for making an accurate diagnosis, but they can be insufficient for an optimal clinical outcome in terms of treatment. Early advocates of narrative medicine insisted that the patient's illness story is indispensable for delivering quality healthcare, especially for the management of chronic diseases (Brody, 2003; Kleinman, 1988; White and Epston, 1990). Today, narrative medicine is attracting attention as a viable approach to medicine and its practice, with the notion of narrative competence as an important skill for delivering quality healthcare (Charon, 2006). In addition to patient's illness narrative, the doctor's story is also tantamount to optimal clinical outcomes (Hunter, 1991). Last, one of the major criticisms of narrative medicine is that the facts associated with a patient's illness story might be compromised by being distorted, embellished, or even fabricated (Solomon, 2015, p. 104). One possible solution to this problem is the integration of EBM with narrative medicine (Meza and Passerman, 2011).

Finally, the traditional cardinal and theological, as well as contemporary, virtues have recently been incorporated into medicine and its practice (Bryan, 2005). After the eclipse of virtue ethics by consequentialist and deontological ethics, virtue theory and ethics reemerged in the first part of the twentieth century. Edmund Pellegrino and David Thomasma (1993) initially championed the role of traditional virtues, especially *phronesis*, in clinical practice. In a subsequent work, they included the theological virtues of faith, hope, and charity (Pellegrino and Thomasma, 1996). Importantly, the motivation for the incorporation of virtues into medicine has been the notion that medicine is a moral enterprise between patients and physicians qua persons who strive to achieve the good. Indeed, virtues have been used to define the "good" physician (Drane, 1995). Besides the role of virtues in the ethical or moral practice of medicine, epistemic virtues have been used to address issues in CR and decision-making (Gupta and Upshur, 2012; Marcum, 2009b). Finally, virtues have also been employed to address two crises in medicine: quality of care and professionalism (Marcum, 2012b).[11]

Conclusion: A Metaphysical Turn

As Stegenga and coauthors note in their chapter on new directions in the philosophy of medicine, contemporary philosophy of medicine took an "epistemological turn" during the second half of the twentieth century, which had important implications not only for its present condition but also for its future. Besides this turn, I propose—based on the discussion in *The Companion*'s chapters—that contemporary philosophy of medicine is also undergoing a "metaphysical turn," which has equally important implications for its future. This turn involves both an ontological and a presuppositional direction.

Just two of the many aspects to the ontological direction of the metaphysical turn are briefly considered here. The first pertains to the fundamental nature of personhood, especially from a humanistic perspective. The nature of the person is critical for fashioning a vigorous contemporary philosophy of medicine, especially in terms of merging both medical scientism and humanism. As noted previously, one of the chief goals of medicine is the relief of suffering,

Being→Having→Doing

Figure 1.1 Relationships among being, having, and doing (see text for details).

whether physical and/or existential or psychological. Both medical scientism and humanism subscribe to this goal, although both approach it differently. For medical scientism the person is a machine and relief of suffering takes the form of a cure, while for medical humanism the person is embodied in a life-world and the relief of suffering involves revising embodiment vis-à-vis the life-world. The notion of personhood provides a common focal point for coalescing them, especially in terms of restoring the person's dignity, which illness compromises. Although medicine cannot often achieve the goal of a cure, it can, or should, manage the harm and humiliation illness often inflicts on a person—and not add to them.

The second aspect encompasses the role of virtues in clinical practice, especially in terms of medical professionalism. The ontological question is who the physician wants to be, that is, a question of being (Figure 1.1). Hopefully, the physician wants to be a "good" professional, which implies having. To that end, the physician must have or acquire the skills to practice medicine competently. But technical skills alone are not enough to be a good physician—interpersonal skills are also required. Only when equipped with both technical and interpersonal competence can the good physician engage in doing or practicing medicine—the delivery of compassionate quality healthcare (Marcum, 2011). Finally, in terms of virtues, both epistemic and ethical virtues are necessary for satisfying this direction of the turn, and philosophers of medicine can play a key role in assisting the medical profession in identifying and appropriating the requisite virtues and values.

The presuppositional direction of the metaphysical turn pertains to the assumptions underlying medicine and its practice. If a practical combination of medical scientism and humanism is going to be achieved, the presuppositions that underlie each need to be reconciled or resolved with one another (Table 1.1). As noted earlier, this is possible as shown for the objective–subjective dyad—in that a subject's authenticity guarantees an object's genuineness. This resolution in terms of authenticity and genuineness is only one way of bridging the gap between presuppositional dyads, and it most likely may not work for all of them. For example, it is not readily apparent how authenticity and genuineness would help to bridge the gap between the positivism–historicism dyad. Alternative ways for bridging the gap between these seemingly contradictory presuppositional dyads need to be developed, and they represent an important challenge to contemporary philosophers of medicine—if medical scientism and humanism are to be coalesced in an operative relationship that delivers the best possible healthcare.

In sum, contemporary philosophy of medicine is a vibrant and growing field that engages more than bioethical issues. It also engages the metaphysical, ontological, epistemological, and methodological issues facing modern medicine, as introduced and discussed in *The Companion*. Finally, to paraphrase a modern song, contemporary philosophy of medicine's "future's so bright . . . [its] . . . gotta wear shades.[12]

Notes

1. For a review of medical pluralism, particularly with the United States, see Kaptchuk and Eisenberg (2001a, b).
2. For example, Miriam Solomon (2015) takes a pluralistic approach to the generation of Western medical knowledge with respect to consensus conferences, evidence-based medicine, translational medicine, and narrative medicine.
3. For a recent and comprehensive overview of the logico-analytical method to the philosophy of medicine, see Sadegh-Zadeh (2015).
4. Interestingly, the notion of personalized medicine is embraced by both advocates of the art and the science of medicine. For the art of medicine, personalized medicine reflects the patient qua person (Miles and Mezzich, 2011) while for the science of medicine the patient qua genomic sequence (Hamburg and Collins, 2010)—which has led at times to confusion over the notion (Ekman et al., 2011).
5. Boenink's observation concerning the technologically mediated nature of health and disease is reminiscent of Heidegger's (1977) concern of technology becoming a means towards distorting reality rather than for revealing nature for what it is.
6. Bragazzi (2013) traces the evolution of medicine, from P0 medicine or paternalistic medicine, which was eventually eclipsed by P3 medicine, to P4 medicine with the addition of participatory, P5 medicine with psychocognitive, and finally P6 medicine with public.
7. For an example of recent discussion in the philosophical literature over the issue of aging, see De Winter (2015).
8. Besides the epistemological issues, ethical issues have also been raised, especially the protection of patients from poorly thought-out research in an attempt to expedite the process from bench-to-bedside (Petrini, 2010).
9. Biomedical informatics, telemedicine, and e-medicine are related topics to translational, integrative, systems, and P4 medicine (Fong et al., 2011; Om, 2015; Shortliffe and Cimino, 2014).
10. Engel's BPS approach to patient care is not the first to take a holistic approach to patient care. Focus on the patient qua whole has been a constant theme throughout medicine's history, especially in the twentieth century in response to efforts to view medicine as a science.
11. Values-based medicine as discussed in chapter 2 is another important approach to healthcare.
12. The song is "The Future's So Bright" by Timbuk 3.

References

Auffray, C., Chen, Z., and Hood, L. (2009). Systems medicine: The future of medical genomics and healthcare. *Genome Medicine* 1(1): 2.

Baer, H. A. (2004). *Toward an Integrative Medicine: Merging Alternative Therapies with Biomedicine*. Oxford: AltaMira Press.

Baglivi, G. (1723). *Practice of Physick*, 2nd edition. London: Midwinter.

Barabási, A. L., Gulbahce, N., and Loscalzo, J. (2011). Network medicine: A network-based approach to human disease. *Nature Reviews Genetics* 12(1): 56–68.

Black, D. (1968). *The Logic of Medicine*. Edinburgh: Oliver & Boyd.

Borrell-Carrió, F., Suchman, A. L., and Epstein, R. M. (2004). The biopsychosocial model 25 years later: Principles, practice, and scientific inquiry. *Annals of Family Medicine* 2(6): 576–82.

Bragazzi, N. L. (2013). From P0 to P6 medicine, a model of highly participatory, narrative, interactive, and "augmented" medicine: Some considerations on Salvatore Iaconesi's clinical story. *Patient Preference and Adherence* 7: 353–59.

Brody, H. (2003). *Stories of Sickness*, 2nd edition. New York: Oxford University Press.

Bryan, C. S. (2005). Medicine and the seven basic virtues. *Journal of the South Carolina Medical Association* 101(9): 327–28.

Cassell, E. J. (1991). *The Nature of Suffering and the Goals of Medicine*. New York: Oxford University Press.

Charon, R. (2006). *Narrative Medicine: Honoring the Stories of Illness*. New York: Oxford University Press.

De Winter, G. (2015). Aging as disease. *Medicine, Health Care and Philosophy* 18(2): 237–43.

Drane, J. (1995). *Becoming a Good Doctor: The Place of Virtue and Character in Medical Ethics*, 2nd edition. Kansas City, MO: Sheed & Ward.

Ekman, I., Swedberg, K., Taft, C., Lindseth, A., Norberg, A., Brink, E., Carlsson, J., Dahlin-Ivanoff, S., Johansson, I. L., Kjellgren, K., and Lidén, E. (2011). Person-centered care—Ready for prime time. *European Journal of Cardiovascular Nursing* 10(4): 248–51.

Engel, G. L. (1977). The need for a new medical model: A challenge for biomedicine. *Science* 196(4286): 129–36.

Fong, B., Fong, A. C. M., and Li, C. K. (2011). *Telemedicine Technologies: Information Technologies in Medicine and Telehealth*. New York: John Wiley & Sons.

Ghaemi, S. N. (2010). *The Rise and Fall of the Biopsychosocial Model: Reconciling Art and Science in Psychiatry*. Baltimore, MD: Johns Hopkins University Press.

Greenhalgh, T., and Wieringa, S. (2011). Is it time to drop the "knowledge translation" metaphor? A critical literature review. *Journal of the Royal Society of Medicine* 104(12): 501–509.

Guoan, L., Yiming, W., Qionglin, L., Yuanyuan, X., and Xuemei, F. (2011). System medicine and translational medicine. *World Science and Technology* 13(1): 1–8.

Gupta, M., and Upshur, R. (2012). Critical thinking in clinical medicine: What is it? *Journal of Evaluation in Clinical Practice* 18(5): 938–44.

Hamburg, M. A., and Collins, F. S. (2010). The path to personalized medicine. *New England Journal of Medicine* 363(4): 301–304.

Hayward, R. (2006). Balancing certainty and uncertainty in clinical medicine. *Developmental Medicine & Child Neurology* 48: 74–77.

Heidegger, M. (1977). *The Question Concerning Technology and Other Essays*, W. Lovitt, trans. New York: Harper & Row.

Hood, L. (2013). Systems biology and P4 medicine: Past, present, and future. *Rambam Maimonides Medical Journal* 4(2): e0012.

Hsu, E. (2008). Medical pluralism. *International Encyclopedia of Public Health* 4: 316–21.

Hunter, K. M. (1991). *Doctor's Stories: The Narrative Structure of Medical Knowledge*. Princeton, NJ: Princeton University Press.

Jones, W. H. S., trans. (1923). *Hippocrates*, Vol. II. Loeb Classical Library. Cambridge: Harvard University Press.

Kaptchuk, T. J., and Eisenberg, D. M. (2001a). Varieties of healing. 1: Medical pluralism in the United States. *Annals of Internal Medicine* 135(3): 189–95.

Kaptchuk, T. J., and Eisenberg, D. M. (2001b). Varieties of healing. 2: A taxonomy of unconventional healing practices. *Annals of Internal Medicine* 135(3): 196–204.

King, L. S. (1978). *The Philosophy of Medicine: The Early Eighteenth Century*. Cambridge: Harvard University Press.

Kleinman, A. (1980). *Patients and Healers in the Context of Culture: An Exploration of the Borderland between Anthropology, Medicine, and Psychiatry*. Berkeley, CA: University of California Press.

Kleinman, A. (1988). *The Illness Narratives: Suffering, Healing and the Human Condition*. New York: Basic Books.

Kligler, B., and Lee, R. (2004). *Integrative Medicine: Principles for Practice*. New York: McGraw-Hill.

Lemoine, M., Darrason, M., and Richard, H. (2014). Where is philosophy of medicine headed? A report of the International Advanced Seminar in the Philosophy of Medicine (IASPM). *Journal of Evaluation in Clinical Practice* 20(6): 991–93.

Lonergan, B. J. F. (1972). *Method in Theology*. New York: Herder and Herder.

Loughlin, M., Bluhm, R., Fuller, J., Buetow, S., Upshur, R. E., Borgerson, K., Goldenberg, M. J., and Kingma, E. (2014). Philosophy, medicine and health care—Where we have come from and where we are going. *Journal of Evaluation in Clinical Practice* 20(6): 902–907.

Luciano, J. S., Andersson, B., Batchelor, C. R., Bodenreider, O., Clark, T., Denney, C. K., Domarew, C., Gambet, T., Harland, L., Jentzsch, A., and Kashyap, V. (2011). The translational medicine ontology and knowledge base: Driving personalized medicine by bridging the gap between bench and bedside. *Journal of Biomedical Semantics* 2(S-2): S1.

Maizes, V., Rakel, D., and Niemiec, C. (2009). Integrative medicine and patient-centered care. *Explore: The Journal of Science and Healing* 5(5): 277–89.

Marcum, J. A. (2009a). *The Conceptual Foundations of Systems Biology: An Introduction*. New York: Nova Scientific Publishers.

Marcum, J. A. (2009b). The epistemically virtuous clinician. *Theoretical Medicine and Bioethics*, 30(3): 249–65.

Marcum, J. A. 2011. Care and competence in medical practice: Francis Peabody confronts Jason Posner. *Medicine, Health Care and Philosophy* 14: 143–53.

Marcum, J. A. (2012a). Medical uncertainty and paradox, and the quality-of-care crisis. *International Journal of Health, Wellness and Society* 2(1): 21–31.

Marcum, J. A. (2012b). *The Virtuous Physician: The Role of Virtue in Medicine*. New York: Springer.

Marincola, F. M. (2003). Translational medicine: A two-way road. *Journal of Translational Medicine* 1(1): 1.

Meza, J. P., and Passerman, D. S. (2011). *Integrating Narrative Medicine and Evidence-Based Medicine: The Everyday Social Practice of Healing*. London: Radcliffe.

Miles, A., and Mezzich, J. (2011). The care of the patient and the soul of the clinic: Person-centered medicine as an emergent model of modern clinical practice. *International Journal of Person Centered Medicine* 1(2): 207–22.

Murphy, E. A. (1997). *The Logic of Medicine*, 2nd edition. Baltimore, MD: The Johns Hopkins University Press.

Om, A. (2015). E-medicine: What it means for patients. *American Journal of Medicine* 128(12): 1268–69.

Pavelić, K., Martinović, T., and Pavelić, S. K. (2015). Do we understand the personalized medicine paradigm? *EMBO Reports* 16(2): 133–36.

Peabody, F. W. (1927). The care of the patient. *Journal of American Medical Association* 88: 877–82.

Pellegrino, E. D., and Thomasma, D. C. (1993). *The Virtues in Medical Practice*. New York: Oxford University Press.

Pellegrino, E. D., and Thomasma, D. C. (1996). *The Christian Virtues in Medical Practice*. Washington, DC: Georgetown University Press.

Petrini, C. (2010). Ethical issues in translational research. *Perspectives in Biology and Medicine* 53(4): 517–33.

Rakel, D. (2012). *Integrative Medicine*, 3rd edition. Philadelphia: Elsevier.

Sadegh-Zadeh, K. (2015). *Handbook of Analytic Philosophy of Medicine*, 2nd edition. Dordrecht: Springer.

Schwartz, G. E. (1982). Testing the biopsychosocial model: The ultimate challenge facing behavioral medicine? *Journal of Consulting and Clinical Psychology* 50(6): 1040–53.

Shortliffe, E. H., and Cimino, J. J., eds. (2014). *Biomedical Informatics: Computer Applications in Health Care and Biomedicine*, 4th edition. New York: Springer.

Smith, C. (2010). *What Is a Person? Rethinking Humanity, Social Life, and the Moral Good from the Person Up*. Chicago: University of Chicago Press.

Solomon, M. (2015). *Making Medical Knowledge*. New York: Oxford University Press.

Sulmasy, D. P. (2002). A biopsychosocial–spiritual model for the care of patients at the end of life. *The Gerontologist* 42(Suppl 3): 24–33.

Wade, C., Chao, M., Kronenberg, F., Cushman, L., and Kalmuss, D. (2008). Medical pluralism among American women: Results of a national survey. *Journal of Women's Health* 17(5): 829–40.

Welch, W. H. (1908). The interdependence of medicine and other sciences of nature. *Science* 27: 49–64.

White, M., and Epston, D. (1990). *Narrative Means to Therapeutic Ends*. New York: Norton & Co.

Woolf, S. H. (2008). The meaning of translational research and why it matters. *Journal of American Medical Association* 299(2): 211–13.

2 Research Problems and Methods in the Philosophy of Medicine

Michael Loughlin, Robyn Bluhm, and Mona Gupta

Introduction

What is the philosophy of medicine? What problems does this discipline solve and how does it go about solving them? There are some, of course, who still maintain that philosophy has no business whatsoever in medicine, the latter being a science, and the former being the sort of idle speculation one engages in when lacking sound research evidence for one's conclusions. As one internet blogger[1] puts it, philosophy is "largely ignored by science." In a characteristically simplistic and dismissive account of the views of two renowned philosophers of science, John Worrall and Nancy Cartwright, on the nature of causality, the blogger quips:

> Many words are spent on defining causality but, at least in the clinical setting the meaning is perfectly simple. If the association between eating bacon and colorectal cancer is causal then if you stop eating bacon you'll reduce the risk of cancer. If the relationship is not causal then if you stop eating bacon it won't help at all. No amount of Worrall's 'serious thought' will substitute for the real evidence for causality that can come only from an RCT.[2]

It is symptomatic of the blogger's disdain for philosophical methods that he sees no reason to defend his own conception of science, and thinks that banal or "common sense" observations about bacon substitute for any efforts to understand, let alone to respond to, the quite extraordinarily detailed arguments on the nature of science and causal explanations developed by the thinkers he swiftly dismisses. On such a view the philosophy of medicine is presumably something one does if lacking the scientific background to do real medicine, and the idea of "research problems and methods in the philosophy of medicine" represents something of an oxymoron.

The willingness to examine critically one's own underlying assumptions is a prerequisite for engaging in philosophical thinking and discourse (Loughlin et al., 2015). It is therefore not unreasonable to expect authors in any area of applied philosophy to have considered the nature and limitations of their activity and its relationship with the practices it hopes to inform. While these anti-philosophical ideas about the relationship between medicine, science, and philosophy do not, we believe, stand up to serious intellectual scrutiny, they do represent a conceptual framework with a lengthy intellectual heritage, and one whose influence needs to be understood if we are to confront the methodological questions facing the philosophy of medicine. Were such responses confined to the blog pages of a bizarre, secular science counterpart to the Reverend Fred Phelps[3] they could perhaps be ignored. But the very fact that they can be articulated—and treated as effectively "just plain obvious"—in such popular media (on a site that apparently commands a large following) is indicative of their pervasive influence.

We return to the issue of causation in medicine later in this chapter, and hopefully say enough to indicate that the issue is not perfectly simple, nor have the significant controversies on this question been resolved.[4] The claim that we need evidence (indeed, real evidence) to answer causal questions in medicine is what is known as a "platitude": no reasonable person could dispute it. In contrast, the assertion that only a randomized controlled trial (RCT) can provide evidence relevant to the causal reasoning that necessarily informs clinical decision-making is not only controversial, but apparently represents what a prominent defender of evidence-based medicine (EBM) describes, in his contribution to this volume, as a "straw man" version of EBM (see Jeremy Howick, chapter 5). In his view, even the more popular and credible position, that RCTs provide better evidence than observational studies and/or mechanistic reasoning, needs modification if it is to be intellectually defensible. Whatever one thinks of this argument, the insertion of the otherwise superfluous qualifier "real" in the earlier quotation is indicative of an implicit philosophical claim. While practitioners in all manner of clinical contexts might treat context-specific features of situations as vital evidence about causal factors affecting the symptoms patients present (Greenhalgh 2012; Macnaughton 2011), the only semantic content supplied by the term "real" here is to imply a contrast, to express the background assumption that such forms of evidence are *not* real—that the information such personal observations embody cannot qualify for the term "evidence" in the way that the results of RCTs can. Of course, the only defense of this claim in the blog derives from running it together with a platitudinous declaration that we need evidence as the basis for causal conclusions, and given the blogger's avowed disdain for philosophy, he is unable to recognize, let alone defend, his own distinctly philosophical commitments.

Ironically, it is from academic philosophy itself that such anti-philosophical ideas originate. The idea that the only source of real knowledge is a fairly narrowly defined conception of empirical science owes its intuitive plausibility to what is sometimes called the "legacy of positivism" (Achinstein and Barker, 1969) and an associated atomistic approach to knowledge that has had a profound effect on the development of biomedicine (Macnaughton, 2011). Logical positivism (or empiricism) bolstered the view that only empirical data acquired in certain specific ways could provide objective evidence, giving rise to an intellectual culture in which judgment, personal experience, and context-specific information were regarded with suspicion as subjective factors (Kirkengen and Thornquist, 2012; Loughlin et al., 2013). While this philosophical position has been subjected to extensive criticism, and the problems it creates for scientific practice have been well documented (Kincaid et al., 2007; Maxwell, 2004; Nagel, 1986), there is no consensus regarding the most appropriate alternative epistemological framework to understand the relationship between science, knowledge, experience, theory, judgment, and value. Indeed, the debate between broadly empiricist and rival rationalist positions in epistemology is far from being resolved, and we discuss the specific implications of this debate for current accounts of medical causality later in this chapter.

What is more, there are serious questions about the nature and status of the philosophy of medicine, and there is by no means a general consensus in the area as to how they are resolved. Two features of philosophy contribute to this situation. First, the already noted characteristic trait of the philosopher to examine underlying assumptions. Second, another required trait of consistency: to be a philosopher is to be willing to follow a line of thinking to its logical conclusion, however uncomfortable or counter-intuitive it may initially appear.

In combination, these two features lead philosophers themselves to ask difficult questions about what philosophy is — what its methods are, what sort of questions it can meaningfully answer, and consequently its limitations as a form of academic enquiry. It was this ruthless consistency that led logical positivists, influenced by ideas inherited from the great empiricist philosophers Locke and Hume, to conclude that it was not the business of philosophy to discover truths, but simply to solve (linguistic) puzzles, so as to assist in the project of empirical science — the only means for discovering genuine, non-trivial truths (Ayer, 1987, pp. 34–35). Arguably, under the leadership of the positivists, academic philosophy became something of a suicidal discipline, dismissing the questions that preoccupied its greatest thinkers over the centuries — about the nature of reality, the value of life, how human beings should live and practice — as either meaningless or purely subjective, in some cases apparently reveling in the practical irrelevance of its increasingly obscure, exclusive, technical discourse (Loughlin, 2002, pp. 119–26).

Key to arriving at this suicidal conclusion was the positivists' model of philosophical methodology, typically characterized as deductivist because it effectively equates rational argument—the presentation of *good reasons* to believe a conclusion—with logical validity. A deductively valid argument is one in which the conclusion follows logically from the premises presented, meaning that to deny the conclusion while asserting the truth of the premises is to be guilty of a formal contradiction. Hume's consistent application of the view of knowledge and reasoning as consisting, strictly, in the processes of observation and deduction led him ultimately to question the rational basis of so many of our everyday beliefs that the plausibility of his own conception of reasoning was itself called into question.

Hume is credited with discovering the problem of induction, noting that our inherent disposition to discover patterns in experience, to see particular conjunctions of events as indicative of broader, general, or universal laws, goes beyond the processes of observation and deduction, and therefore would seem to be non-rational. While we may be happy to regard the patterns observed by the witch-doctor (or perhaps the homeopath) as unwarranted generalizations lacking any rational basis, as Russell (1967, p. 38) famously notes, unless we regard induction as an inherently rational process, we must "forego all justifications of our expectations about the future," in which case we would have to admit that "we have no reason to expect the sun to rise tomorrow, to expect bread to be more nourishing than a stone, or to expect that if we throw ourselves off the roof we shall fall."

No one denies that rationality *minimally* requires the avoidance of contradiction and compatibility with empirical evidence. But if we limit our conception of reasoning to these essential characteristics, then we risk regarding as non-rational the human capacities and dispositions that make us able to distinguish good generalizations from bad (and consequently science from prejudice and superstition) and that enable us to be both good reasoners and good observers in practice:

> Consider the claim that "my mother is unhappy today." I might come to believe this on the basis of certain evidence: her facial expressions, the tone of her voice, her mannerisms as she goes about certain mundane tasks. The fact that someone who does not know her so well might encounter the same behaviour but fail to come to the same conclusion shows that the evidence for the claim does not logically entail the conclusion. (Loughlin, 2002, pp. 40–41)

Does it follow that such evidence does not provide us with a good reason to believe the conclusion, that it is not real evidence? Would a principled refusal to accept such evidence make us better, more rigorous thinkers or bad practitioners and (more generally) practically inept human beings? If a theory about rationality causes us to reject the use of our interpretive and other human faculties that in fact make practical reasoning possible, then we have reason to reject that view of rationality.[5]

Despite these problems, deductivism in its various forms has had a huge influence on thinking about clinical reasoning, effectively determining the methodological assumptions of dominant approaches to both medical epistemology and medical ethics. Tonelli (2014) points out that, in EBM, the results of empirical research function as the major premises from which conclusions about particular cases are deduced, while in biomedical ethics, the approach called "principlism" attempts to derive particular conclusions from the application of general principles, whose justification is presumably either self-evidence or just their general acceptability. (Though for the positivist, no major moral premise, however widely accepted, can claim anything other than "subjective" justification, rendering the whole idea of "moral reasoning" inherently problematic.)

Though overused and misused by some authors,[6] the phrase associated with Toulmin (1982), that medicine "saved the life" of philosophy, has more than a ring of truth about it. Toulmin argued that by returning their attention to the concrete—to the problems of particular, real cases in medical discourse— philosophers had found their subject "coming alive again" and had regained the sense of engagement with practical matters that had characterized the discourses of Socrates and Aristotle. Toulmin's specific focus was on the revival of moral philosophy: "By reintroducing into ethical debate the vexed topics raised by particular cases, they [medicine and law] have obliged philosophers to address once again the Aristotelian problems of practical reasoning, which had been on the sidelines for too long" (p. 749). Instead of regarding moral philosophy as a body of theory, and then raising skeptical questions about how, if at all, this body could be applied to the real world, (what practical conclusions, if any, could be deduced from its major premises, etc.), philosophers engaging in interdisciplinary debate treated philosophy as an activity—a style of thinking that enables us to describe the logical structure of arguments, to identify and analyze key assumptions and concepts, and to clarify debates by exposing ambiguities and errors of reasoning. As Toulmin notes (with practical illustrations), in making this contribution to a genuine *dialog* with practitioners, philosophers were sometimes able to assist in discovering a level of consensus about the (non-trivial) truth in particular cases that would astonish the positivists and ethical subjectivists.

It was not only ethics that stood in need of revival, nor could its revival be achieved in artificial separation from other aspects of philosophical thinking. Ethical questions—about what we should do in any given situation—are embedded within whole understandings of the situation, inseparable from our beliefs about what is the case (the traditional concern of those areas of philosophy termed "ontology" or "metaphysics"), what it is that we feel we can claim to know (epistemology), and our broader beliefs about reasoning (logic), as well as the meaning we ascribe to different aspects of the situation or to our perception of it (phenomenology) (Loughlin et al., 2015, p. 358). Since the publication of Toulmin's paper, medicine and healthcare have raised a host of pressing problems about the nature of health, disease, care, clinical judgment, evidence, causation, reasoning, and knowledge in clinical practice and the relationships between scientific explanations of disorder and human experience. Just as Socrates found in the marketplace scope to explore with his interlocutors the vast range of questions that formed the canon of philosophy, so, by applying their critical and analytical skills to debates in medicine and healthcare, contemporary philosophers have regained what Toulmin (1982) characterized as "a seriousness and human relevance" for their discipline.

Toulmin's case-based approach to practical reasoning is often labeled casuistry, and its contemporary defenders note that it challenges some of the most entrenched assumptions of traditional analytical philosophy. In particular, it has been argued that casuistry problematizes the sharp distinction between fact and value, which owes its origins to the work of the empiricists (again, most notably Hume) and via the positivists has massively influenced the understanding of evidence in clinical medicine—in particular in the EBM movement. Tonelli (2014, pp. 238–40) argues that the fact–value dichotomy is a theoretical construct that can distort clinical reasoning. This is because, in real cases, there is no necessarily clear divide between factual and evaluative aspects of a situation: even our characterization of particular observed facts is bound up with explicit or implicit value-judgments. Whether or not we agree with this specific claim, it reminds us that the dialog between medicine and philosophy must be a genuine one, not a one-way process in which something called philosophical theory is applied to the resolution of practical problems, whose nature is (by implication) philosophically unproblematic (Loughlin, 2002, pp. 143–46). Even our description of a background situation, and the identification of some features of it as representing the problem, embodies assumptions that can be questioned (see later) and theoretical distinctions can be called into question if they fail to serve some useful purpose: the way to defend them (if they are defensible) is to show that they do, in fact, contribute to a way of understanding a real situation that can help us to deal with it more adequately.

Critics of casuistry have focused on its ability, celebrated by Toulmin, to drive consensus in particular cases, arguing that this consensus can reflect implicit shared values among the participants in a dialog—for instance, on what represents an adequate characterization of a problem and what it means to respond adequately to that problem (Kopelman, 1994). Unless these shared, underlying values are identified and subjected to critical scrutiny, the process runs the risk of "self-confirming bias" (Fulford, 2014, p. 159). This criticism raises serious and unresolved philosophical questions about the relationship between the consensus of belief in a given group, the truth of the matter and what individuals have good reasons to believe. No credible defender of casuistry (certainly not those we have cited) would wish to defend the idea that the correct answer in any given case is defined with reference to an uncriticized consensus. The very idea of intellectual progress seems to depend on the willingness of individuals to challenge the consensus on a given issue, to recognize that our shared assumptions at any given point in time may simply be wrong. To fail to consider this possibility is to become the sort of unreflective dogmatist criticized at the beginning of this chapter, to adopt the standing assumption that "intellectual history came to an end . . . at just the point that we arrived on the scene" (Loughlin et al., 2013, p. 136).

This is precisely why we stated the willingness to examine critically one's own assumptions as a prerequisite of philosophical thinking. All thinking, in any area of life and practice, requires us to conceptualize the data of experience in some way, categorizing data according to different types or patterns, and a great virtue of philosophical thinking is that it enables us to focus on the *way* we do this, to bring our background assumptions and theories into the foreground of thought, to understand how they help us to frame our experience. That way, we can at least come to consider alternative ways of framing experience, alternative ways of seeing the world and characterizing problems. Advocates of what is sometimes called the "therapeutic" view of philosophical method (Hutchinson, 2008) argue that, even when presented with an apparently compelling argument for a given conclusion, we sometimes have a "suspicious sense"—the idea that there is something wrong that we cannot quite put our finger on. The explicit reasoning may be valid, but the object of our suspicion may not be what is said as much as the assumptions that underlie it. It may not have occurred to us to identify, let alone question, these assumptions until now. But until we do so, we cannot free ourselves from their influence, so we cannot release our potential to think creatively, to explore alternative conceptualizations of our circumstances, ones that may prove more valuable (Loughlin, 2002, p. 18). Consider the arguments in Rachel Cooper's contribution in this volume (chapter 11), on the nature of disability. A lot hinges on what we see as the problem for the disabled person: whether we see that problem as located in the person herself, or in the social world in which she is required to live her life. Is her difficulty in moving about in that world a consequence of the fact that she is inherently damaged, or is it because that world has been designed and constructed without reference to, without due consideration for, the need to accommodate her specific mode of being? Whatever conclusion we come to, we can hardly be said to have given the issue serious consideration if we have not even tried out the alternative ways of framing the problem and at least started to explore some of their implications for its solution.

Clinical Practice and Theory

Returning then to our original questions, we can at least now begin to give some qualified answers, to say something about what the philosophy of medicine must be if it is to be worth doing. On the one hand, it must not consist in the application of preconceived theoretical perspectives to practice, with the goal of correcting the perceptions and practices of those involved from an epistemically privileged position. The problems it investigates must be problems that arise within practice, within the lived experiences of practitioners and patients. On the other hand, it cannot take the current consensus on any particular issue— be it the nature of medical evidence or clinical reasoning, or the role of value-judgments in the diagnosis of medical problems—as an unchallenged given. Usual practice may be the necessary starting point for the philosophy of medicine, but that does not mean that this starting point is somehow beyond criticism. Indeed, the more radical movements in the philosophy of medicine have been those that took it upon themselves to critique common practices, and to argue that the goals of medicine were better served by significant—sometimes revolutionary—changes in the methods employed by practitioners in diagnosing and treating illness.

Any perceived tension between these two constraints upon research methods in the philosophy of medicine may be resolved by reminding ourselves of the point made in the previous section—that our current thoughts and practices exist within a history that is ongoing. We are not at the end of this history, in a place where all problems and puzzles have been eliminated. At times within the history of medicine, there have been problems arising from within practice that have not been entirely resolved by the application of business as usual, giving rise to a sense that all was not well—a frustration with how things are. Theoretical innovation has been one aspect of the continued intellectual evolution of clinical practice: movements to transform or revolutionize practice have been declared by their advocates to be natural responses to medicine's failure to practice consistently, with reference to its own avowed values and standards— be they of scientific rationality or compassionate humanity. So it was that early exponents of EBM appealed to the language of a paradigm shift, a term taken from Thomas Kuhn (1970). They appealed to this language because in Kuhn's work a paradigm shift occurs when those working within a tradition begin to recognize that it no longer makes sense in its own terms and that it gives rise to problems that it cannot solve. "When defects in an existing paradigm accumulate to the extent that the paradigm is no longer tenable, the paradigm is challenged and replaced by a new way of looking at the world" (EBM Working Group 1992, p. 2420). Medicine's desire to treat patients in a way that maximized the likelihood of achieving the best outcomes was inconsistent with a failure to utilize the growing evidence-base made possible by "developments in clinical research over the last 30 years" and its continued reliance instead on sources of evidence that were (the authors claimed) inferior (p. 2420).

More recently, advocates of "person-centered" approaches to medicine and healthcare have argued that contemporary medicine faces "a crisis of knowledge, care, compassion and costs" because "the exaltation of the biomedical model of clinical practice has led to a fascination with the molecular and cellular basis of disease and organ dysfunction" (Miles and Asbridge, 2013, p. 1). While they acknowledge that "pharmacological and technological innovations have mediated huge shifts in individual and population health," they argue that, having at one point facilitated progress, the current dominance of this "biomedical reductionism" now stands in the way of the progress that is needed (p. 1).

[T]here is a growing sense of unease that all is not well, with observations increasingly made that medicine has lost sight of the human dimension of illness. An exclusionary participation with the physical and a consequent neglect of the psychological, emotional and spiritual dimensions of patient care, together with the ongoing shift towards superspecialization, are pushing healthcare services into compartmentalization, fragmentation and reduction. (p. 1)

In each case, problems arising from within clinical practice have (according to the authors) required a radical shift in the nature of practice itself. They have inspired critical reflection on the underlying assumptions that frame conventional practice, which give practitioners their sense of what they are doing—the purposes, values, and methods of their own practices. These problems have caused some to question and re-evaluate at least some of those assumptions, and to conclude that business as usual needs to be altered in accordance with some new framework. To think in this way about medical practice is to think philosophically about medicine.

It follows that a fundamental research problem for the philosophy of medicine has been understanding the nature of practice itself. What is clinical practice? And, what should it be? Different understandings of practice can be characterized in terms of different models, but how should we choose between competing models of practice? Even that question contains an assumption worth interrogating, that distinct models of practice are in competition, such that we must choose between them. Do these models represent alternative and mutually incompatible conceptions of practice—of what it is or what it should aspire to be—or do they represent distinct but compatible aspects of the correct characterization of what clinical practice is or should be?

In this section, we tackle each of these questions in turn (returning to the final one in the concluding section of the chapter). We discuss what clinical practice is and what it should be, by examining the evolution of three influential models of clinical practice: EBM, patient-centered medicine (PCM), and values-based practice (VBP). Each of these approaches offers a new model of clinical practice and in so doing, locates fault within some aspect of usual clinical practice (UP). By examining these models' portrayals of UP, we can begin to sketch out what clinical practice is, and then compare it to at least three versions of what it should be. This exercise requires reflection on what criteria should be used to judge UP and these or any other models.

What Is Clinical Practice, and What Should It Be?

We take UP to be what doctors do in the course of providing care to patients. Its goal is the cure or, if not possible, the palliation of disease, accomplished through two main objectives: diagnosis and treatment of patients' problems. Over the past 30 years, a variety of new approaches to medical practice or specific aspects of medical practice have emerged from different corners of the health professional world. These include EBM, whose origins reflect synergies between clinical epidemiologists and researchers in internal medicine and critical care; PCM, authored by scholars and practitioners in family medicine; and VBP, inspired by a specific application of philosophy to psychiatric care. In addition, approaches to specific aspects of clinical practice have also been developed. These include shared decision-making, which aims to strengthen the active participation of patient and clinician in clinical decision-making; relationship-centered care, which emphasizes the importance of the quality of the clinician–patient relationship for both clinical care and on health outcomes; and the patient–partner movement, which aims to increase patient participation and leadership in individual care as well as to incorporate patients' voices into clinical service development, health professional education, and research planning.[7]

In this section, we focus specifically on EBM, PCM, and VBP, because they represent models of clinical practice, which—if not complete—are intended to be comprehensive.[8] In addition, these models are well-known and influential: their theoretical foundations and practical applications have been well-documented, enshrined in policy documents and guidelines in health services across the globe.

Evidence-based Medicine

The phrase "evidence-based medicine" first appeared in the published medical literature in the early 1990s and since then has become a dominant discourse in clinical practice. Although it can count at least a few distinct sources of intellectual inspiration, the principles of its current iteration (1992 onward) were articulated through the application of the methods of clinical epidemiology to clinical problems. It has been taken up across the medical specialties and has even expanded into health services and policy evaluation. EBM has also generated enormous debate because, in part, of its portrayal of UP. Compared to "the traditional paradigm of medical practice," EBM's proponents place lower value on unsystematic clinical experience, pathophysiologic rationale, and authority (Guyatt et al., 2008, p. 10). These proponents characterize UP as a situation in which practitioners engage in clinical decision-making about patient care, often guided by sources of information of dubious epistemic value, or even to the detriment of patients' health.

Why would clinicians practice in such a manner? EBM's advocates located the fault both in medical training and in UP. Traditionally, medical training did not teach trainees how to understand clinical research studies, interpret their data, and then apply these data to clinical decisions. These trainees would then go on to the milieu of UP, which lacked mechanisms to require or even to promote these activities. By contrast, EBM teaches physicians that decisions about diagnostic tests, prognostication, which treatments to offer, and the prediction of harm should be guided by research studies; that certain types of research studies produce data that are more valid (defined as "closeness to truth") than others; and that research methods and the data they yield can therefore be ranked hierarchically. The specific steps involved in practicing EBM include:

1. Converting the need for information (about prevention, diagnosis, prognosis, therapy, causation, etc.) into an answerable question;
2. Tracking down the best evidence with which to answer that question;
3. Critically appraising that evidence for its validity (closeness to the truth), impact (size of the effect), and applicability (usefulness in our clinical practice);
4. Integrating the critical appraisal with clinical expertise and with the patient's unique biology, values, and circumstances; and
5. Evaluating the effectiveness and efficiency in executing steps 1 to 4 and seeking ways to improve them for the next time. (Strauss et al., 2011, p. 3)

By learning the principles of EBM and the skills needed to put them into practice, practitioners would be able to achieve two things:

1. Base their own clinical decisions on valid sources
2. Argue against ill-founded practices being used by others

EBM does not question the goal of medicine (cure or palliation of disease). Instead, it reminds readers that the physician's job is to ensure that patients are presented with valid research data in the service of meeting these objectives, during the process of clinical decision-making. Nor does EBM question the objectives of clinical practice (diagnosis and treatment of disease); but, it contends that following its rules enables practitioners to meet these objectives more effectively. According to EBM, clinical practice should be evidence-based practice in equipping clinicians with the skills to practice in accordance with its rules. Thus, EBM offers an epistemic remedy to UP.

Patient-centered Medicine

There are now several movements that go by similar names: PCM, patient-centered care (Berwick, 2009), and person-centered medicine. The relationships between them are still a matter for debate, with some exponents stressing the similarities and others arguing that the language of *person*-centeredness represents a broader approach than PCM. Historically, the concept of a patient represented a semantic contrast to that of an agent, and so the traditional distinction in medicine between practitioner and patient arguably reveals philosophical presuppositions that may be questioned.[9] As James Marcum notes (in chapter 10 of this volume) "person-centred" approaches are influenced by philosophical work on personalism, emphasizing the "agency" and "inter-subjectivity" of all parties to the clinical encounter. In this section, we focus primarily on PCM since it is an important historical point of reference for other related movements (Suchman, 2005; Mezzich, 2011).

PCM was born in the milieu of Canadian family medicine, which was, and remains, a key entry point for accessing health services. Many of these patients have complex psychosocial needs falling outside the boundaries of UP. PCM is by its own terms "a new clinical method." The term "patient-centered" stands in contrast to the characterization of UP, which PCM advocates argue is disease-centered. By this is meant that the goals of clinical practice should be to go beyond those of UP, in order to address some of these additional needs. PCM advocates aim to improve clinical practice by expanding UP's objectives of diagnosis and treatment to include understanding the person, meaning the patient's experience of illness, concept of good health, and social context. PCM places the patient's account of health and illness on an equal footing with the doctor's and with UP's. This means that the formulation of the problem and appropriate targets for therapeutic intervention ought to be negotiated with patients. PCM does not aim to abandon the goal of UP—to cure or palliate disease—but instead asserts that patient-centered clinical practice may be more successful in achieving this goal than UP itself (Stewart et al., 2014, p. 12).

Clinicians are to carry out PCM through a series of four complementary spheres of action when working with patients:

1. Exploring health, disease and the illness experience;
2. Understanding the whole person;

3. Finding common ground; and
4. Enhancing the patient–clinician relationship. (Stewart et al., 2014, p. 7)

At the same time, PCM's advocates are committed to EBM, believing that PCM is compatible with it, and indeed incorporates it. They do not view EBM as a clinical method as such but instead as a method for "acquiring the best available evidence" about issues in healthcare that can then be used in the practice of PCM (p. 15). Yet, it is not clear how this compatibility works in practice. For example, one of PCM's four components is finding common ground with the patient, including formulation of the problem and identifying the goals of treatment. EBM is oriented toward determining which interventions are most effective toward achieving certain outcomes, both the interventions and outcomes having been preselected by researchers of the studies that clinicians are meant to consult. But what if patients want an intervention that is not evidence-based or to pursue unstudied outcomes? How does the physician practicing PCM, seeking to find common ground, reconcile his or her approach to EBM at that point? Does the PCM practitioner practice EBM until the patient rejects something that EBM promotes? Does this mean PCM practitioners can take or leave EBM depending on the particular circumstances?

This is no doubt one reason why some contemporary exponents of the approach write under the label person-centered medicine (see chapter 10 by Marcum) and prefer the terminology of evidence-informed to evidence-based medicine (Miles and Loughlin, 2011). These exponents note that the concept of evidence in EBM has been modified from a very broad, common-language conception (where evidence simply refers to any piece of information that gives us a reason to believe a conclusion—such as your mother's facial expression and mannerisms giving you reason to believe she is unhappy) to a more specialist, scientific conception of evidence, closely associated with the findings of clinical research. They prefer to treat medicine as a human practice "informed by" science, and not as a science or a practice "based on" scientific evidence, and they maintain that "excellence in clinical practice will remain out of reach until clinicians apply advances in biomedicine and technology within a humanistic framework of care" (Miles and Ashbridge, 2014, p. 3).

Values-based Practice

VBP builds on the work of the philosopher and psychiatrist Bill Fulford, who developed the approach in the United Kingdom in the early 2000s. While Fulford initially targeted mental health practice, he believes that VBP can apply across specialties and health professions. VBP's central idea is that patients and practitioners alike hold diverse values that may come into conflict in the course of clinical decision-making. VBP finds fault in UP's lack of recognition of this diversity of values and portrays decision-making in UP as a process through which physicians may impose professional, institutional, social, or even personal values on patients' decision-making. At best, patients might be able to accept or refuse physician-recommended interventions through legal mechanisms, such as the requirement for informed consent. But Fulford does not see a legalistic approach as serving the needs of the ongoing, collaborative process of clinical decision-making that is required in the domain of mental health, where there is greater diversity about such value-laden questions as what constitutes good health. According to Fulford (2011, p. 977), VBP is a tool whose goal is to facilitate balanced judgments in individual cases where values are complex and conflicting. While VBP does not reject diagnosis and treatment as the objectives of clinical practice, it adds its own objective, which is to recognize the diversity of individual values and to incorporate this diversity through its specific approach to clinical decision-making. But apart from seeking to implement its decision-making process, VBP does not promote any specific goal. The goals of practice arise in clinical encounters from VBP deliberation.

Like EBM and PCM, VBP offers a series of elements that comprise the practice. These include four practice skills:

1. Awareness of values
2. Reasoning about values
3. Knowledge of values and facts
4. Communication

They also include six claims or principles:

1. Services ought to be user-centered
2. Multidisciplinarity
3. EBM and VBP work together
4. We only notice values when there is a problem
5. Increasing scientific knowledge increases choices that can demonstrate divergence in values
6. VBP involves providers and users making decisions in partnership

Fulford (2014) notes that there are other tools for working with diverse and potentially conflicting values in clinical encounters, such as the methods of clinical ethics, but he sees clinical ethics as allocating moral authority to rules. By contrast, VBP believes that moral authority for a given decision can only be achieved on a case-by-case basis by giving any and all values a fair hearing through an open-ended, deliberative process (pp. 151–52).

Fulford states that VBP works alongside EBM. The complementarity of the two approaches is emphasized by the claim that medicine rests on the "two feet" of evidence (as characterized by EBM) and values (as revealed by the processes explained in the literature on VBP) (Peile, 2014, pp. 24–25). While VBP recognizes the pervasiveness of values in health practice, it claims that EBM represents the facts of medicine. As noted in the previous section, this attempt to divide practical reasoning in medicine into two distinct components (albeit both needed for decision-making)—regarding the facts, as revealed by scientific research and regarding the values of the parties involved, ascertained through the processes of VBP—is contentious, with some arguing it represents a false dichotomy (Tonelli, 2014). This categorization also seems to ignore the values that underlie EBM, such as the values underlying the process of knowledge production and its products, including the research data that are the basis of evidence-based practice. If values are pervasive in all areas of practice, why would EBM be exempt? Furthermore, EBM already offers its own process for working with values in clinical decision-making (Gupta, 2014). VBP does not discuss how these two work together. Does it propose that in using the VBP method, the clinician should set aside EBM's method for incorporating values? The meaning of the two models working alongside each other is not clear.

Choosing between Models: Assessment Criteria

Each of the three models discussed here offers itself as a candidate to replace or modify UP. Which, if any, of these models should be chosen? And, on what basis? Each model criticizes UP for failing to achieve its goals or for having the wrong goals. Because of these failures, each model implies that UP does not meet the ends of medicine. While a serious discussion of the ends of medicine lies beyond the scope of this chapter, they have traditionally been related to preserving life, relieving suffering, and promoting flourishing. The third of these is more contentious than the others, with some claiming that promoting flourishing (an Aristotelian term related to the idea of "the good life") equates to health enhancement, when the goal of medicine should more modestly be disease prevention (Kottow, 2002, pp. 78–79) and others suggesting that, at least in some areas (notably mental health) the goal of promoting "the good life" can be a recipe for authoritarian practice (Fulford, 2014, p. 157). Even the first two goals may of course be called into question in specific cases, for instance, when they are thought to be in conflict. Thus, the debate about the ends of medicine cannot be neatly separated from wide-ranging debates about what kind of life is worth living, what kinds of suffering are worth relieving, and what kinds of flourishing should be targeted (if at all).

Do all or any of the three models discussed here achieve the ends of medicine better than UP? Do any of the models achieve these ends better than any other? The models do not concern themselves directly with the question concerning the ends of medicine. Instead, they leave this question untouched but rather offer perspectives on how it might be answered in daily clinical practice and by whom. EBM would leave this question to the researchers who produce the data to be applied to clinical decisions. By offering patients evidence-based options, researchers determine what medicine should be about, for whom, and under what circumstances. It is not clear where PCM and VBP stand on this point. Because of their commitment to EBM, it seems that PCM and VBP accept the same state of affairs, allowing individuals to negotiate and debate their values regarding the evidence-based options on offer. Or, it may be that practicing in a patient-centered or values-based manner means precisely that EBM can be overridden under certain circumstances.

If the aforementioned models do not differentiate themselves by their ability to achieve the ends of medicine, then by what criteria should we judge them and assess their ability to serve as models of clinical practice? To compete with UP, a candidate model should be comprehensive (cover all the tasks of clinical practice), effective (be able to achieve what it says it will achieve), and feasible. Given that there are practitioners who state that they are practicing according to each of the three models, we accept that they are feasible. Here we discuss comprehensiveness and effectiveness.

UP is comprehensive by definition as it includes everything that doctors do in patient care. Any model of clinical practice should be able to offer guidance on this same terrain. Let us consider one example of an important area of practice in which guidance by the different models may prove to be insufficient or confusing, namely, the interface between clinical practice and legal requirements. In many jurisdictions, there are aspects of practice framed by law (e.g., informed consent). In UP, legal requirements must be respected. Does the same stand according to the models? And if so, is this consistent with their own logic?

Suppose researchers could conduct a clinical trial to evaluate the effectiveness of obtaining informed consent (defined as better informed and more health-promoting clinical decision-making) in a specific patient group (patients with generalized anxiety disorder). In the trial, the patients who participate in the informed consent process find it anxiogenic, refuse treatment, and end up feeling worse (more anxious), while those who do not participate in the process accept the treatment and get better. How should the evidence-based practitioner handle this situation? Should the practitioner advocate against informed consent for such patients because the evidence-based option seems to lead to better health, or opt to ignore the evidence because that is what is legally required? The patient-centered practitioner would come to understand that the patient feels overwhelmed by too much information about risk and would prefer to accept the doctor's recommendation rather than engage in the informed consent process. Does this give the patient-centered practitioner warrant to omit the informed consent process? Or would the physician have to default to UP, because PCM does not cover this aspect of practice? Meanwhile, the values-based practitioner would encourage an open discussion of the values at stake: the patient's trust in the physician's recommendation versus the physician's duty to respect the law. But before any true deliberative process could occur, the practitioner would simply have to overrule the patient's values due to the legal prescription. The point here is that if a model of clinical practice is *not* comprehensive, the practitioner has no choice but to default to UP for those areas that are not covered. Therefore, in order to evaluate a model, we need to know which areas of practice are covered, and under what circumstances.

Any model of practice should also be effective, that is, it should achieve what it claims to be able to achieve. Here we refer back to the goals of each model. Are they able to achieve their goals? How do we tell? EBM proponents state that its effectiveness cannot be evaluated according to its own standards of evidence, but point to certain RCTs that demonstrated that treatments previously thought to be effective were actually harmful (Gupta, 2014, p. 125). Alternatively, they claim that the ultimate goal of EBM is to be good at implementing the five-step procedure outlined earlier (Strauss et al., 2011, p. 3). PCM's exponents, meanwhile, report on the evaluation of their model through various research methods (Stewart et al., 2014, pp. 333–75) including the standards of EBM (pp. 346–52). They argue that systematic reviews show that training practitioners in patient-centered interaction improves elements of practitioner communication and patients' health outcomes (pp. 346–51). VBP's proponents agree that this kind of empirical base is necessary for VBP as well (Fulford, 2013, p. 543). UP can meet its goal—cure or palliate disease—sometimes. Whether or not the models do the same, do it better, or do something altogether different remains to be seen.

Summary

In the past few decades, numerous commentators have surveyed the domain of clinical practice and found it lacking in its goals, its objectives, or its methods for achieving them. Various new models of practice have been developed, and the three models discussed here have received considerable attention and resources from the clinical community, health policy-makers, and clinical researchers. Their emergence and influence raise a number of philosophical questions including what clinical practice is, what it should be, and how we can know if any new model is a good model of clinical practice or not. The models cannot be adequately assessed in isolation from broader assumptions about the ends of medicine, and it is also worth noting that they embody conceptions of the relationship between medicine and science, as well as the nature of science as applied to medical practice.

Science and Medicine

We have seen that some authors argue that medicine is not a science but a value-laden practice informed by science, and that this distinction is crucial to the right understanding of medicine. Although the role that science can play in medicine, and the specific sciences that are most useful and relevant, are both open to debate, there is no doubt that medicine relies on the results of scientific research. This section sketches some of the scientific areas that are of current interest to philosophers, briefly outlining some of the questions being addressed, and then turns to the broader question of what philosophy of science can say about the contribution that science can and should make to clinical practice and to health policy.

There are two major kinds of medical research: (1) population-level research, including clinical research that draws on epidemiological methods to examine the relationship between risk factors and/or interventions, on the one hand, and clinical outcomes, on the other; and (2) pathophysiological research, which involves investigating disease processes (and, to a lesser extent, the mechanism of action of interventions). Different disciplines and research areas tend to focus on one or the other of these approaches, though, as we show later, the extent to which they incorporate information from the other approach, and/or assumptions about what is occurring at the other (population or mechanism) level, will vary.

Two sets of related philosophical questions can be asked about the biomedical sciences. One set focuses on the sciences themselves, while the other looks at the role of the sciences in clinical medicine. We begin with the second set of questions. Philosophers of medicine have distinguished between rationalist and empiricist approaches to medicine. Medical rationalism focuses on understanding disease mechanisms and is therefore closely aligned with the physiological research described earlier. Medical empiricism, by contrast, is described as being concerned with patient outcomes (Newton, 2001), independent of examining and understanding the mechanisms that give rise to those outcomes, and with the careful description and categorization of clinical phenomena (Wulff et al., 1990, p. 33). Although many areas of biomedical research that take an empiricist approach focus on populations, the link between medical empiricism and population-level research is not as close as that between physiological research and medical rationalism, as we show later.

Wulff et al. (1990) describe historical approaches to medicine in terms of this dichotomy, though they use the term "realism" instead of "rationalism."

They suggest that historically, medicine has been dominated by speculative realism. This philosophical approach to medicine has involved the development of theories regarding the causes of disease. The most famous of these is the Hippocratic system, according to which diseases were understood as imbalances in the body's four humors. This system is realist, because it posits the existence of an underlying disease mechanism, and it is speculative because its followers believed that "it was possible by armchair reasoning alone to ascertain the nature of that disease mechanism" (p. 31). Similarly, some forms of medical empiricism do not take sufficient account of medical rationalism; Wulff et al. point to attempts in the eighteenth century to categorize diseases without reference to the underlying disease mechanisms. The classification systems amounted to "no more than divisions and subdivisions of ill-defined symptoms, and they had no lasting effect on the development of modern medicine" (p. 34). Wulff et al. describe the ideal approach as one of "realism under empirical control" (p. 32); when this occurs, the search for disease mechanisms is not speculative, but is based on careful observation and often also on experimentation.

Both the empiricist concern with observation and the realist concern with mechanisms can be observed in contemporary medicine and medical research. Until very recently, medical research took a rationalist approach by focusing on physiological knowledge. Newton (2001) attributes this in part to the influence of the Flexner report, published in 1910. Although the purpose of the report was to examine medical education, Flexner's emphasis on the importance of understanding the mechanisms of disease "created a template of medicine, in which the high priests are scientists who illuminate the basic processes of disease" (p. 303). Medical school curricula and clinical training were both focused on understanding disease mechanisms.

As we have seen, our understanding of what it means to have a scientific understanding of medical causation has, since the early 1990s, been massively influenced by medical empiricism, in the form of EBM. One of the most famous definitions of EBM is "the conscientious, explicit, and judicious use of current best evidence in making decisions about the care of individual patients" (Sackett et al., 1996, p. 71)—a definition that might well lead us to assume that EBM considers any form of evidence to be relevant, when in practice, the relevant evidence comes from well-designed studies that rank high on EBM's hierarchy of evidence. Moreover, most of what has been written about EBM, by its proponents in both medicine and philosophy, has focused on studies that examine treatments (as opposed, e.g., to prognosis, or to diagnostic tests).

According to the evidence hierarchy for treatment studies, the best evidence comes from systematic reviews or meta-analyses of RCTs, or, where only one study is available, a single RCT. Nonrandomized studies (reviews of multiple studies, then a single study) fall below this on the hierarchy. Note that all of the top levels of the hierarchy look at treatment outcomes in groups of patients;

the methods here are similar to those used in epidemiology (we return to this point later). Below these studies come case reports and case series (reflecting the unsystematic observations of a single clinician or a small group of clinicians) and then research from laboratory studies that examines physiological processes or outcomes.

Philosophers have both defended and criticized EBM.[10] Here, we use the hierarchy of evidence to introduce questions about the potential contributions of population-level research and physiological research to medicine. As noted, EBM's hierarchy of evidence claims that the best research evidence comes from population-level studies that examine outcomes in large groups of people who receive an intervention of interest, comparing them with outcomes in a similar control group. This basic study approach—examining the relationships between potential causal factors and health effects in populations of patients—comes from epidemiology. As we have seen, the roots of EBM lie in an earlier movement called "clinical epidemiology" (Feinstein, 1985; Sackett et al., 1985), which explicitly aimed to use the techniques of epidemiology in clinical research.

Yet there are important differences between epidemiology and clinical research. First, clinical research tends to focus specifically on one cause, the intervention being tested, while epidemiology takes into account the effects of a number of different factors on disease outcomes. Second, epidemiology is closely related to public health, which aims to improve outcomes in populations, rather than in individuals, while clinical research is intended to inform decision-making in the care of individual patients. Because of this, Last (1988) claims that "clinical epidemiology" is an oxymoron.

Philosophical discussions of epidemiology, therefore, share some issues with discussions of clinical research, but also address distinct questions. Alex Broadbent's chapter in this volume (chapter 4) surveys current work in philosophy of epidemiology, suggesting that a central issue for both philosophers and epidemiologists themselves involves questions about causation. He also notes that epidemiology is highly unusual among the sciences, because it does not develop a body of theory. While epidemiology may draw heavily on theories relevant to a specific condition or question being investigated, it operates via a piecemeal approach, helping itself to whichever theoretical background is relevant to the problem at hand. So instead of being defined by its specific body of theory, the defining features of this young science are to be found in its methods.

Given that so much work in the philosophy of science concerns theory development, developing a philosophical account of epidemiology raises specific and interesting challenges for philosophy. Broadbent also notes that epidemiology has limitations, that "having identified a disease 'vector' or an exposure of interest, epidemiology needs to hand over to laboratory sciences which can tell us more about how exactly the exposure works." This suggests that epidemiology is a purely empiricist approach to medicine, with no interest in understanding physiological mechanisms. But because epidemiology does draw on work from other sciences, it incorporates the knowledge obtained from a rationalist approach, as well. For example, epidemiological studies may examine the effects of sex/gender, age, socioeconomic status, comorbidities, or genetic/genomic make up on health outcomes. All of these characteristics presumably are linked to differences in the underlying physiological mechanisms, though we can recognize the influence of the characteristics even without understanding the mechanisms themselves. It is worth noting that the interaction with rationalist research is another characteristic that distinguishes epidemiology from EBM, at least when it comes to research on the effects of treatment. Since EBM focuses on differences between average outcomes in treatment and in control groups, and does not tend to address questions about the effects of social, demographic, or biological characteristics on outcomes within study groups, it can be characterized as a shallow form of empiricism, compared with a deeper form of empiricism that uses knowledge of mechanisms to help to understand the sources of variability in outcomes.

In fact, there are areas of medical research that are defined by the specific health-related factors on which they focus; two chapters in this volume look more closely at specific factors that are relevant to health. Tania Gergel (in chapter 9) examines gender medicine and Marianne Boenink (in chapter 3) assesses personalized medicine. Gender medicine has recently become an area of great interest among medical researchers. It was inspired in part by the recognition that much of the research being done in biomedicine used only male subjects. While clinical trials have been required to enrol both women and men for some time now, these studies still do not always investigate whether there are differences in treatment outcomes for the two groups. Personalized medicine aims toward an ideal in which knowledge about individual genetic/genomic characteristics and differences in molecular biology permit the refinement of estimates of health risks and prognosis, and the tailoring of treatment to an individual's biological characteristics. While both Gergel and Boenink raise important questions about the assumptions that underlie their respective topics, as well as their potential implications for health and medicine, from the perspective of Wulff et al. (1990), gender medicine and personalized medicine both have promise as approaches that represent "realism under empirical control." Both areas of research take into account knowledge of physiological differences and their effects on outcomes.

Another area of recent interest in biomedical research, one that focuses mainly on population-level explanations, is evolutionary or Darwinian medicine. Evolutionary medicine draws on evolutionary biology to understand human health and disease. Its central tenet is that pathophysiology and the vulnerability to disease should be understood in terms of trade-offs that secured other evolutionary advantages. Moreover, it claims that contemporary health problems are often the result of changes in our environment and lifestyles, which of course change much more rapidly than our genome, so that there is a mismatch between the environment to which the human genome was adapted and the one in which it currently functions.

Pierre Méthot (2011, 2015) distinguishes between (a broad conception of) evolutionary medicine and a narrower Darwinian medicine. He describes the former as a "forward looking" attempt to predict the effects of evolutionary processes on human health; it considers not just human evolutionary history but ongoing evolutionary changes in microorganisms that are relevant to infectious disease and antibiotic resistance. This approach overlaps in interest with epidemiology, since it examines current patterns of disease. By contrast, Darwinian medicine is "backwards looking" in that it "applies evolutionary principles from the vantage point of humans' distant biological past in order to assess present states of health and disease" (Méthot, 2015, pp. 587–88).

Although evolutionary medicine looks at populations and at variability in outcomes, it also has an interest in explaining how these outcomes came about. It therefore has some rationalist and some empiricist tendencies. But instead of seeking the specific causes of an outcome at a physiological level, it focuses on processes that underlie evolutionary change in general. Darwinian medicine, as the name suggests, focuses primarily on the processes of adaptation and natural selection. Valles (2012) has criticized the focus on adaptation, arguing that it distorts research in the field (see also Cournoyea, 2013). Evolutionary medicine, by contrast, considers a wider range of biological processes relevant to evolution, including symbiosis and epigenetics (Méthot, 2015). It may therefore not be subject to these criticisms.[11]

This section has surveyed a number of important areas of biomedical research and has briefly discussed some of the philosophical questions they raise. Two key aspects of the discussion have been that (1) biomedical research tends to focus on either health outcomes in populations or on the physiological mechanisms that produce these outcomes; and (2) there are two distinct orientations to medicine: empiricist and rationalist. While these are, at least to some extent, naturally allied with one of the two broad approaches to research (empiricism with population level research, and rationalism with research on physiological mechanisms), we have suggested that most areas of biomedical research do (and should) incorporate some aspects of both rationalism and empiricism.

Philosophy of Science and Philosophy of Medicine

The previous section discussed a number of current trends in medical research, addressing some of the philosophical questions they raise and pointing out their philosophical commitments. In this section, we turn to developments within philosophy itself, in particular to the ways in which recent work in philosophy of science is beginning to be used in philosophy of medicine.

Over the past decade or so, there has been a resurgence of interest in medicine among philosophers of science. We outline briefly several areas of research in philosophy of science that are particularly relevant to philosophy of medicine. These include both traditional questions (including the nature of scientific theories, the confirmation of theories by evidence, and the establishment of causal relationships) that are relevant to assessing biomedical research, regardless of its specific methods or discipline. In addition, there are some areas of philosophy of science that have developed more recently and are relevant to medicine, specifically the focus on scientific pluralism and questions about the nature and roles of values in science.

The distinction between population-level research and research on physiological mechanisms is relevant in philosophy of science, as well as in medical research itself. We noted earlier that the philosophy of science has traditionally been centrally concerned with theories. While this is true, it is an oversimplification, as there are a variety of approaches to understanding what a theory is, and how theories are related to other concepts, such as laws of nature, or models. The syntactic view of theories, which dates back to logical empiricism, views theories as a set of statements (many of which represent laws of nature), while the semantic view sees theories as a set of models. A more recent development is the focus on mechanisms, which are usually described as explanations, rather than as theories (Craver, 2002). The basic idea underlying this approach is that scientists working in the life sciences do not primarily attempt to develop theories, but rather to elucidate physiological mechanisms.

Although there are a number of ways of describing what a mechanism is, one prominent view is that "[m]echanisms are entities and activities organized such that they are productive of regular changes from start or set-up to finish or termination conditions" (Machamer et al., 2000, p. 3). Another important feature of mechanistic explanations is that they are inherently multilevel. The entities that make up one level of the mechanism are themselves composed of other entities, which work together in a mechanism to allow the higher-level entity to contribute to the function of the higher-level mechanism. That is, an entity itself can be viewed as a mechanism, the output of which is the activity of the higher-level entity. For example, a cell is composed of a number of molecular components that contribute to the activity of the cell, allowing it to take its place in a mechanism.

Although the new mechanism has been very influential in philosophy of science, relatively little work on mechanisms has been done to date in the philosophy of medicine itself. One question has to do with the nature of mechanisms of disease: for example, Mauro Nervi (2010) has argued that these should be considered as distinct mechanisms, while Sara Moghaddam-Taheri (2011) has argued that pathological mechanisms should be understood as broken normal mechanisms. This question is still not entirely settled. One interesting way that the question might be answered is by linking discussion of physiological mechanisms to other questions in philosophy of science/philosophy of medicine. For example, Justin Garson (2013) has drawn on work in philosophy of biology that examines biological functions in evolutionary terms; the idea is that a mechanism has a normal function in virtue of its evolutionary history. This suggestion seems to weigh in favor of the broken normal view.

To date, however, most of the discussion of mechanisms in philosophy of medicine has been influenced by work on EBM and has addressed the question of the extent to which physiological research on mechanisms (which is near the bottom of the hierarchy of evidence) can inform treatment decisions, whether instead of, or as a supplement to, clinical trials (Andersen, 2012; Bluhm, 2013; Howick, 2011; Howick et al., 2013). Recall that EBM, with its focus on RCTs and meta-analyses, is an empiricist approach to medicine, while the elucidation of physiological mechanisms is rationalist. Contemporary rationalism is not like the theory-heavy, armchair speculative realism criticized by Wulff et al. (1990). Rather, it is based on experimentation and careful observation. Yet, it is still not clear what kind or amount of physiological knowledge is required to support predictions of clinical outcomes.

The question of predicting outcomes is related to the question of what kind of research evidence is necessary to establish causal claims in medicine. The ability to make claims about causality is important in all areas of science. As described earlier, physiological research focuses primarily on understanding the causes of disease in terms of the mechanisms that lead to the signs and symptoms of it (and, to a lesser extent, on elucidating the mechanism of action of treatments). Epidemiological studies examine the influence of potential risk factors (i.e., causes) on disease occurrence. Using similar methods, clinical trials aim to determine whether a therapeutic intervention causes improvement in patient outcomes. Philosophical discussions about causality in medicine have attempted to clarify the contributions that each of these kinds of research can make to our knowledge of causes.

One debate centers on whether RCTs can provide any information about causes. Proponents argue that RCTs, as opposed to observational studies, are necessary to show that a treatment causes an outcome of interest, because only RCTs can control appropriately for the influence of confounding factors. Cartwright argues, however, that RCTs can only support causal claims if we build knowledge of causes (or assumptions about what causal factors are relevant) into our experimental design, and that mere statistical associations can only be taken to be evidence of causal relations if we already have some idea of what the causal relationships are (e.g., Cartwright and Hardie, 2012).

Recent discussions have been strongly influenced by what has come to be known as the "Russo–Williamson thesis"—after the arguments presented in Russo and Williamson (2007)—which claims that both knowledge of mechanisms and knowledge of the statistical relationship between risk factors/interventions and outcomes are necessary to obtain causal knowledge in the health sciences. Statistical evidence linking causes and effects is required to show that the occurrence of an effect does depend on the presence of the cause. Mechanisms give us knowledge that a statistical relationship observed in a study sample is not merely limited to that sample, or to the specific circumstances in which the statistical relationship was observed.

In addition, it is important to realize that, to some extent, causal claims are always limited to specific circumstances. This fact has important implications for the use of biomedical and clinical research to inform policy and practice. Scientific research is designed to isolate specific causal factors of interest, whether in the carefully controlled conditions of a laboratory, or in social science and epidemiological research that uses statistical controls. This research does not, however, give sufficient information to predict how these causes operate in the very different contexts in which the policy is implemented. Cartwright, for example, cautions that while scientific studies can show that a policy "works somewhere," much more information is needed to warrant the claim that the policy also "works here" (Cartwright and Hardie, 2012).

Pluralism, Science, and Values

Ultimately, the sciences described claim that they can contribute to improved health, whether by directly influencing patient care and/or by contributing to the development of public health policies. But within each of these sciences, as we have shown, there are disagreements and controversies. These issues take on additional complexity when we look at all of the sciences together, since they use very different methods and focus on distinct aspects of biology or medical intervention. One of the most pressing problems in contemporary philosophy of science is understanding how to integrate the findings of different sciences and scientific approaches.

During the mid-twentieth century, the heyday of logical empiricism, philosophy of science was guided by the assumption that, as science progressed and provided more knowledge of the natural and social worlds, scientific theories would converge to provide a unified body of knowledge. By contrast, many contemporary philosophers of science accept some form of scientific pluralism, emphasizing the diversity (both among and within scientific disciplines) of methods, theories, scientific models, and background assumptions about the nature of the phenomenon being studied. This diversity influences both the results of research and its interpretation, leading some philosophers to conclude that it is impossible to draw any general conclusions that transcend the myriad specific scientific contexts within which a phenomenon is investigated (Longino, 2013).

Related to this point are questions about the different sorts of value-judgment that underlie and motivate scientific research. An obvious focus for this approach in philosophy of medicine has to do with the role of commercial interests, e.g., pharmaceutical and biotech companies, in shaping medical research and its uptake in clinical practice. However, even leaving aside commercial issues, a host of social, cultural, and political values may influence medical research at numerous stages, including questions about which areas become priorities and receive research funding, about what kinds of studies are considered to provide good evidence, and about how much evidence is needed before clinical practice should be changed.

Conclusion: The Search for the Base or Center

It seems clear then that medicine is informed by a broad variety of approaches in science, and no one methodology can claim to be definitive of the whole range of studies, theories, and practices that legitimately qualify for the descriptor "medical." This is hardly surprising given the richness and diversity of medical research and practice, and the vast range of problems we are prepared to characterize as "medical." There are also well-defended claims that medicine should be informed by a broader range of sources and methods than can sensibly be classified as scientific, and/or that our notion of scientific reasoning needs to be expanded to incorporate a role for the sort of human capacities and dispositions that would qualify as subjective and non-rational in the writings of the logical positivists. Several authors in this volume[12] argue that the philosophy of medicine has been impoverished to the extent that it has failed to make a systematic study of the humanistic aspects of medical practice, including the role of intuitive and tacit knowledge in medical epistemology and phenomenological approaches to understanding illness and associated problems of meaning, suffering, and embodiment. It is therefore perhaps no greater a surprise that, as noted in our opening comments, there is a diversity of methodological approaches within the philosophy of medicine itself, and no one, unifying meta-methodology to tell us what the different approaches have in common.

Should this strike us as a problem? Apart from being various ways of thinking about medical problems, research, and practices, should areas as different as the philosophy of epidemiology, medical humanities, and virtue epistemology (to name just a few of the distinct and developing areas of medical philosophy) have anything in common? If there need be no general, methodological thread linking all of these different approaches, then this does of course create a problem when it comes to distinguishing legitimate from illegitimate approaches to the subject matter. It means we need to assess each alternative approach as it comes, making up our own minds as to its validity and usefulness. We do not yet have (nor, arguably, may we ever have) a definitive set of rules that simply tell us which approaches are legitimate and which are not.

It is not, however, clear that this is a problem any rational person should expect ever to be solved. Is phenomenology an intellectually respectable and practically useful way to inform and enhance our understanding of medical problems and practices? The only way to answer that question is to make a serious study of work in the area of medical phenomenology, applying one's critical faculties to form a judgment about the quality of the arguments and analyses presented. (The reader might begin by studying in detail the chapters by Fredrik Svenaeus (chapter 8) and Tania Gergel (chapter 9) in this volume.) To think that there must, somewhere, be a list one can consult to bypass this process of critical engagement with the specifics of the area is to adopt a "repair manual" approach to thinking (Loughlin, 2002, p. 4), to seek exemption from the responsibility to form one's own conclusions, and thus to opt out of the processes of reasoning.

There are, however, other problems presented by the diversity of methods in the medical philosophy. We have seen, in our discussion of the relationship between EBM, PCM, and VBP, that there are legitimate questions about the extent to which different approaches in the philosophy of medicine are complementary or embody incompatible assumptions. In that discussion, a key problem concerned the status of these approaches as distinct models of clinical practice, each claiming to be comprehensive accounts of what UP should be. The very idea that such a comprehensive account should be the goal of the philosophy of medicine may strike many readers as natural, but there are also those who question why the giving of a complete account of an area should be the goal of all and any serious theoretical enterprise. Considering the names of the three approaches mentioned in this paragraph, Ross Upshur (2014a, p. 989) comments that in medical philosophy "[t]he persistent desire to name some concept or idea as the base or the centre strikes me as misguided in some fundamental way. We have seen little attention or discussion about the near mania for appellations of this sort."

As we noted earlier (cf. the comments on Toulmin in the opening section), philosophy can be construed as either a body of theory or as an activity. We argued that its value, certainly in an area such as the philosophy of medicine, appears to be as an activity, an engagement with common ideas and practices in the area. The philosopher asks critical questions to expose and interrogate underlying assumptions that frame debates, with the goal of assisting the protagonists in understanding their own assumptions and considering possible alternative conceptual frameworks. In medicine this means engaging in dialog with practitioners and patients, taking up problems that arise directly from their accounts of the problems of practice, and exploring ways of conceptualizing the problems, relevant evidence, and potential solutions. But for many theorists, the ultimate goal of such an activity must be the production of a complete body of theory, a philosophy of the area. The attraction of this idea may in part lie in a comparison with the view of scientific progress noted in the closing comments of our previous section, that theoretical unity is the ultimate goal of science.

Whatever its appeal, it explains the motivation to present an account of the "base" or "center" of all medical practice, as though explaining an entire and extremely diverse area via a single, underlying concept. But as Upshur (2014b, pp. 214–15) notes:

> Basing or centring medicine on any one thing, be it evidence, persons or patients, seems to be a mistaken enterprise. I am not sure what motivates the requirement for this and why, for example, evidence, values and persons or patients cannot be seen as mutually constitutive. In some circumstances evidence, however conceived, may hold more weight than values and vice versa. There are contexts where the interests of persons or patients, always deserving of respect, may take a subordinate role to the needs of a community.

Social practices rarely come into existence because some person or group sits down, decides we need a practice called X, sets out its defining characteristics, and then rounds up a group of people whose qualifications suggest they are the best qualified to create the needed practice. Practices evolve, so there is indeed something bizarre about searching retrospectively for their base or foundation. If they emerged without having to be at any point founded, then why try to create a foundation, center, or unifying concept for them? It may be that theorists think that is the only way to explain or make sense of these practices, but in that case we need to examine the theorists' own assumptions about what it is to explain or make sense of a practice.

Wittgenstein's (1958, p. 31) instruction "Don't think, but look!" sounds like the sort of anti-philosophical declaration we might expect from the blogger cited in our opening section, but it is meant to serve as a warning about philosophical methodology that may have relevance to future debates in medical philosophy. As Cooper notes in chapter 11 of this volume, a great deal of work in the "philosophy of" medicine has been done attempting to define such key concepts as health and disease, but it is possible that no definition is ever going to capture all legitimate uses of these terms in the various contexts in which they operate. They may be what Wittgenstein calls "family resemblance terms," such that understanding their meaning is a matter of tracking their uses in the range of contexts in which people employ them, understanding their contribution to the forms of life this employment facilitates. To attempt to abstract an overall, definitive meaning of the term (to stop, as it were, looking and to theorize in the sense meant in the quotation by "thinking") involves taking terminology out of its specific context of use when analyzing its meaning, and there are dangers associated with this.

So, a practitioner might have a very clear sense of what it means for an aspect of her practice to be patient-centered, and may be able to explain in a particular case how she has applied this idea to the benefit of her patients. But when she fills in a management survey aimed at producing more patient-centeredness in her area or institution, via the production of general policy documents and practice guidelines, she may find that the answers she has given lead to policies and regulations that, far from facilitating her efforts in this area, actually inhibit them. This may not be because the survey's respondents are being inconsistent or "don't know what they're doing," nor need it be a result of incompetence or malice on the part of the managers attempting to base their polices on the responses. When language "goes on holiday" (Wittgenstein, 1958, p. 19), moving out of the context that gave it meaning, only to be recycled, in a different context and then fed back to practitioners as an application of some more general insight, there can be slippages of meaning, and one role of the philosopher of medicine should be to track these possible changes and the problems they create for the communication processes in organizations.

So if PCM and EBM really do want to demonstrate their mutual compatibility (cf. our discussion of these models in the section "Clinical Practice and Theory"), then they may need to moderate their claims about their own status. Instead of presenting themselves as comprehensive clinical practice models, or general theories of medicine, they might instead regard themselves as distinct ways of conceptualizing practice that bring to light otherwise neglected or deemphasized aspects, leaving it to the judgment of the informed reader of their theories to work out which approach makes sense of the specific situation she is facing. This more modest, but still important, aspiration may be a more realistic goal of theory than the attempt to provide a definitive theory of any given area of practice, and it fits with the model of philosophy as an activity, a dialog with practitioners, patients, and anyone else with a stake in the practices analyzed.

Such an approach might arguably be part of a solution to the crisis for EBM some of its prominent exponents have recently highlighted (Greenhalgh et al., 2014). This methodological concern might well be relevant to the developing movement for person-centered medicine, discussed at various points in this chapter. The last thing this movement needs, we suspect, is a definitive account of the meaning of the term "person" (which, if it is to be at all plausible, and to serve the declared purposes of the movement, must incorporate the idea of rational agency) followed by a discussion of what precisely it means for medical practices to be centered on such persons—followed swiftly by accusations that the movement risks condemning human beings that do not fit this model of personhood to the margins of medical concern and care (Loughlin, 2014). The movement's wholly legitimate efforts to reestablish the importance of certain aspects of practice (those deemphasized by the approaches it condemns as "reductionist") will not be served by its declaring itself to be the new candidate for the definitive "philosophy of" or new "foundation for" the practice of medicine. Nor does it need to make such a claim to argue that its proposals for framing discussions about medicine in the future represent significant progress with regard to what has gone before. (James Marcum takes up these concerns, and the use of "base" and "center", in more detail in chapter 10.)

One factor affecting which of the two alternative methodologies the philosopher of medicine adopts was touched on in the conclusion of the previous section—the values being served by research. If one sees one's role as a philosopher as serving the needs of the policy-maker, then the appeal of a new, revolutionary insight, the discovery that all of medicine is in fact based on or centered in factor X, and a complete definition of what X is may well serve the purposes of the audience for whom one is writing. But if the purpose is to assist "a broader audience" (Loughlin, 2002 p. 151), including practitioners and the public, to make sense of a complex and challenging environment, then the more modest goal may well also be the more useful one to adopt.

Notes

1. David Colquhoun, self-styled "defender of science" and crusader against quackery, religious belief, and all things "unscientific." Probably one of the few people on earth who actually wants the Westboro Baptist Church to picket his funeral.
2. Why philosophy is largely ignored by science: http://www.dcscience.net/2011/10/28/why-philosophy-is-largely-ignored-by-science/ (accessed May 8, 2015).
3. Founder of the Westboro Baptist Church, self-styled religious controversialist and crusader against all things "ungodly." Also of the view that critical examination of one's underlying assumptions is a waste of time.
4. The issue is a central preoccupation of several chapters in this volume. See in particular Marianne Boenink (chapter 3), Alex Broadbent (chapter 4), Jeremy Howick (chapter 5), and Brendan Clarke and Federia Russo (chapter 12).
5. A good illustration of a much richer conception of reasoning can be found in Hillel Braude's chapter 13 on clinical decision-making, appealing to the Aristotelian idea of practical wisdom to give an account of what good clinical reasoning consists in.
6. Including some of those who, to use Toulmin's (1982, p. 749) term, "barbarously" embraced the label "ethicists" (Loughlin, 2004).
7. See http@//medicine.umontreal.ca/doc/PPS_Rapport_2011-2013.pdf (accessed May 7, 2015).

8. Some authors, such as Jeanne Daly (2005), refer to EBM as a science of clinical practice rather than a model, but its authors envision its role as going beyond science and offering techniques to guide actual practice.
9. The defenders of PCM also reject the construal of the patient as the passive recipient of treatment and the practitioner as bearing sole responsibility for the decisions and outcomes of the process.
10. Jeremy Howick's chapter 5 in this volume provides an overview of this literature and presents his own analysis.
11. The issues in this area are taken up in much greater detail in Michael Ruse's chapter 6 to this volume.
12. See in particular the chapters by Alfred Tauber (chapter 7), Lydie Fiolová (chapter 7a), Fredrik Svenaeus (chapter 8), Tania Gergel (chapter 9), and Hillel Braude (chapter 13).

References

Achinstein, P., and Barker, S. F. (1969). *The Legacy of Logical Positivism: Studies in the Philosophy of Science*. Baltimore, MD: The Johns Hopkins Press.

Andersen, H. (2012). Mechanisms: What are they evidence *for* in evidence-based medicine? *Journal of Evaluation in Clinical Practice* 18(5): 992–99.

Ayer, A. J. (1987). *Language, Truth and Logic*. Harmondsworth: Penguin Books.

Berwick, D. M. (2009). What patient-centered should mean: Confessions of an extremist. *Health Affairs* 28: 555–65.

Bluhm, R. (2013). Physiological mechanisms and epidemiological research. *Journal of Evaluation in Clinical Practice* 19(3): 422–26.

Cartwright, N., and Hardie, J. (2012). *Evidence-Based Policy: A Practical Guide to Doing It Better*. Oxford: Oxford University Press.

Cournoyea, M. (2013). Ancestral assumptions and the clinical uncertainty of evolutionary medicine. *Perspectives in Biology and Medicine* 56(1): 36–52.

Craver, C. F. (2002). Structures of scientific theories. In *The Blackwell Guide to the Philosophy of Scinece*, eds. P. Machamer and M. Silberstein. Wiley-Blackwell, pp. 55–79.

Daly, J. (2005). *Evidence-Based Medicine and the Search for a Science of Clinical Care*. University of California Press-Milbank Memorial Fund.

Evidence Based Medicine Working Group (1992). Evidence-based medicine: A new approach to teaching the practice of medicine. *JAMA* 268: 2420–25.

Feinstein, A. R. (1985). *Clinical Epidemiology: The Architecture of Clinical Research,* 2nd edition. Philadelphia PA: W. B. Saunders Company.

Fulford, K. W. M. (2011). The value of evidence and evidence of values: Bringing together values-based and evidence-based practice in policy and service development in mental health. *Journal of Evaluation in Clinical Practice* 17: 976–87.

Fulford, K. W. M. (2013). Values-based practice: Fulford's dangerous idea. *Journal of Evaluation in Clinical Practice* 19: 537–46.

Fulford, K. W. M. (2014). Living with uncertainty: A first-person plural response to eleven commentaries on values-based practice. In *Debates in Values-Based Practice: Arguments For and Against*, ed. M. Loughlin. Cambridge: Cambridge University Press, chapter 13, pp. 150–70).

Garson, J. (2013). The functional sense of mechanism. *Philosophy of Science* 80(3): 317–33.

Greenhalgh, T. (2012). Why do we always end up here? Evidence-based medicine's conceptual cul-de-sacs and some off-road alternative routes. *Journal of Primary Health Care* 4(2): 92–97.

Greenhalgh, T., Howick, J., and Maskery, N. (2014). Evidence based medicine: A movement in crisis? *British Medical Journal* 348: g3725.

Gupta, M. (2014). Values-based practice: A new tool or a new package? In *Debates in Values-Based Practice: Arguments For and Against*, ed. M. Loughlin. Cambridge: Cambridge University Press, pp. 85–95.

Guyatt, G., Haynes, B., Jaeschke, R., Meade, M. O., Wilson, M., Montori, V., and Richardson, S. (2008). The philosophy of evidence-based medicine. In *Users' Guides to the Medical Literature: A Manual for Evidence-based Clinical Practice*, eds. G. Guyatt, D. Rennie, M. Meade, and D. Cook. Chicago: AMA Press, pp. 9–16.

Howick, J. H. (2011). *The Philosophy of Evidence-Based Medicine*. Chichester, West Sussex: BMJ Books, Wiley-Blackwell.

Howick, J., Glasziou, P., and Aronson, J. K. (2013). Problems with using mechanisms to solve the problem of extrapolation. *Theoretical Medicine and Bioethics* 34(4): 275–91.

Hutchinson, P. (2008). *Shame and Philosophy: An Investigation in the Philosophy of Emotion and Ethics*. Basingstoke: Palgrave.

Kincaid, H., Dupre, J., and Wylie, A. (eds.). (2007). *Value-Free Science? Ideals and Illusions*. Oxford: Oxford University Press.

Kirkengen, A. L., and Thornquist, E. (2012). The lived body as a medical topic: An argument for an ethically informed epistemology. *Journal of Evaluation in Clinical Practice* 18(5): 1095–101.

Kopelman, L. M. (1994). Case method and casuistry: The problem of bias. *Theoretical Medicine* 15(1): 21–38.

Kottow, M. H. (2002). The rationale for value-laden medicine. *Journal of Evaluation in Clinical Practice* 8(1): 77–84.

Kuhn, T. S. (1970). *The Structure of Scientific Revolutions*. Chicago: University of Chicago Press.

Last, J. M. (1988). What is "clinical epidemiology"? *Journal of Public Health Policy* 9(2): 159–63.

Longino, H. (2013). *Studying Human Behaviour: How Scientists Investigate Aggression and Sexuality*. Chicago: University of Chicago Press.

Loughlin, M. (2002). *Ethics, Management and Mythology*. Oxford: Radcliffe Medical Press.

Loughlin, M. (2004). Camouflage is still no defence: Another plea for a straight answer to the question "what is bioethics?" *Journal of Evaluation in Clinical Practice* 10(1): 75–83.

Loughlin, M. (2014). What person-centred medicine is and isn't: Temptations for the "soul" of PCM. *European Journal of Person-Centred Health Care* 2(1): 16–21.

Loughlin, M., Bluhm, R., Fuller, J., Buetow, S., Borgerson, K., Lewis, B. R., and Kious, B. M. (2015). Diseases, patients and the epistemology of practice: mapping the borders of health, medicine and care. *Journal of Evaluation in Clinical Practice* 21(3): 357–64.

Loughlin, M., Lewith, G., and Falkenberg, T. (2013). Science, practice and mythology: A definition and examination of the implications of scientism in medicine. *Health Care Analysis* 21(2): 130–45.

Machamer, P., Darden, L., and Craver, C. (2000). Thinking about mechanisms. *Philosophy of Science* 67(1): 1–25.

Macnaughton, J. (2011). Medical humanities' challenge to medicine. *Journal of Evaluation in Clinical Practice* 17(5): 927–32.

Maxwell, N. (2004). *Is Science Neurotic?* London: Imperial College Press.

Méthot, P. (2011) Research traditions and evolutionary explanation in medicine: How do they differ and how to benefit from them. *Medical Hypotheses* 74: 746–49.

Méthot, P. (2015). Darwin, evolution, and medicine: Historical and contemporary perspectives. In *Handbook of Evolutionary Thinking in the Sciences*, eds. Thomas Heams,

Philippe Huneman, Guillaume Lecointre, and Marc Silberstein. Dordrecht: Springer, pp. 587–617.

Mezzich, J. (2011). Building person-centered medicine through dialogue and partnerships: Perspective from the International Network for Person-Centered Medicine. *The International Journal of Person Centered Medicine* 1(1): 10–13.

Miles, A., and Asbridge, J. (2013). Editorial. *European Journal of Person Centred Healthcare* 1(1): 1–3.

Miles, A., and Asbridge, J. (2014). Editorial. *European Journal of Person Centred Healthcare* 2(1): 1–15.

Miles, A., and Loughlin, M. (2011). Models in the balance: Evidence-based medicine versus evidence informed individualised care. *Journal of Evaluation in Clinical Practice* 17: 531–36.

Moghaddam-Taheri, S. (2011) Understanding pathology in the context of physiological mechanisms: The practicality of a broken-normal view. *Biology and Philosophy* 26(4): 603–11.

Nagel, T. (1986). *The View from Nowhere*. Oxford: Oxford University Press.

Nervi, M. (2010). Mechanisms, malfunctions and explanation in medicine. *Biology and Philosophy* 25(2): 215–28.

Newton, W. (2001). Rationalism and empiricism in modern medicine. *Law and Contemporary Problems* 64(4): 299–316.

Peile, E. (2014). Values-based clinical reasoning. In *Debates in Values-Based Practice: Arguments For and Against*, ed. M. Loughlin. Cambridge: Cambridge University Press, chapter 2, pp. 20–36.

Russell, B. (1967). *The Problems of Philosophy*. Oxford: Oxford University Press.

Russo, F., and Williamson, J. (2007). Interpreting causality in the health sciences. *International Studies in the Philosophy of Science* 21(2): 157–70.

Sackett, D. L., Rosenberg, W. M. C., Muir Gray, J. A., Haynes, R. B., and Richardson, W. S. (1996). Evidence-based medicine: What it is and what it isn't. *British Medical Journal* 312: 71–72.

Sackett, D. L., Tugwell, P., and Haynes, R. B. (1985). *Clinical Epidemiology: A basic science for clinical medicine*, 2nd edition. Little Brown & Co.

Stewart, M., Brown, J. B., Weston, W., McWhinney, I., McWilliam, C., and Freeman, T. (2014). *Patient-Centred Medicine: Transforming the Clinical Method*, 3rd edition. London: Radcliffe Publishing.

Strauss, S. E., Glasziou, P., Richardson, W. S., and Haynes, R. B. (2011). *Evidence-Based Medicine: How to Practice and Teach It*, 4th edition. Edinburgh: Churchill Livingstone.

Suchman, A. L. (2005). A new theoretical foundation for relationship-centered care: Complex responsive processes of relating. *Journal of General Internal Medicine* 21: S40–44.

Tonelli, M. (2014). Values-based medicine, foundationalism and casuistry. In *Debates in Values-Based Practice: Arguments For and Against*, ed. M. Loughlin. Cambridge: Cambridge University Press, chapter 19, pp. 236–43.

Toulmin, S. (1982). How medicine saved the life of ethics. *Perspectives in Biology and Medicine* 25(4): 736–50.

Upshur, R. (2014a). Conventions or foundations? A response to Miles Little's ex nihilo nihil fit? Medicine rests on solid foundations. *Journal of Evaluation in Clinical Practice* 20(6): 988–90.

Upshur, R. (2014b). A critique of modest foundationalism. In *Debates in Values-Based Practice: Arguments For and Against*, ed. M. Loughlin. Cambridge: Cambridge University Press, chapter 17, pp. 209–19.

Valles, S. (2012). Evolutionary medicine at twenty: Rethinking adaptationism and disease. *Biology and Philosophy* 27(2): 241–61.

Wittgenstein, L. (1958). *Philosophical Investigations*, G. E. M. Anscombe, trans. Oxford: Basil Blackwell.

Wulff, H. R., Andur Pedersen, S., and Rosenberg, R. (1990). *Philosophy of Medicine: An Introduction*, 2nd edition. Oxford: Blackwell Scientific Publications.

Part II

Current Research and Future Directions

3 Disease in the Era of Genomic and Molecular Medicine

Marianne Boenink

Introduction

Science and technology have been playing a crucial role in medicine for several centuries, but in the past decennium developments in biomedical technoscience seem to have accelerated. New tools in molecular biology, information and communication technologies, and nanotechnology are emerging in rapid succession and have enabled new types of research into the genetic and molecular basis of disease, in particular when converging. Such developments are associated with a strong promissory discourse: the new tools are claimed to produce unprecedented insights into diseases and revolutionary possibilities to counter them effectively. Visions of a genomic medicine suggest that sequencing a person's DNA early on may enable prediction of health problems later on, and that knowledge of a patient's genomic profile may help to choose the most effective treatment. In a similar vein, visions of molecular medicine suggest that if only we could regularly examine bodily functioning at the molecular level (which is becoming possible anywhere, anytime), prediction and prevention, as well as personalizing and close monitoring of treatment, are feasible.

Such visions suggest that genomics and molecular medicine, even though they offer revolutionary instruments, just help us to realize a long-standing and widely shared value: health. Many philosophers of technology point out, however, that technology is much more than a (supposedly neutral) instrument to achieve a preset goal (Verbeek, 2005; Ihde, 1990; see also Hofmann, 2001). Technology shapes the way we perceive and experience reality, as well as the values we pursue. This is confirmed by research in history of medicine, showing that what counts as disease or health coevolves with technological possibilities and scientific frameworks (Reiser, 1978; Rosenberg, 1989, pp. 5–10, and 2003, pp. 502–503). It makes sense, then, to investigate what view of disease and health is implied in genomics and molecular medicine. What exactly is pursued in these visions and in the research meant to contribute to realize them?

This chapter presents an overview of the shifts and continuities visible in the way disease (and to a lesser extent health) has been conceptualized in biomedical discourse in the past decennium. In doing so, I more or less follow the scientific and technological developments in their order of appearance. To set the stage, I start with a brief discussion of "classical medical genetics," and the promises and visions surrounding the Human Genome Project (HGP) that was developed in the mid-1980s. With the completion of the HGP at the beginning of the new millennium, genetics made way for a "genomic" approach, focusing on interactions among genes. Soon after, the attention of biomedical researchers broadened from genes to various kinds of molecules. In the second section, I discuss how these shifts affected thinking about disease. In the third section, I (again, briefly) go into recent developments in epigenetics and systems biology approaches, which suggest that another shift in thinking about disease and health may be at hand. Before I start this philosophical analysis of recent history, however, let me say a few words about the philosophical approach pursued here.

Philosophical debates about the character of disease and health (illness unfortunately has not received as much attention) often take place on an abstract level. Many philosophers aim to develop a generally valid concept of disease and/or health, and examples from clinical and/or scientific practice are then used to corroborate one or the other theory (examples are Boorse, 1975, 1977; Nordenfelt, 1995; Reznek, 1987; Wakefield, 1992). Their ultimate aim, however, is not to provide an empirically adequate description of disease and/or health, but to provide a coherent definition and theory, which may subsequently serve as a referee to indicate what doctors, patients, scientists or policy makers should (not) label as "disease." In this chapter, however, I do not aim at such a normative epistemology and ontology of disease. What I offer is a hermeneutical reconstruction and clarification of concepts of disease circulating in recent biomedical discourse. By focusing on subsequent types of biomedical research and their aims (and not on specific diseases) I attempt to highlight how such research both builds on and invites specific ways of thinking about disease.

Although the chapter follows a chronological order, this does not imply that in a specific period just one approach is in use. In practice, several types of research and several concepts exist next to each other, which do not necessarily cohere. By distinguishing among them and teasing out their implications, I strive to contribute to a better understanding of how disease is framed in different types of research, and where this might lead us with regard to medical practice and the role of disease in human life. Such an analysis, I claim, is crucial if we want to deal reflexively with the way biomedical technoscience is shaping the future of medicine, instead of passively responding to the next new thing in biomedical technoscience.

From Medical Genetics to the Human Genome Project

The Century of the Gene

As philosopher of science Evelyn Fox-Keller (2000, pp. 1–7) has noted, the twentieth century was the century of the gene. The century started with a renewed interest by biologists for the rules of inheritance, which Mendel had discovered 40 years earlier. The term "genetics" was introduced in 1906, and the concept of gene first emerged in 1909. For some time, it was not clear what a gene actually is, and whether the term refers to a real entity. It was only when deoxyribonucleic acid (DNA) was identified as the substance of genetic material (in the 1940s and 1950s) and Watson and Crick revealed its double helix structure (in 1953) that genes became a reality. Genetics then became a discipline rooted in molecular biology, and the role of genes in human life could be investigated with biochemical tools. A wide array of new insights in the workings of DNA and genes followed, with the most spectacular advances in the 1970s when recombinant DNA technology first enabled genetic modification. At the end of the century, the HGP promised to open up the genetic basis of human life, bringing genes centre stage, not only in molecular biology but also in the public imagination.

The HGP was developed in the mid-1980s as a "big science" project in molecular biology. As such, it was considered comparable to endeavors in particle physics or space research, where huge sums of money and years of work were dedicated to pursuing a specific goal. Such grand ambitions were unprecedented in biology, and needed justification that would convince not only those involved in the sciences of genetics and biology, but also those outside: funding institutions, politicians, citizens. One line of justification stressed that the genome is what distinguishes one species from another; thus, the human genome is the key to what makes us human. The identification of the complete human genome was presented as the "holy grail" of the science of human life. Molecular biologist Walter Gilbert, one of the founders of the HGP, even linked the pursuit of the human genome to the classic injunction "Know thyself" (Kevles and Hood, 1992, p. 19). In addition to this line of justification, however, proponents of the HGP stressed the potential benefits of human genome knowledge. And the *biomedical* benefits were mentioned most frequently.

For most of the twentieth century, genetics had been a marginalized field in medicine. Yoxen (1982, p. 152) describes it as "ghetto-ized," referring to its low status compared to other fields of medicine. Medical geneticists studied the set of (often rare) hereditary and congenital diseases, that is, diseases occurring in several members of the same family and/or manifest at birth or soon after. Sorting out whether a newborn baby suffers from a congenital disease or whether different individuals within a family do indeed suffer from the same disease involved careful clinical work. The field was therefore strongly focused on diagnosis, and much less on the underlying pathology. Once a medical geneticist established the hereditary character of a disease, s/he focused on counseling the families (e.g., about the risk of conceiving another child with the disease), rather than on technological intervention or cure. Hereditary disease was usually incurable disease.

In the second half of the twentieth century, however, the interest in the pathology underlying hereditary diseases gradually increased. By the 1980s, genetic factors had been shown to play a role in diseases like Huntington's disease, Down's syndrome, and familial hypercholesterolemia. But genetic factors were also thought to play a role in diseases that were not considered hereditary historically. Several common forms of cancer had, for example, been linked to "oncogenes" that seemed to influence the emergence and development of the disease. Francis Collins (1999, p. 28), one of the directors of the HGP, stated: "[S]ince the 1970s, nearly all avenues of biomedical research have led to the gene." Even though this may have been a strategic exaggeration, genes and genetic defects at this point in biomedical research definitely started to be seen as important factors in the explanation of disease more generally.

The biomedical interest in the human genome also built on and gave new form to two long-standing trends in biomedical research. First, subsequent technologies had enabled biomedical researchers and physicians to view and analyze the human body at ever more detailed levels. Molecular biology and genetic sequencing technologies made it possible to zoom in one step further and to discover what the body looks like at the level of genes and DNA. In addition, the central tenet of modern medicine has been that scientific insight in bodily causes of disease enables the development of rational, disease-modifying treatments. Both tendencies came together in the framing of genes as *ultimate causes* of disease. Understanding which genes are causing bodily processes to go wrong, it was reasoned, helps to address pathology at its root cause.

The sequencing of the complete set of human DNA promised by the HGP, then, was presented as the groundwork for the subsequent linking of genes with diseases. To see how this hope both built on and shifted specific views of disease, we have to go back to the concept of disease in medical genetics, prior to the HGP. Some of the ideas common in what I will call classical medical genetics carried over into the discourse surrounding the HGP.

Disease in Medical Genetics Prior to the HGP

Genetic disease in classical medical genetics was a subset of disease in general. This subset is delineated first and foremost by the hereditary or congenital character of its manifestation, and only secondarily by its (supposedly) genetic explanation. If the disease is hereditary, there should be a genetic element that is transferred from one generation to the next. If it is congenital, there should be a genetic defect that is present from birth. Although for some diseases, such as Down's syndrome, the defect had been identified (i.e., trisomy 21), for many others, such as phetylketonuria, Huntington's disease, or cystic fibrosis, it remained obscure. Whether or not the pathology was known, however, classical medical genetics assumed a strong link between the genetic defect and the disease. The defect was thought of as the *necessary and sufficient cause of disease*, meaning that having a genetic defect necessarily leads to the disease (Lindee, 2000). Because of this strong, deterministic linkage, disease is easily *reduced* to the genetic defect. Down's syndrome, for example, is thought to be caused by trisomy 21. Anyone with this trisomy displays the clinical features typical for the syndrome. Conversely, if the defect could (hypothetically) be repaired, the disease would not emerge. So it is a small step only to think of the trisomy as the disease.

As anthropologist Monica Konrad (2005) points out, geneticists tend to talk about genes in a "spatialized" way. Genes are perceived as very small parts of the body, presences in bodily space (pp. 54–56). They have specific places or loci on chromosomes, which themselves are also clearly thought of as occupying space in the cell's nucleus. During cell division, chromosomes move, cross, split, and merge. As a result, genes are rearranged in space, both within the person and between persons. In this process of recombination, they may become misplaced or lost, resulting in errors—and these errors are the pathology underlying genetic disease.

The conception of disease in medical genetics is, then, largely "ontological" (a term coined by Owsei Temkin; see Rosenberg, 2003, p. 493; see also Whitbeck, 1977). Genetic disease is localized as an entity in bodily space, where it is waiting to be discovered. Such ontological thinking (or localization theory, as it is also sometimes labeled) usually presupposes that the pathological entity automatically leads to the clinical signs and symptoms characteristic of the disease: it is deterministic. Moreover, it is reductionist in that it reduces the phenomenon of the disease to the entity, ignoring other factors that might play a role. In general, it invites thinking about medical treatment in terms of removal or destruction of the entity, for example, by surgery or drugs. However, since genetic defects are often present in the body's cells, this option is hardly feasible in the case of genetic disease. The ontological framework thus clarifies why medical genetics had difficulty in developing treatments. Ontological thinking would suggest gene therapy, replacing faulty genetic material with normal genes, but this option was (and remains) largely speculative and problematic.

The HGP: One Gene-One Disease

As noted earlier, the interest in the connection between genetics and disease radically shifted from the 1970s onward. In the last quarter of the twentieth century, it became common to assume that *all* diseases had a genetic component (Yoxen, 1982). With that shift, some of the ontological thinking about the relationship between genetic material and disease carried over into biomedical thinking in general (Fox-Keller, 1992). Of course the ontological way of thinking had been playing a role in nongenetic factors earlier in biomedical research as well, but now the locus of pathology was relocated to the gene. The gene was conceptualized as *the* entity ultimately causing disease. As discussed earlier, this view played an important role in justifying the investments in the HGP.

Both the mapping of genes as spatial entities in the HGP and the deterministic thinking of classical medical genetics stimulated thinking in terms of a one gene-one disease model. Hypotheses about a gene for X abounded, with X ranging from eye color, via various forms of cancer and Alzheimer's disease, to aggression. Whether or not the relationship between genes and disease should be conceptualized in a deterministic way was actually under contestation from the origins of the HGP (Lewontin, 1991). In many justifications for and much communication about the HGP, however, disease was reframed as genetic in essence. Genes were thought of as the *ultimate* cause of disease, ignoring other steps of and influences on the process. The implied view of disease can be called neo-ontological: although the one gene-one disease model suggests the existence of a process to get from gene to manifestations of disease, this process is then reduced to its supposed ultimate cause—the gene, which is conceptualized as an entity with a clear location. The neo-ontological view, that is, is not only reductive (singling out one element) but also reifies disease by constructing it as an entity, not as a dynamic process.

The neo-ontological view of disease also manifests itself in the emergence of the category of presymptomatic disease. If specific genetic mutations lead to disease, individuals carrying that mutation—but without complaints or symptoms—can be thought of as diseased nonetheless. And this verdict might even justify medical intervention, whether in the form of regular examinations, medication, or preventive surgery. Identifying a genetic mutation then equals a diagnosis, showing how the ontological view brings along (and may even broaden) the division between subjective experience of illness and objective observations of disease.

Implications of the One Gene-One Disease Model: Geneticization

The shift in conceptualization of disease described earlier is more than a matter of language or semantics. After all, the terms and frameworks adopted to

diagnose and interpret disease imply directives for how to deal with that disease. Moreover, both the disease label itself and the practice it invites often
have an impact not only at the individual level but also at the social level. The
question what this impact is and how to evaluate it has been extensively discussed by social scientists and ethicists performing ethical, social, and legal
implications research. Here, I highlight only one of the observations made in
this field: the claim that increasing interest in genetics during the 1980s and
1990s led to geneticization.

The sociologist Abby Lippman (1991, p. 19) coined the term "geneticization" to label "an ongoing process by which differences between individuals
are reduced to their DNA codes, with most disorders, behaviours and physiological variations defined, at least in part, as genetic in origin." Geneticization,
then, indicates a general cultural tendency to interpret societal issues in genetic
terms. Lippman argued that focusing on genetic explanation of differences
between human beings, whether such differences concern diseases, deviant
behavior (like alcoholism or criminal behavior), or personal differences (race,
sexual orientation), is problematic for at least two reasons. First, it attributes
these differences to biological causes, implying that the differences are innate
and therefore hard to change. Second, genetic explanations invite biological
remedies, whereas other interventions might be more fitting. For example, if
a certain type of cancer is interpreted as a genetic disease, attention will be
redirected toward possibilities for gene therapy, and away from possibilities to
change the environment by decreasing pollution or alleviating poverty.

The geneticization thesis has attracted considerable attention and generated
extensive debate. Philosophers have used it to describe the shifting meaning of
specific diseases in the wake of genetic research (Hoedemakers and ten Have,
1998; Sherwin and Simpson, 1999; ten Have, 2001; Stempsey, 2006). However,
it has also been criticized as empirically inadequate (for an overview, see
Hedgecoe, 2009). First, the phenomenon of geneticization may be less ubiquitous than Lippman suggested. More importantly, the actual effects of the
increasing attention for genetics may be more heterogeneous than geneticization suggests.

It is not my aim here to settle this debate. It should be noted, however, that
the geneticization thesis is closely associated with a specific interpretation of
genetics and genetic causation. Genetic explanations of disease (to focus on
what is most relevant here) do indeed single out biological causes. However,
these causes are only considered as innate and hard to change if we assume that
genetic mutations necessarily lead to disease. In a similar vein, they draw attention away from nongenetic options for intervention only if genes are considered
as the only and ultimate factor in disease causation. Underlying the geneticization thesis, then, is not so much a criticism of a genetic bias per se, but of a
specific view of genetics: a monocausal and determinist view of the relationship

between genes and disease (or, for that matter, any other trait or behavior). Lippman's thesis thus presupposes the validity of the neo-ontological view of disease; in this respect, it was a child of its time.

Genomics and Molecular Medicine

From Genes to Genome to Omics

While the HGP was completed, the idea that each disease is caused by defects in just one gene was increasingly criticized. It became clear that humans have fewer genes than originally anticipated (about 30,000 instead of 100,000), and the one gene-one disease (or trait) model became untenable. Research in common diseases showed that often several genes are implicated. Moreover, specific genetic mutations did not automatically lead to disease: many genes apparently have what is called low penetrance. This led biomedical researchers to conclude that several causal factors must interact in the emergence of disease. This shift is indicated by the term "genomics," which increasingly replaced "genetics." Where the latter focused on gene *substance*, the former targets *functioning* genes. Guttmacher and Collins (2002, pp. 1512–13) define "genetics" as "the study of single genes and their effects," and genomics as "the study of the functions and interactions of all the genes in the genome, including their interactions with environmental factors." With the start of the new millennium and the publication of the draft sequence of the human genome, genomics became booming business.

The first step away from the hegemony of the one gene-one disease model and toward a genomic paradigm is the distinction now made between diseases that are thought to have a clear genetic basis (so-called monogenetic disease or single gene disorders) and those that are either polygenetic (involving several genes) or multifactorial (involving genes, environment, and their interaction). Monogenetic diseases appear to satisfy more or less the deterministic model of disease, but they are now thought to constitute a small minority of all diseases. For many common diseases, like different forms of cancer, COPD, or Alzheimer, researchers now distinguish a genetic and a multifactorial variant, with the latter again forming the majority of cases (Khoury, 2003).

New forms of research emerged, which were enabled by the increasing speed and decreasing costs of scanning a number of genes or even the whole genome. During the first decade of the twenty-first century genome-wide association (GWA) studies became very popular. These studies map small genetic variations (often single-nucleotide polymorphisms or SNPs) between individuals in large populations, with the aim to link these with differences in disease outcome. In this way, researchers tried to identify whether people with (multifactorial) diabetes 2 or asthma, for example, have a specific genetic profile: a combination of SNPs that correlates with the disease. Unlike the isolated genetic mutations looked for earlier, such genomic profiles are not seen as causes of or even the substance of the disease, but as markers. Since the GWA studies are correlational, it is quite unclear whether the variations are actually implicated in the disease process, and if so, how. This cannot be determined without further experimental and/or pathological research.

Genomic profiles may have different functions. They could indicate an increased risk for future disease (and thus enable prediction and possibly prevention), contribute to diagnosis, predict how the disease may develop (prognosis), predict whether it will respond to specific therapies (therapy selection), and monitor the effects of the chosen therapy. In the area of risk prediction, GWA studies have not been very successful; ten years after completion of the HGP they have hardly revealed substantial risks groups (Varmus, 2010, p. 2028; see also Lander, 2011). There are, however, a number of genomic tests on the market that contribute to prognosis and therapy selection. Early examples are micro-arrays producing genomic profiles of breast cancer patients, which help to determine whether a patient is likely to profit from hormone therapy (Kohli-Laven et al., 2011). Increasingly, moreover, combinations of diagnostic kits and treatment (so-called companion diagnostics) are available. A new drug for cystic fibrosis, for example, can be prescribed only when a patient tests positive on the concurrent genomic test (European Science Foundation (2012) offers a list of companion diagnostics available). Both types of applications actually differentiate among subsets of patients to select the most effective therapy.

The rejection of the one gene-one disease model led to increased attention for the interactions among genes and between genes and environment. The shift toward the functioning of genes also brought nongenetic molecules into view. How does DNA actually translate into RNA, and RNA into proteins, metabolites, neurotransmitters, and so on? If genes do not determine everything that follows, it makes sense to find out what happens in between genetic code and clinical outcome. Disease is now often framed in terms of a pathway, and a whole range of different molecules possibly implicated in the pathway became a focus for research. This brought about an explosion of omics fields: proteomics, metabolomics, transcriptomics, microbiomics, and so on. The -omics suffix indicates that these fields explore the huge number of molecules and interactions that might be at play by collecting large sets of specimens (e.g., in biobanks) and analyze these with tools from the new field of bioinformatics. The goal is to reveal something about the structure, role, and function of particular molecules in human beings. A recurring aim is to identify "molecular biomarkers": molecules that indicate medically relevant events in the body. Such biomarkers, like the genomic markers mentioned earlier, may serve several functions varying from prediction, to prognosis, treatment selection, and monitoring.

Overall, then, the landscape of biomedical research has shifted significantly since the HGP's completion. These changes were accompanied by visions of molecular medicine: the idea that medicine should be based on insights in bodily functioning and pathogenesis at the molecular level, and also strive for intervention at that level (Freitas, 2007; Boenink, 2009, 2010). This vision built not only on developments in molecular biology, but it also gained traction because of developments in information and communication technologies and nanotechnology. As indicated earlier, the combination of the first two made it possible to generate, collect, and analyze large amounts of data at the molecular level of bodily functioning. Nanotechnology contributes by enabling the miniaturization of instruments to measure and to intervene in bodily processes, possibly in vivo and at any location. Sensors may be worn, implanted in, or ingested by the person to be examined, making more frequent measurements possible. Thus, visions of molecular machines sensing, diagnosing, and repairing the body nonstop promise continuous and ubiquitous care for a person's health, from the cradle to the grave.

Biomarkers and the Cascade Model of Disease

Did the shift from genetics to genomics and the subsequent broadening toward molecular medicine also bring about a different conception of disease? Some have argued that it did not. Melendro-Oliver (2004, p. 30), for example, responding to the shift from genetics to genomics, argues that this shift has not eliminated the deterministic view of disease. In her view, genes are still thought of as the most important causal factor of disease, both in scientific (genomic) and social discourse. Biomedical research in the era of genomics, as before, is searching for specific causes by focusing on internal, rather than external factors, and assuming that bodily functioning is mechanistic—nothing new, she claims.

Although this may have been true for genomic research right after the HGP's completion, since then biomedical research has branched out beyond genes. Thinking about disease in terms of "a gene for X" seems to have been gradually replaced by thinking in terms of "a biomarker for X." This shift is more than linguistic; it has implications for the way disease is framed. Although the concept of biomarker has received much less philosophical attention than the concept of gene, it warrants further philosophical analysis.

The general definition of the term "biomarker" is "a characteristic that is objectively measured and evaluated as an indicator of normal biological processes, pathogenic processes, or pharmacologic responses to a therapeutic intervention" (Biomarkers Definition Working Group, 2001; see also Metzler, 2010). The term is used for bodily characteristics (often molecular) that are thought to signify something about the state of health of the body. So biomarkers are signs or more specifically, *indexical* signs (Bell, 2013). An indexical sign refers to the signified because it is thought to be causally linked to the latter, like a foul smell signifies the burning of potatoes. This is also evident in the metaphors used to explain the role of biomarkers: they are called footprints or fingerprints. They are thought to enable the discovery of something that might have remained hidden; they betray what is going on. Another metaphor used for biomarker is "signature of disease," which stresses the capability of the biomarker to unveil the unique characteristics of the disease. Both metaphors share the implication that biomarkers enable us to see something that might otherwise be invisible or go unnoticed; they act, as some argue, as windows into health and disease (Hood et al., 2004).

Such metaphors make us forget, however, that the signs themselves are not neutral; they are technologically constituted. The "window," to stick with this metaphor, may appear to consist of transparent glass, but it actually frames our view in a specific way. To understand how biomarkers mediate our view of disease and health, we have to analyze their technological constitution. This happens in two ways. First, the tools of molecular biology and nanotechnology mediate how we access the body. They zoom in on the *molecular level of bodily functioning* and *quantify* what is happening there. Embedded in the measurements is, moreover, the idea of a *dynamic* body that changes in real time. Measurements of molecular functioning are, however, not necessarily markers of something else. They may simply reveal bodily functioning as such. The results of the measurements become biomarkers only if they are linked to reports on someone's state of health. For this, a second set of technologies is necessary, from biobanks collecting both medical records and results of bodily testing to software for storing and analyzing the data and to algorithms showing patterns in the data. These technologies incorporate data not only produced by the molecular tools, but also data on clinical states of health and disease. As with the first set of technologies, biobanks and bioinformatics usually require that variations in health status are entered in numerical form, using clear-cut categories to describe disease and health.

Overall, then, the double technological mediation of biomarkers encourages what Canguilhem (1991, p. 42) labeled a "quantitative view of disease." Disease in this view is a quantitative deviation from a population mean. Such deviations are not necessarily pathological; they become so only beyond a certain threshold, if the body produces either too much or too little of a specific substance. The quantitative view also implies that disease and health form a continuum, and that the boundary between the two is relative and arbitrary. Treatment, by implication, is thought of as restoring a normal level of bodily functioning. The first and foremost aim of biomedical research is, in this view, to explore normal functioning. Molecular biology will subsequently enable more insight into clinical pathology, and the development of rational therapies.

Although Canguilhem traced the quantitative view of disease in the context of the rise of physiology in the nineteenth and early twentieth centuries, most of its characteristics can be easily recognized in current molecular medicine research. By investigating quantities of specific substances and comparing them in different populations, cut-off points for normal and deviant biomarker results are established, usually with a grey zone in between. These markers are thought of as snapshots of the disease process, and as such they are thought to offer valuable clues for how to modify this process. Repeated biomarker measurements enable monitoring the effects of a chosen intervention; if the results go in the direction of "normal" values, treatment is considered successful.

Different biomarkers, strictly speaking, reveal *states* at a certain moment in time. By connecting the dots between different biomarkers, researchers often try to reconstruct the pathway between genetic roots and ultimate clinical phenomena. Such reconstructions frequently imply what I have elsewhere labeled a "cascade model" of disease (Boenink, 2010). The disease process is framed as a stepwise, steadily growing cascade. Deviations in molecular functioning, for example, when a genetic mutation leads to different RNA levels, are supposed to lead to changes in protein production, which may lead to changes in cell functioning, and so on to the level of tissues, organs, and the body as a whole. This framing is in line with what Francis Crick labeled the central dogma of molecular biology, which claims that information flows from DNA to RNA and proteins, but never in the reverse direction (Fox-Keller, 2000, p. 53; Dupre, 2010, p. 26).

This cascade model of disease invites pleas for early diagnosis and intervention. After all, if the pathological process is supposed to become progressively serious, it will also become more difficult to stop, divert, or even counter the stream. It need not surprise, then, that the development of biomarker tests is often accompanied by promises of prediction and prevention. Such promises are not new; they were voiced already in the discourse surrounding the HGP. The rhetorical force of more recent promises of prediction and prevention stems from the claim that molecular medicine, in contrast to genetics, brings into view *real-time* disease processes. Both the miniaturization of the tools to measure the body (enabling more frequent measuring) and the ever-increasing amount of detail in which bodily substances can be sensed have led to claims of, for example, single cell or even single molecule diagnostics, catching disease when it just starts. Prediction in such cases is actually more like prognosis; in view of observed bodily changes, we suspect that a pathological process is at work, and it will ultimately lead to the experience of complaints and symptoms. The process may be stopped or reversed by timely intervention, thus preventing the disease from becoming manifest.

Disease, Dynamics, and Determinism

In contrast with the static view of disease implied in the expectations surrounding the HGP, research in both genomics and molecular medicine increasingly focuses on the dynamics of bodily functioning. As a result, disease is now conceptualized in a *physiological*, rather than a neo-ontological way. It is approached as a process in time, in which functioning can be more or less normal—whatever normal may be. This shift from a neo-ontological to a physiological framing of disease does not necessarily solve the philosophical difficulties inherent in the neo-ontological approach; it may even raise new ones. I discuss two issues that seem particularly challenging for the physiological view of disease, as it is implied in current research in molecular medicine. First, by focusing on the disease process and on quantitative variations in bodily functioning, the boundary between disease and health becomes ever fuzzier. Second, the cascade model of disease easily invites claims of prediction and prevention, but these presuppose causal relationships between different disease elements that may not be warranted on the basis of current research.

As for the boundary between disease and health, this issue raised significant philosophical reflection already in the context of the HGP. If genetic mutations indicate an increased risk of disease, does this mean that people who experience themselves as healthy are diseased after all? The increasing awareness that mutations do not necessarily lead to disease has brought several commentators to observe that "being at risk" has become a third category, in between disease and health. Labels like susceptibility or predisposition are not just neutral descriptions, however, they can have real implications. They may serve to justify regimes of medical surveillance. Several critics charge this as another form of medicalization, which may disempower the individuals involved. Others, however, have argued that this last conclusion is too hasty. The new identities, roles, and responsibilities created by these labels are also actively taken up by the individuals to whom they are applied.

Novas and Rose (2004) have coined the term "biocitizenship" to indicate that molecular technologies create new bonds between individuals, with which individuals then may explicitly identify themselves to take social and political action. They rally for funding of research for their particular disease, and meet at web fora where they share experiences and exchange advice. A striking example is that some women who tested positive for BRCA1 or 2, the genes predisposing for an increased risk of breast and ovarian cancer, have started identifying themselves as "previvors." As Rose (2007, p. 85) points out in the context of genetic susceptibility testing, the philosophical question of whether predisposition amounts to a disease may be leading us astray, because this question suggests that there is a clear-cut ontological criterion to distinguish between these two. In practice, the reasons to accept that persons are labeled (and perceive themselves) as diseased in the absence of symptoms may be linked to social and ethical advantages (see also Rose, 2009).

Similar questions resurface in molecular medicine, because biomarker measurements may also reveal deviant functioning in asymptomatic individuals. Part of the problem for both genomics and molecular medicine is that definitions of disease based on pathology may not neatly align with diagnoses based on subjective experiences. Genomic and molecular medicine thus tend to widen the gap between disease and illness and between subjective experience and objectively measured manifestations of disease. In the context of molecular medicine, however, an additional issue comes to the fore: even if we stick to objective observations, the boundary between disease and health (or nondisease) becomes rather vague. This is a direct consequence of the increased focus on disease dynamics and the use of a quantitative view of disease. As I indicated earlier, this view of disease implies that normal and abnormal bodily processes are gradually distinct only. In practice, the boundary hinges on cut-off points, often embedded in clinical guidelines and protocols. Such cut-off points are ultimately epistemologically arbitrary, even though there may be very good practical and social reasons for drawing the line in a specific way.

Although arbitrary boundaries between disease and nondisease have been part of medicine, at least since the introduction of physiology, they seem to have become a ubiquitous feature in molecular medicine. They are not independent from the boundary between disease and illness, however. As Canguilhem (1991) reminds us, a quantitative approach of disease always hinges on the distinction between illness and health. Researchers determine what is quantitatively normal by comparing different populations, often by way of biobanks. When grouping individuals into populations, they actually distinguish between those who saw fit to see a doctor and received a diagnosis and those who did not. The clinical diagnosis, and before that the experiential distinction between health and illness (or unhealth), are both, then, epistemologically prior to any quantitative distinction. That being said, we should realize that genomics and molecular medicine continuously redraw the boundaries between disease and nondisease, as well as between health and illness. Although it may not be productive to search for general foundations to warrant these distinctions, we should critically question what is lost and won by shifting boundaries of specific disease categories and by the creation of new labels.

As the earlier discussion shows, novel biomarkers are usually considered informative to the extent that they produce knowledge of real-time bodily processes, which apparently tell something about future health. Here we touch on the second issue I want to address: molecular medicine in particular seems to (re-) introduce time as a crucial dimension of how we consider and deal with disease. The snapshots biomarker testing produces are meaningful because they are linked with the individual's future functioning. However, the dynamics ascribed to disease processes are often constituted in a specific, limited way. Modeling pathology as a cascade suggests a linear, unidirectional course of events, from genetic mutation, via RNA and proteins, to clinical symptoms. It also suggests that events in the cascade are linked in an automatic way. Once the stream has started to flow, it develops into an ever-growing torrent. The chain may not be completely determined, but with each step, the likelihood of subjective health problems increases.

In practice, however, the subsequent steps in the chain are less closely linked than the cascade model suggests. This is particularly true in case of early, or "upstream," markers. These more often than not have low predictive value. Apparently pathological processes are much more complex and varied than the cascade model allows for. The lack of predictive power suggests that causal relations are not as simple as assumed in the cascade model. And the weakness cannot be repaired by dividing what was first seen as one pathway into many distinct pathways. First, the assumption of unidirectionality may be misguided. The direction of events may sometimes be reversed. For example, critics of the central dogma of molecular biology argue that interaction with the surrounding cell may affect epigenetic changes in the genome (Dupre, 2010, p. 26). Likewise, pathological processes may include feedback loops, dead ends, or complex interactions. Second, molecular medicine focuses completely on the molecular events in the body. Many potential (co-)causes and mitigating or reversing factors outside the body are left out of the picture. Food intake, work stress, housing, and the like are usually not taken into account. Both the unidirectional assumption, and the reductionist scope of most biomarker research, then, severely limit the predictive capability of molecular medicine.

As a result, molecular medicine may open up bodily functioning in real time, but it is not clear what these real-time snapshots tell about what comes next. Against this background, much biomarker discourse is imprecise, to say the least. "X is a biomarker for Alzheimer's disease" is often shorthand for "X indicates that you have an increased risk of amyloid plaques in your brain, although unknown factors may protect you against building up these plaques, or prevent them from leading to clinical symptoms and subjective experiences." Admittedly, the second message is a rather complicated one. By "black boxing" presuppositions of and unknowns in the underlying research, however, molecular medicine seems to be overplaying its hand, and this may ultimately be counterproductive for maintaining public trust and funding.

Personalized Medicine: Fragmenting the Normal

Molecular medicine is frequently associated with promises not only of prediction and prevention, but also of personalization (Hood et al., 2004; Tian et al.,

2012). The preceding section explained why we should not take the claim of prediction (and by implication prevention) at face value. The same is true for the promise of personalization. As in the case of prediction and prevention, the recent surge of interest in personalization started in genetic and genomic medicine. In the expectations surrounding the HGP, personalization (or tailoring) of treatment was often put forward as an important future application of the knowledge gained by the HGP (Collins, 2010; Hedgecoe, 2004). By investigating how genetic variation is linked to drug response (including nonresponse), researchers hoped to be able to explain why a specific drug works for one person but not for another. Such insights might help to select the right drug for the right person, and even to develop new drugs tailored to specific genomic profiles. Promises of personalized medicine thus were first and foremost linked to the emerging field of pharmacogenomics. They were construed, moreover, in opposition to a "one-size-fits-all" strategy aiming for blockbuster drugs, which was retrospectively ascribed to past pharmacological research.

Similar promises are now attached to molecular biomarkers more generally. Biomarkers are thought to differentiate between different disease types (or pathways), and thus to offer good clues for selecting (or developing) the treatment that matches this particular pathway. This broadening has not fundamentally altered the concept of personalization implied. The general meaning of personalization in pharmacogenomics, as in molecular medicine, is that treatment is (and should be) tailored to the biological characteristics unique to an individual. This ideal actually fits well with older ideas of a rational, scientific medicine, in which knowledge of disease pathology is the basis for treatments that can modify the pathological process.

As several authors have noted, there is a profound irony in the recent use of the term "personalized medicine" (Dickenson, 2013; Tutton, 2014; Boenink, 2013). Since the first decade of the twentieth century, the term "person-centered medicine" has been used to criticize the emergence and consolidation of science-based medicine. The latter was perceived as overrelying on technological tools and the numbers they produce, and it was accused of treating disease, instead of people (Rosenberg, 2002; Lawrence and Weisz, 1998). Such critics usually argued that good doctors care for the individual and his or her needs, meaning that they take into account a patient's life story, values, and social and material context in a holistic way. Often this implied that (cold) technology obstructed a good (warm, human) patient–physician relation, rather than facilitating it. In the recent discourse on personalized medicine, however, technology is actually a crucial vehicle for "personal care." Moreover, the "person" targeted here is not a person with a life story, but a body with specific, quantifiable characteristics. No wonder some proponents of personalized medicine in the older meaning feel the concept has been hijacked and turned into something completely different. The reductionist and mechanistic approach of disease in biomedicine that was the target of earlier critics now poses as the peak of personalization.

There is another reason why "personalized medicine" may be a misleading term. In the visions of personalized medicine treatments are not tailored at the level of the individual person, but at the level of a subpopulation. Increased knowledge of genomic or biomarker profiles enables the differentiation of more and more subgroups, that is, improved stratification. Detailed molecular profiling may produce precise, molecular cues for developing effective treatments. This is why some have proposed to use "stratified medicine" (European Science Foundation, 2012) or "precision medicine" (National Academy of Sciences, 2011), rather than personalized medicine. The first term indeed fits better with the shifts currently brought about by genomic and molecular research. The second terms covers the ambitions and hopes associated with such research.

One might wonder whether the search for personalization, by continuously narrowing down subpopulations, might ultimately lead to a full individualization of the boundary between the normal and the pathological. In my view, such a development would sit very uneasily with some of the fundamental assumptions guiding genomic and molecular medicine.

Personalized medicine actually amounts to the latest manifestation of what Rosenberg (2002, p. 240) has called the "specificity revolution" in medicine (Mulinari, 2014). This revolution dates back to the nineteenth century and refers to the growing intellectual and social significance of specific disease categories. Influenced by the rise of modern pathology and the development of technologies to investigate the body, diseases came to be seen as specific, mechanism-based ailments with a characteristic clinical course, while "idiosyncrasies of place and person," according to Rosenberg (2002, p. 243), became less and less important. Specifying disease, that is, helped to purify our view of disease from personal details. In the wake of the search for specificity, an increasing number of technologies entered diagnostic practice as "instruments of precision," promising an ever more precise understanding of disease (p. 243). In its most recent version, then, specificity is found at the molecular level and in quantification of bodily functioning. Zooming in on this level, the boundaries between normal and abnormal are redrawn, but only at the level of subpopulations. The idea of personalizing in the meaning of individualizing what is and is not normal would be at odds with the objectivist view of disease underlying the specificity revolution. This view claims, after all, that "disease" exists independent of its manifestation in individual subjects.

Epigenetics and Systems Approaches

From One-way Process to Mutual Interaction and Complexity

The shift from genetics to genomics and molecular medicine broadened the number of substances looked at in biomedical research and increased attention for their interactions. As we have seen earlier, this entailed an approach toward disease as *process* and a renewed interest in the role of real time. Most biomarker research, however, still focuses on snapshots of this process, which are then more or less explicitly connected into mechanistic cascades. Even though the number of different disease pathways has exploded in recent years, thinking in terms of a cascade continues to reduce bodily processes to their molecular constituents and to a unidirectional connection between them.

There are, however, fields of biomedical research that critically question the reductionist and deterministic stance taken in molecular medicine, and these have gained recent notoriety: epigenetics and systems biology approaches. Epigenetics is the field studying the expression and regulation of genes during an organism's development, as well as in evolution. The crucial starting point here is that gene expression is *not* predetermined or automatic; it thus departs from the central dogma of molecular biology that processes flow only from DNA to RNA, proteins, and upward, and not the other way round. Whether and how genetic mutations lead to changes in bodily functioning depends on interactions between genes and nongenetic factors, both inside and outside the body. Such factors may, moreover, have lasting, and sometimes even transgenerational, effects on genomic functioning. Systems approaches, in addition, plea for the inclusion of different levels of bodily functioning (cell, tissue, organ, organ system, body), as well as environmental, social, and lifestyle influences in biomedical (and more generally in biological) research. Both fields continue the shift in attention from genome structure to genome functioning, which originated in genomics and molecular medicine. They distance themselves from earlier approaches, however, by stressing that genes (or any other molecules) are neither static nor isolated entities. Molecules do not function independently from context. These contexts, whether internal or external to the body, vary widely. It is crucial, then, to pay attention to the dynamics, complexity, and variety of bodily functioning in general and of disease process in particular.

Epigenetic research has shown, in part, how maternal stress during pregnancy can have lasting effects on the health of offspring (McGowan et al., 2009; Meaney, 2010), or how early-life adversity mediates forms of DNA methylation that seem to contribute to depression, suicide, and other mental disorders (Nada et al., 2012). In systems biology, attention is, for example, drawn to the way gut bacteria (the microbiome) form an interface among lifestyle factors such as nutrition, genomic characteristics, and pathological events like the emergence of intestinal cancer (Rawls et al., 2004). The number of factors that contribute to health and disease is huge, and possible interactions are even more daunting. Nonetheless, systems biology aims for an approach in which information from many different technologies is combined into what some call a holistic, comprehensive medicine (Tian et al., 2012).

Rethinking Body and Environment: Disease as Entanglement

Attempts to acknowledge the complexity of disease processes suggest that it is insufficient to simply multiply the number of disease pathways, as implied by the vision of stratified medicine. The idea of a pathway itself should be reinterpreted by rethinking its constituents. John Dupre (2011, p. 125) argues that both epigenetics and systems approaches imply that molecular bodily processes do not develop in an endogenous manner. That is, molecules do not develop in and of themselves. They always function (and can function only) in a context (of the cell, the organ, the body, but also of that body's behavior, its social and material setting). There is no essence in DNA or any other molecule that is necessarily realized in development, and which is juxtaposed to its environment (whatever that may mean). This implies that we should not conceive of bodies as passive and stable, something only acted upon by humans and their technologies (Dupre, 2010). Moreover, it raises fundamental questions regarding the common juxtaposition of molecules (or bodies) and environment, or between nature and nurture.

According to Fox-Keller (2010), the juxtaposition between nature and nurture took off only in the late nineteenth century. Francis Galton coined the phrase "nature and nurture," claiming that heredity is only in the body (thus also justifying his eugenic program). The question whether disease is caused by one or the other, or what percentage of disease is explained by genes and environment, respectively, has been nagging biomedical researchers ever since. In view of the findings of epigenetics and systems biology, Fox-Keller and others argue that it may be much more fruitful to think of nature-nurture in terms of a *symbiosis*. Admittedly, it may be hard to stop talking about and thinking in terms of body and environment, or nature and nurture altogether. We should be aware, however, that each of these can function only in interaction with the other. Body and environment are continuously interfacing, as the example of the microbiome indicates.

Both epigenetics and systems biology, then, offer insights that invite another reconceptualization of disease. Disease is still viewed as a process, and in that respect the view remains physiological. It is no longer modeled as a cascade, however, but as a complex and evolving "entanglement" (Lock, 2013). Particularly in systems approaches, the reconstruction of such entanglements or networks usually involves much computational work because of the large number of elements involved. Algorithms are developed to make sense of the network of relations and simulation models employed to explore different possibilities. As both Lock (2013) and Niewöhner (2011) have argued, however, doing justice to all the different elements in a network proves difficult. There is a serious risk that the sociohistorical forces are conceptualized in an impoverished way.

> We may be in danger of embracing a new form of somatic determinism. Although the contribution of environments (social and environmental) to human development, health and illness is beyond dispute, there is a distinct possibility that it is the apparent molecular endpoints of such variables will capture the most attention, without shedding light on the complex factors implicated in the perturbations of these molecular barometers. (Lock, 2013, pp. 1896–97)

In other words, influences of lifestyle and social environment may be taken into account in a molecularized way only.

And even when due attention is given to social factors, a bias with regard to how accessible certain elements are may play a role. Parental behavior and socioeconomic status may be retrieved and measured relatively easily, but it is much harder to find out how, for example, experiences of discrimination or social injustice are implicated in disease processes. Lock (2013, p. 1897) argues that we should not shy away from including subjective accounts (as produced in ethnographic research) in healthcare research. Anyway, a critical look at methods in biomedical research is paramount, and we may need to develop novel methods and combine existing ones in unprecedented ways if we want to reconstruct the complex dynamics of disease processes.

Disease and Contingency: Personalized Medicine Revisited

The entanglement view of disease not only broadens the types of influences included in the view of disease, it also affects the way the process character of disease is thought of. As noted earlier, in genomic and molecular medicine disease pathways are thought of as law-like events, mechanisms in which one step determines what happens next. In epigenetics and systems biology, however, disease processes come to the fore as fundamentally *contingent*. Because of the large number of elements involved and the complexity of the interactions, we cannot automatically assume that state A at moment t1 will always be followed by state B at t2. Causal processes may be much more irregular than presupposed in past biomedical research. This has, of course, enormous implications for prediction and prognosis and also for thinking about intervention. It is questionable whether a population approach, however stratified, will ever provide sufficiently strong evidence for predictions on the level of the individual.

As Tian, Price, and Hood (2012) have suggested, however, systems approaches to medicine are less focused on identifying the disease (and thus on diagnosis), and more interested in frequent (or even continuous) monitoring of an individual's functioning. This would be enabled not only by developments in molecular biology, but also by the growing number of devices to sense regularly and to analyze continuously bodily parameters, as well as one's lifestyle and environment. Participants of the Quantified Self Movement are already experimenting with such forms of monitoring. The collection of an ever-growing set of data about their own functioning enables them to determine what is normal (or abnormal) *for them*. Comparison with the data of others helps to interpret further what might be going on and which interventions could improve functioning. Conclusions with regard to health and disease are based, then, on a complex comparison of individual functioning over time, as well as with the functioning of others who are considered comparable.

The European Science Foundation in its 2012 report on Personalised Medicine conjures up a similar vision of ubiquitous and continuous monitoring and data analysis.

> The goal would be to generate ongoing descriptions of an individual's phenotype, including all the molecular, morphological, physiological and psychological information that characterises a person in health and disease, and to be able to assess it in relation to environmental exposures, history and psychosocial context in order to identify appropriate preventive or therapeutic measures to promote continued health. (p. 43)

By including a large number of parameters, focusing not only on the body but on the body in interaction, both the complexity and the contingency of the functioning of this "embedded body" would be tackled (Niewöhner, 2011). In principle, this would allow the individual to decide personally when deviant test results and/or subjective experiences are a reason to start worrying and to seek help.

This is, again, easier said than done. An interesting attempt at individualizing medicine appeared in the journal *Cell* (Chen et al., 2012). The authors monitored the "integrative personal omics profile" of one person (the principal investigator). During 14 months, they measured twenty times the same set of parameters, including DNA, RNA, proteins, metabolites, and autoantibodies. In this period, the research subject contracted a viral infection twice. In the first set of measurements, a genetic predisposition for type 2 diabetes was discovered. After the second virus infection, the researchers saw diabetes "emerge" (they claim) in the test subject. As a result, the subject was able to make lifestyle adjustments and to start treatment early on.

This example raises interesting issues about the concept of disease implied by the aim of individualizing. It is a typical example, because the researchers did indeed focus completely on the molecular barometer (as Lock suspects most biomedical researchers are inclined to do). They did not include information on lifestyle and environment, let alone on history and social relations. The collected data nonetheless, in principle, allow for the individualization of the boundary between disease and health. In this case, however, the definition of what is normal or abnormal was firmly rooted in traditional medical knowledge of molecular pathology. Diabetes was recognized as such only because of existing (population-based) definitions of the disease. Diagnosis was envisioned, moreover, as an objective verdict about a state of affairs, not as a normative judgment regarding the undesirability of potential developments for this person. The subject, even though a biomedical researcher, apparently did not feel competent to diagnose and decide what to do; he reported that he was grateful for all the medical advice he received when presenting the results at scientific conferences (Dennis, 2012).

As this example shows, it is questionable whether it will ever be possible to conceive a radically personalized medicine in a coherent way. Can we ever fully individualize the boundary between disease and health? It seems that distinguishing between the two requires comparisons, and even if individual functioning is continuously measured, the results may not provide a sufficient basis for action. In particular when *anticipatory* knowledge is desired, indicating how functioning is likely to develop in the time to come with and without intervention, comparison with other individuals is indispensable. The promise of epigenetics and systems approaches is that by collecting, analyzing, and comparing data about bodily functioning in a wider sense, we should be able to interpret the patterns and deviations in an individual's data in a more informed way. This will not remove the fundamental contingency of disease processes, however, nor will it allow for complete control. Disease processes may always evolve in surprising directions, and interventions may always remain experimental: that a treatment works in one person does not guarantee that it will work in others, as doctors and patients know too well. The irony of current developments in biomedical research, then, is that they help to understand why this is the case, without necessarily offering ways to remedy this predicament.

Conclusion

Developments in biomedical technoscience shape and are shaped by the way we think about disease. Since the initial completion of the HGP, much biomedical research has been driven and justified by visions of a medicine that will be predictive, preventive, and personalized. This apparent consensus on what future medicine (or healthcare more broadly) should look like disguises marked differences between the way different types of biomedical research conceptualize disease. Such differences are salient to what prediction, prevention, and personalization actually mean in clinical practice.

Medical genetics and the expectations surrounding the HGP tend toward a neo-ontological view of disease, in which genetic defects are identified with the disease. Prediction and prevention in this case involves counseling about reproduction and, if possible, forms of gene therapy. Personalization means stratification of individuals to subpopulations with specific mutations. Genomics and molecular medicine have brought along a shift toward a physiological view of disease, which includes a renewed focus on disease as process. This process is modeled as a cascade of subsequent changes in molecular functioning, of which biomarker measurements provide quantified snapshots. The mechanistic and unidirectional character ascribed to this cascade is crucial for prediction and prevention, goals that involve frequent monitoring of bodily parameters. Such monitoring, however, is also likely to blur the boundary between disease and health. Moreover, the identification of additional biomarkers is producing a wide array of supposed disease pathways, leading to a fragmentation of diseases. This fragmentation is the basis for claims of personalization, which in practice reduce to more detailed stratification of patient groups.

Both epigenetics and systems biology, however, approach disease as a process of dynamic and complex entanglements of many different variables. Researchers from these fields stress that molecules interact within a context, and they contest the one-way cascade model. The complex and contingent character ascribed to the disease process suggests that it may be hard to sustain any predictive claim, except by applying complex algorithms to massive data sets. Interestingly, possibilities for prevention may increase if more variables influencing the dynamics of the process are taken into account. Systems approaches, then, seem to encourage thinking of personalization in terms of an "individualization of the normal." However, the tendency to identify ever more specific disease categories, by distinguishing particular underlying pathological processes that may be countered by specific treatments, appears to meet its Waterloo. To recognize patterns in individual functioning as a particular disease, comparison with others is unavoidable. Disease categories can be specified, but never fully individualized.

Does this mean that the subject and his or her experience of illness is completely excluded from the way disease is viewed in the fields of biomedical science and technology? Yes and no. The increasing molecularization and quantification of disease certainly deflect attention from subjective experience in favor of an outsiders' objective view. However, as I pointed out earlier,

Canguilhem is right in claiming that such objective knowledge is always dependent on individuals who think they have good reason to visit a doctor. As the Quantitative Self Movement shows, new technologies also open up possibilities to play an active role in monitoring one's functioning and to connect measurements with more subjective experiences. In systems approaches, there is a tension between the use of algorithms that distances the identification of disease from individuals' own experience of their health and possibilities to engage actively these individuals in decisions about what to monitor and how to interpret the results. Even though it may not be common in most of the field, it is possible to imagine forms of systems medicine in which objective measurements and subjective experiences are combined and in which both patients and medical experts have a role.

Finally, all this suggests that we should not accept at face value any vision or promise of the direction that medicine is taking. Analyzing and comparing how different scientific fields using different technologies frame disease in (sometimes slightly, but sometimes radically) different ways helps to anticipate how fruitful a particular approach might be, even if we cannot know what disease is independent from these technological and scientific mediations. Equally important, a philosophical reconstruction of evolving disease concepts in biomedicine helps to get a better idea of what practices of treating disease and promoting health along the lines of these visions would look like, what activities, roles, and experiences would be involved. In both roles, philosophical analysis enables critical reflection on visions and promises conjuring a future you cannot refuse. If we do not want to succumb to technoscientific developments, but want to shape our treatment of disease and promotion of health in the future, such philosophical analysis is a crucial first step.

References

Bell, K. (2013). Biomarkers, the molecular gaze and the transformation of cancer survivorship. *BioSocieties* 8(2): 124–43.

Biomarkers Definition Working Group (2001). Biomarkers and surrogate endpoints: Preferred definitions and conceptual framework. *Clinical Pharmacology and Therapeutics* 69(3): 89–95.

Boenink, M. (2009). Tensions and opportunities in convergence: Shifting concepts of disease in emerging molecular medicine. *Nanoethics* 3(3): 243–55.

Boenink, M. (2010). Molecular medicine and concepts of disease: The ethical value of a conceptual analysis of emerging biomedical technologies. *Medicine, Health Care and Philosophy* 13(1): 11–23.

Boenink, M. (2013). Van confectie naar maatkleding? "Personalized medicine" en het onderscheid normaal—pathologisch. In *Komt een filosoof bij de dokter. Denken over gezondheid en zorg*, eds. M. Schermer, M. Boenink, and G. Meijnen. Amsterdam: Boom.

Boorse, C. (1975). On the distinction between health and illness. *Philosophy and Public Affairs* 5: 49–68.

Boorse, C. (1977). Health as a theoretical concept. *Philosophy of Science* 44: 542–73.

Canguilhem, G. (1991). *The Normal and the Pathological*. New York: Zone Books.

Chen, R. et al. (2012). Personal omics profiling reveals dynamic molecular and medial phenotypes. *Cell* 148: 1293–307.

Collins, F. S. (1999). Shattuck lecture—medical and societal consequences of the Human Genome Project. *The New England Journal of Medicine* 341(1): 28–37.

Collins, F. (2010). *The Language of Life: DNA and the Revolution in Personalized Medicine*. London: Harper Collins.

Dennis, C. (2012). The rise of the "narciss-ome." *Nature*, March 16, 2012, http://www.nature.com/news/the-rise-of-the-narciss-ome-1.10240, accessed February 22, 2015.

Dickenson, D. (2013). *Me-Medicine vs. We-Medicine: Reclaiming Biotechnology for the Common Good*. New York: Columbia University Press.

Dupre, J. (2010). The polygenomic organism. In *Nature after the Genome*, eds. S. Parry and J. Dupre. Oxford: Blackwell, pp. 19–31.

Dupre, J. (2011). Emerging sciences and new conceptions of disease; or, beyond the monogenomic differentiated cell lineage. *European Journal of Philosophy of Science* 1: 119–31.

European Science Foundation (2012). *Personalised Medicine for the European Citizen. Towards More Precise Medicine for the Diagnosis, Treatment and Prevention of Disease (iPM)*. http://www.esf.org/fileadmin/Public_documents/Publications/Personalised_Medicine.pdf, accessed August 23, 2015.

Fox-Keller, E. (1992). Nature, nurture and the Human Genome Project. In *The Code of Codes. Scientific and Social Issues in the Human Genome Project*, eds. D. J. Kevles and L. Hood. Cambridge: Harvard University Press, pp. 281–99.

Fox-Keller, E. (2000). Decoding the Genetic Program. In *The Concept of the Gene in Development and Evolution: Historical and Epistemological Perspectives*, eds. P. Beurton, R. Falk, and H. J. Rheinberger. Cambridge: Cambridge University Press.

Fox-Keller, E. (2010). *The Century of the Gene*. Cambridge: Harvard University Press.

Freitas, R. A. (2007). Personal choice in the coming era of nanomedicine. In *Nanoethics: The Ethical and Social Implications of Nanotechnology*, eds. F. Allhoff, P. Lin, J. Moor, and J. Weckert. Hoboken: John Wiley, pp. 161–72.

Guttmacher, A. E., and Collins, F. S. (2002). Genomic medicine: A primer. *New England Journal of Medicine* 347(19): 1512–20.

Have, H. ten. (2001). Genetics and culture: The geneticization thesis. *Medicine, Health Care and Philosophy* 4(3): 295–304.

Hedgecoe, A. (2004). *The Politics of Personalised Medicine: Pharmacogenetics in the Clinic*. Cambridge: Cambridge University Press.

Hedgecoe, A. M. (2009). Geneticization: Debates and controversies. In *Encyclopedia of the Life Sciences*. Chichester: Wiley.

Hoedemakers, R., and ten Have, H. (1998). Geneticization: The Cyprus paradigm. *Journal of Medicine and Philosophy* 23(2): 274–87.

Hofmann, B. (2001). The technological invention of disease. *Journal of Medical Ethics: Medical Humanities* 27: 10–19.

Hood, L., Heath, J. R., Phelps, M. E., and Lin B. (2004). Systems biology and new technologies enable predictive and preventative medicine. *Science* 306: 640–43.

Ihde, D. (1990). *Technology and the Lifeworld: From Garden to Earth*. Bloomington: Indiana University Press.

Kevles, D. J., and Hood, L. (eds.) (1992). *The Code of Codes: Scientific and Social Issues in the Human Genome Project*. Cambridge: Harvard University Press.

Khoury, M. (2003). Genetics and genomics in practice: The continuum from genetic disease to genetic information in health and disease. *Genetics in Medicine* 5(4): 261–68.

Kohli-Laven, N., Bourret, P., Keating, P., and Cambrosio, A. (2011). Cancer clinical trials in the era of genomic signatures: Biomedical innovation, clinical utility, and regulatory-scientific hybrids. *Social Studies of Science* 41(4): 487–513.

Konrad, M. (2005). *Narrating the New Predictive Genetics: Ethics, Ethnography and Science.* Cambridge: Cambridge University Press.

Lander, E. S. (2011). Initial impact of sequencing of the human genome. *Nature* 470: 187–97.

Lawrence, C., and Weisz, G. (eds.) (1998). *Greater Than the Parts: Holism in Biomedicine, 1920–1950.* Oxford: Oxford University Press.

Lewontin, R. C. (1991). *The Doctrine of DNA: Biology as Ideology.* London: Penguin.

Lindee, M. S. (2000). Genetic disease since 1945. *Nature Review Genetics* 1: 236–41.

Lippmann, A. (1991). Prenatal testing and screening: Constructing needs and reinforcing inequalities. *American Journal of Law and Medicine* 17(1/2): 15–50.

Lock, M. (2013). The lure of the epigenome. *The Lancet* 381: 1896–97.

McGowan, P. O. et al. (2009). Epigenetic regulation of glucocorticoid receptor in human brain associates with childhood abuse. *Nature Neuroscience* 12: 342–48.

Meaney, M. J. (2010). Epigenetics and the biological definition of gene x environment interactions. *Child Development* 81: 41–79.

Melendro-Oliver, S. (2004). Shifting concepts of disease. *Science Studies* 17(1): 20–33.

Metzler, I. (2010). Biomarkers and their consequences for the biomedical profession: A social science perspective. *Personalized Medicine* 7(4): 407–20.

Mulinari, S. (2014). The specificity triad: Notions of disease and therapeutic specificity in biomedical reasoning. *Philosophy, Ethics and Humanities in Medicine* 9: 14.

Nada, B. et al. (2012). Association with early-life socio-economic position in adult DNA-methylation. *International Journal of Epidemiology* 41: 6–74.

National Academy of Sciences (2011). *Toward Precision Medicine: Building a Knowledge Network for Biomedical Research and a New Taxonomy of Disease.* Washington: National Academics Press.

Niewöhner, J. (2011). Epigenetics: Embedded bodies and the molecularization of biography and milieu. *BioSocieties* 6: 279–98.

Nordenfelt, L. (1995). *On the Nature of Health: An Action-Theoretic Perspective.* Dordrecht: Kluwer.

Novas, C., and Rose, N. (2004). Biological citizenship. In *Blackwell Companion to Global Anthropology*, eds. A. Ong and S. Collier. Oxford: Blackwell.

Rawls, J. F., Samuel, B. S., and Gordon, J. I. (2004). Gnotobiotic zebrafish reveal evolutionarily conserved response to the gut microbiotia. *Proceedings of the National Academy of Sciences* 101(3): 4596–601.

Reiser, S. J. (1978). *Medicine and the Reign of Technology.* Cambridge: Cambridge University Press.

Reznek, L. (1987). *The Nature of Disease.* New York: Routledge.

Rose, N. (2007). *The Politics of Life Itself: Biomedicine, Power, and Subjectivity in the Twenty-First Century.* Princeton: Princeton University Press.

Rose, N. (2009). Normality and pathology in a biomedical age. *The Sociological Review* 57(s2): 66–83.

Rosenberg, C. E. (1989). Disease in history: Frames and framers. *The Milbank Quarterly* 67(suppl. 1): 1–15.

Rosenberg C. E. (2002). The tyranny of diagnosis: Specific entities and individual experience. *The Milbank Quarterly* 80(2): 237–60.

Rosenberg, C. E. (2003). What is disease? In memory of Owsei Temkin. *Bulletin of the History of Medicine* 77(3): 491–505.

Sherwin, S., and Simpson, C. (1999). Ethical questions in the pursuit of genetic information: Geneticization and BRCA1. In *Genetic Information: Acquisition, Access and Control*, eds. A. Thompson and R. Chadwick. New York: Kluwer, pp. 121–28.

Stempsey, W. E. (2006). The geneticization of diagnostics. *Medicine, Health Care and Philosophy* 9: 193–200.

Tian, Q., Price, N. D., and Hood, L. (2012). Systems cancer medicine: Towards realization of predictive, preventive, personalized and participatory (P4) medicine. *Journal of Internal Medicine* 271: 111–21.

Tutton, R. (2014). *Genomics and the Reimagining of Personalized Medicine*. Farnham: Ashgate.

Varmus, H. (2010). Ten years on—The Human Genome and Medicine. *New England Journal of Medicine* 362(21): 2028–29.

Verbeek, P. P. (2005). *What Things Do: Philosophical Reflections on Technology, Agency and Design*. University Park, PA: Penn State University Press.

Wakefield, J. C. (1992). The concept of mental disorder. *American Psychologist* 47: 373–88.

Whitbeck, C. (1977). Causation in medicine: The disease entity model. *Philosophy of Science* 44(4): 619–37.

Yoxen, E. (1982). Constructing genetic diseases. In *The Problem of Medical Knowledge: Examining the Social Construction of Medicine*, eds. P. Wright and A. Treacher. Edinburgh, Edinburgh University Press, pp. 144–61.

4 Philosophy of Epidemiology

Alex Broadbent

What is Epidemiology?

Definitions of epidemiology vary, but include some common elements, especially the phrase "distribution and determinants of disease." I define "epidemiology" as the study of the distribution and determinants of disease and other health states in human populations by means of group comparisons, for the purpose of improving population health (Broadbent, 2013, p. 1). Most epidemiologists will accept the elements of my definition.

Epidemiology is a discipline that essentially involves documenting the way health states occur in human populations, and trying to explain the documented patterns of occurrence. The comparison of different groups within a population is key, and was an essential development in the history of the discipline, distinguishing epidemiology from the much older medical use of the case history (which need not involve a comparison). Most epidemiologists, though not all, will also accept that the purpose of epidemiology is to improve population health. There are some who would prefer to see it as a coldly scientific pursuit of knowledge. But without the purposive element of the definition it is hard to make sense of the restriction of epidemiology to human populations, in one dimension (as opposed to ecology, or biology, for example), and to health states in another (as opposed to demography, geography, economics, and other human sciences). Moreover, the history of epidemiology definitely links it to both medicine and public health.

Definitions on their own are not as informative as a survey of some of the paradigm-shaping historical episodes, as they are recited in epidemiology textbooks and classes. While accounts in these locations are sometimes painfully Whiggish from the perspective of a true historian of science, they do tell us how the contemporary epidemiologist conceptualizes her profession.

Epidemiology did not emerge as a distinct field until the latter part of the twentieth century, and indeed teaching approaches and career paths are still not finalized. (Perhaps they will never be.) Nonetheless most epidemiologists will be familiar with at least two nineteenth-century "grandfathers" of the contemporary discipline. One is Ignaaz Semmelweis, who worked in the general hospital in Vienna in the mid-1800s.[1] He noticed that the mortality rate differed sharply between two maternity wards in the hospital. Childbed fever (puerperal fever) was much more prevalent in one ward than in another. To Semmelweis's mind, this could not be explained by the then-dominant theory of disease, the miasma theory, according to which diseases were caused by a "miasma" or bad air sweeping across a district. Crucially, for Semmelweis, the difference between the two wards could not be explained in this way. Thus he set about trying to establish the cause of the difference between the two wards. He identified a number of differences between the wards, and used either experimental intervention or background knowledge to rule most of them out as causes. He asked the priest to desist from walking through the afflicted ward on his way to administer last rites to the dead, in case that was depressing the mothers; he arranged for delivery positions to be the same across the two wards; and so forth. None of these changes made a difference. In the end, he settled on the fact that medical students examined mothers in the afflicted ward but not in the other. They came straight from an autopsy class. He got the students to wash their hands (not a standard practice at the time), and the incidence of childbed fever in the two wards became comparable. He concluded, then, that something on the hands of the medical students, "cadaveric matter," was causing the difference in childbed fever incidence between the two wards.

Clearly, we have here a comparison of groups, and an investigation of the observed difference between two groups to determine a cause of disease. The key elements that come out of this narrative are not only methodological. They also set up epidemiology as a pioneer discipline, pointing the way toward discoveries that have not yet been made—in this case, the discovery of bacteria. They also set epidemiology up as a challenge to established medical thought, and this slightly maverick feel remains a feature of epidemiology. Semmelweis famously failed to persuade the authorities to accept his theory about the transmission of puerperal fever. In contemporary life, the rise of evidence-based medicine (EBM) is in part an attempt to shift the social hierarchy of the medical profession and replace it with an "evidence hierarchy," deriving primarily from epidemiological thinking.

Another important feature of the Semmelweis story is that it illustrates the limits of epidemiology. Semmelweis's theory was strictly incorrect, or at least only part of the truth. Precisely, puerperal fever was caused not by bits of dead flesh but by bacteriological infection. One of the difficulties Semmelweis faced in convincing the authorities of his hypothesis was explaining why washing hands reduced infection rates but did not completely eliminate the disease. This is hard to explain if the disease is caused by cadaveric matter (he hypothesized some sort of internal event in the mothers that caused cadaveric matter to occur inside them naturally on some occasions) but much easier if one has the idea that something in the cadaveric matter, but which can also be found elsewhere, is causing the disease. This aspect of the episode illustrates the thought that epidemiology can get us only so far, and that, having identified a disease "vector" or an exposure of interest, epidemiology needs to hand over the matter to laboratory sciences, which can tell us more about how exactly the exposure works. One of the persisting debates in the philosophical life of epidemiologists concerns the extent to which they need to concern themselves with disease mechanisms, or to which they may treat diseases as "black boxes" when studying their distribution and hypothesizing their determinants.

Semmelweis's story, however, does not illustrate another important feature of epidemiology—its heavy reliance on what is known as "observational data." This terminology is odd from a philosophical point of view, since the contrast is experimental data, and philosophers traditionally call such data "empirical" (or even observational). The distinction, however, is not between the a priori and the a posteriori, but between data that has been obtained by observation alone, and data that has been obtained by (observing the results of) intervention on the population. Semmelweis conducted an intervention to test his hypothesis— an intervention that, today, he would probably not have obtained approval for until he had considerably more evidence.

Another nineteenth-century figure who relied much more heavily on observational evidence is John Snow, the English physician, who is also famous for his work as an anesthetist. Snow lived in London at a time when cholera epidemics were a regular and dreaded occurrence. He collected a great deal of data to support the view that dirty water was causally implicated in the transmission of cholera by going door-to-door, in some cases, to find out which water company supplied each house, and how many cholera victims had lived there. The pattern provided evidence that, in due course, was sufficient to persuade the authorities to limit access to water drawn from heavily polluted parts of the Thames (by removing the handle of the "Broad Street pump"). Like Semmelweis, Snow had to fight prevailing miasma theories of disease; but unlike Semmelweis, his key evidence came not from an intervention of his own, but from a "natural experiment" that circumstances had set up.[2]

These historical figures are important in the teaching of epidemiology, but they lived before the modern discipline had taken shape. The events that led to epidemiology becoming a science, with university departments and career epidemiologists, were the debates about the relation between smoking and lung cancer. These events epitomize the features that the nineteenth-century historical episodes illustrate. They involved heavy reliance on observational data: there was some evidence from the laboratory that tar painted on the ear of rats is carcinogenic, but the difference between painting tar on a rat's ear and breathing it in to a human lung are substantial. They involved overturning established popular and medical beliefs and the vested financial interests of tobacco companies. They involved defeating, in public, some of the most eminent scientists of the day (notably R. A. Fisher, one of the foundational figures of modern statistics, and Paul Berkson, an eminent mathematician and statistician).

A key feature of this episode, which deserves emphasis, is the contextual importance assumed by data which, on their own, would have been quite weak. For example, time trend data is not strong evidence for causation on its own.[3] However, in the smoking and lung cancer case, it was key in ruling out the main contender hypothesis, which was that a genetic predisposition underlay both the tendency to smoke and vulnerability to lung cancer. No such genetic trait could have spread through the population as fast as lung cancer did in the early twentieth century. However, with a time-lag of 20 years or so, it mapped the uptake of smoking very closely; and it also reflected the lag in women taking up smoking compared to men, with incidence of lung cancer also peaking correspondingly later in women. Thus observational data of a kind that, on its own, would have been little use supporting a causal hypothesis became crucial in ruling out a contender hypothesis, and thus crucial for indirectly supporting the causal hypothesis.

This kind of outside-the-box thinking gives epidemiology a detective-like feel, and makes it a great case study for philosophers of science and methodologists. While the received philosophical picture of science, shared by thinkers as diverse and Popper and Kuhn, is of an activity of developing an overarching theoretical framework into which empirical data either fit or fail to fit, epidemiologists work on problems piecemeal, using the theoretical background supplied by whichever established science is relevant to the field. Much has been written about scientific theory as if the development of theory were the goal of all science, but that simply is not an accurate picture of epidemiology. Again, much has been written about experiment as if that were essential to science, but that picture, too, seems a poor fit for epidemiology (as for a number of other sciences). Epidemiology's emphasis on method over theory, the peculiar restrictions on the kinds of data that are commonly available, and the relative youth of this science make it a fascinating and fruitful object of philosophical study. These features of epidemiology would also make it an excellent object of sociological study, but I will not be discussing sociological questions in this brief introduction to the chief philosophical issues that epidemiology throws up.

Causation in Epidemiology: Separating the Issues

The single most obvious philosophical topic in epidemiology is causation. It is obvious because epidemiologists themselves have written about it, and continue to debate it, sometimes hotly. Yet it is less obvious exactly what epidemiologists worry about when they ask questions about causation, and exactly why they worry.

I think that there are, in fact, several slightly different ways in which causation poses philosophical challenges for epidemiology.

(i)   Disease classification systems based on defining causes were dominant in the era in which epidemiology became prominent (the mid-twentieth century). Yet these classification systems, and this way of thinking about disease, were somewhat at odds with the methods, results, and in some ways the whole idea of epidemiology. Hence there was a felt need to defend, or at least situate, epidemiologists' causal claims about disease against the dominant paradigm for thinking about disease. I will refer to this as the question of "multifactorialism."

(ii) Measures of association are used as evidence from which causal inferences might be drawn, but they are also used to express the conclusions of those inferences, and to measure the "strength" of a causal effect. This raises a question as to how these measures are to be interpreted when they are used to express causal facts. What does it mean to say that a relative risk, for example, is "causally interpreted?" The problem here is understanding what more is meant by using a measure of association to express a causal claim, besides the (usually fairly simple) mathematical definition. I will refer to this as the causal interpretation problem.

(iii) The theoretical framework within which causal inferences are drawn, and on the basis of which statistical tools are used, has been a topic of interest across all the statistically driven disciplines in the second half of the twentieth century. In epidemiology, too, there was a felt need to understand what exactly these tools were doing, what their limitations and conditions of correct application are, and what, if anything, this tells us about the kinds of inferences that can be drawn from various kinds of evidence. I will refer to this as the causal inference problem.

(iv) Cutting across all these issues is the need for clear pedagogy, especially in a discipline that is so young and, arguably, still in its formative stage.

The next three sections are devoted to each of the problems (i)–(iii). I will not be concerned with pedagogical matters here, since they do not raise substantial philosophical questions that are specific to epidemiology (at least, not that I am aware of).

Multifactorialism

When epidemiology textbooks introduce causation, they usually mention two metaphors. One is the web of causation, a phrase originating in a textbook by B. MacMahon and T. F. Pugh, the first edition of which appeared in

1960 (MacMahon and Pugh, 1960), and the most recent (and, presumably, last) edition of which appeared in 1996 (MacMahon and Trichopoulos, 1996). The point of the metaphor is to emphasize that the causes of disease are very varied and may also stand in causal relations to each other. A case of lung cancer will feature certain genetic traits, exposure to cigarette smoke over a period of time, along with—perhaps—an upbringing in a low-income household (which, in this instance, might have been a factor in smoking in the first place), and unemployment as an adult (contributing both to continued smoking and a small number of visits to the doctor, who might have discouraged smoking). These events, too, have causes: a prolonged dip in the economy, warfare in the region, and so forth.

The other metaphor commonly employed is quite different: it is the causal pie. This term was introduced by Kenneth Rothman, and originates in a paper rather than in a textbook (Rothman, 1976). The metaphor was subsequently developed and linked to various statistical concepts in a textbook by Rothman, Sander Greenland, and Timothy Lash, the first edition of which appeared in 1986, and the most recent edition of which appeared in 2008. This book, *Modern Epidemiology* (Rothman et al., 2008), is arguably the definitive textbook of the contemporary field. Rothman's idea is that a case of disease is a whole pie, and the various "slices" of the pie are the component causes. All these have to be present for the disease to occur. When they are present, the disease does occur. This is very close to J. L. Mackie's insufficient but necessary part of an unnecessary but sufficient condition (INUS) analysis (although Rothman is (unsurprisingly) not as sensitive to the senses of "necessary" and "sufficient" as Mackie, and probably does not intend a reading of those terms strictly in terms of regularities, as does Mackie [1974]).

The point of these metaphors is not immediately obvious. Both seek to illustrate the point that any given case of disease has many different causes, and thus that any different kind of disease is the result of a constellation of causal factors, which may be present in some individual cases of the disease but absent in others. But why should this point be worth delivering to epidemiology students?

The answer, I think, is that the prevailing view of disease at the time was what I call the "monocausal model of disease" (Broadbent, 2009a, 2013). This is the view that diseases must be classified according to a single defining cause, without which, the case is not a case of that disease (but perhaps of some other disease). This view fits certain diseases very well. For example, without the presence of *Vibrio cholerae* in the small intestine, fever and diarrhea do not amount to cholera, no matter how violent they are. This way of thinking about diseases rose to prominence in the nineteenth century, driven by the rise of the germ theory of disease. Thus Robert Koch (1876; quoted in Evans, 1993, p. 20), who identified *Vibrio cholerae* through a microscope, wrote: "[E]ach disease is caused by one particular microbe—and by one alone. Only an anthrax microbe causes anthrax; only a typhoid microbe can cause typhoid fever."

The turn of phrase "caused by one particular microbe—and by one alone" calls for explanation. Koch cannot have been unaware that there would always be other causes of any case of disease: for example, the causes of the victim's exposure to the microbe in the first place. He was probably operating with an intuitive notion of causation, and for most of us our intuitive notion is clearly "selective" in picking out certain events in the causal history as salient or relevant, at the expense of others. Philosophers for the most part do not accept that selection is a fundamental part of the causal concept[4]; but even if they did, we would still be left with a question as to what sort of salience or relevance Koch believed the microbes had.

The obvious thing to say about these causes is that they are necessary for the diseases in question, as we have already noted. But this necessity is no empirical discovery. It is a matter of definition. There are cases of diarrhea and fever where *Vibrio cholerae* is absent. Nothing stops us calling those "cholera" too, if we choose to classify them that way. Koch's insistence is not on the empirical and descriptive claim that, for every group of symptoms currently gathered under one disease entity, a single common causal factor differentiating, present in cases of that disease and absent otherwise, can be identified. It is the conceptual and normative claim that such a factor should be identified for each disease entity, even if this means revising the extension of that disease so that cases that previously were considered cases of the disease are excluded, while others that were not are included.

The monocausal model rose to prominence because of the prospect of actually applying it successfully to diseases, driven by the discovery of small organisms that seemed to satisfy the model for many of the most terrible infectious diseases. In the twentieth century, however, epidemiology mediated the rejection of the monocausal model by almost exactly the reverse process. Epidemiologists studied exposures that, on the one hand, clearly seemed causally implicated in diseases, and were of public health relevance, while on the other hand, clearly were not suitable candidates for defining a disease. Smoking greatly increases the chance of lung cancer, but lung cancer does occur among nonsmokers. Unlike in the diarrhea/cholera case, it does not seem propitious to divide lung cancer up into smoking-itis of the lung and a small remainder of cases. Exactly why it does not seem propitious is the interesting philosophical question, of course; but for practical purposes, the main task for epidemiologists of the mid-twentieth century was freeing medically trained minds of the idea that diseases properly deserving of the name must be classified according to a single defining cause. This is a large part (at least so I surmise) of the motivation behind the otherwise somewhat curious use of metaphors such as "web" and "pie." These are designed to emphasize something—multicausality, the fact that cases of disease have multiple causes—which, without the intellectual background of the monocausal model, would presumably be reasonably obvious.

The interesting philosophical challenge that contemporary epidemiology faces concerning multifactorialism is that of not throwing the baby out with the bathwater. The monocausal model is clearly unsatisfactory for a number of reasons: the restriction to a single defining cause seems arbitrary; and even if classification by multiple causes is allowed, there is no a priori guarantee that the most fruitful way to classify diseases is by their causes. However, there is no doubt that classification systems are of great practical importance. They are not empirically determined, but they have empirical import. We have as many instances of grue emeralds as of green ones (where a grue thing is green and first observed before some future time t, otherwise blue). But the inductive generalizations, "All emeralds are green" and "All emeralds are grue," cannot both be true (assuming there are emeralds to be found after t). Our ability to latch on to classifying features of a domain of study that are "projectible" or "natural" is central to our ability to make good inductive inferences, and thus to intervene on the world to bring about outcomes we desire. A "grue-like" classification of disease would be disastrous. Clearly, then, medical science must care deeply about the way that diseases are classified, even though there is no easy way to simply "read off" correct classification systems from empirical data.

The difficulty with the multifactorial model of disease is that it is too permissive. The monocausal model imposed restrictions on disease classification which seemed unjustified, in the sense that fruitful research on the distribution and determinants of disease seemed to be possible only if the diseases being investigated are allowed to deviate from the strictures of the model. Had the model been strictly applied, lung cancer would not have formed a legitimate topic of study, since it is not defined by a single cause. The trouble with the multifactorial model, on the other hand, is that it relaxes all causal strictures on classification of disease. This raises the prospect that conditions that really do not have a lot in common become objects of study.

Obesity may be one example of this. To see obesity as a single disease might be to lump together the result of various factors that have little to do with each other, some psychological, some cultural, some social, some genetic. South Africa and the United States of America are two countries with high prevalence of obesity; but it would be reasonable to adopt a cautious attitude when generalizing about causes identified in one of these countries to the other, and especially when projecting the likely effectiveness of an intervention that has worked in one of these countries to the other.[5]

The central philosophical challenge that multifactorialism poses to contemporary epidemiology, then, is working out whether there is any benefit to classifying diseases according to their causes. The grandfathers of epidemiology were part of a movement that revolutionized medical thinking by pushing the monocausal model to prominence. Snow and Semmelweis both fought to claim some special status for the causal vector that they had identified, against a prevailing climate that saw these vectors as predisposing conditions at best, perhaps part of a complex causal story, but not an especially privileged part. A century later, the prevailing climate was one that saw the identification of defining causes as central to medical science and practice, and epidemiologists who wanted to study the relation between smoking and lung cancer, beef burgers, and heart disease, or internet usage and suicide rates have had to push against a view that their intellectual ancestors were instrumental in establishing. This tension within the intellectual history of the discipline suggests that it is still an unresolved question what role causes should play in the proper classification of disease, when it is appropriate to insist on causal classification and when merely symptomatic classification will do, and why causal classification seems to have been so fruitful in some eras and so fruitless in others.

The Causal Interpretation Problem

I turn now to a different philosophical problem, also concerning causation, but in a quite different way. The causal interpretation problem concerns the correct interpretation of measures of association when they are used to express causal facts. This problem can only be illustrated with some actual epidemiological measures. Two of the simplest are relative risk and attributable risk.

The term "risk" in this context is strictly a statistical concept and does not imply danger, nor does it transfer readily from the population to the individual. The risk of a disease is the number of new cases within a given time interval, as a proportion of the population at the start of that interval. Risks are always related to a time interval. A synonymous term is incidence, or incidence rate. It is helpful to have the distinction between risk and prevalence in mind. Prevalence is not a rate: it is the number of cases of a disease as a proportion of the population at a given point in time.

Relative risk, RR, is simply the risk in an exposed population as a proportion of the risk in an unexposed population. For example, we can calculate the lifetime RR of lung cancer among smokers compared to nonsmokers by dividing the lifetime risk of lung cancer among smokers (the exposed population) by the lifetime risk among nonsmokers. Suppose the exposed risk, $R(e)$, is 0.1, and the unexposed risk $R(u)$ 0.05.

$$RR = R(e)/R(u) = 0.1/0.005 = 20.$$

This tells us that twenty times as many smokers as nonsmokers contract lung cancer, as proportions of their respective populations. In this sense, it tells us that smokers are twenty times as likely as nonsmokers to develop lung cancer during their lives.

What an RR of 20 does not tell us, however, is whether smoking causes lung cancer, and thus whether the claim that smokers are more likely to develop lung cancer is merely a statistical fact about these two populations, or whether it tells us something about the health effects of smoking. Part of the issue here is how one can make a justified causal inference, and that is the topic of the next section of this chapter. But another, perhaps more subtle issue concerns the way a measure like RR is understood after a causal inference has been made. In that situation, it is very natural to see the RR as expressing something about the causal effect of smoking on the population. If we conclude that smoking does cause the difference (the whole difference) between exposed and unexposed groups, then it is very natural to see measures of the size of the difference as measures of the effect of smoking. Yet the mathematical formula for RR clearly has no implications at all. The question, then, is what, besides the mathematical definition, is meant when we causally interpret measures of association such as RR.

Measures including the word "attributable" illustrate the problem especially clearly, since "attributable" has clear causal connotations. There are a number of different measures that use this word (and an unfortunate variation in terminology) but the difference between exposed and unexposed risks as a proportion of the exposed risk. In this sense, attributable risk measures how much of the risk in the exposed population—as a proportion—can be "attributed" to the putative cause. For example, using the same figures as before, we could calculate the risk of lung cancer attributable to smoking as follows:

$$AR = [R(e)\text{-}(Ru)]/R(e) = [0.1\text{-}0.005]/0.1 = 0.095/0.1 = 0.95.$$

In other words, 0.95, or 95 percent, of the lung cancer among smokers is "attributable" to smoking.

The difficulty is understanding the word "attributable." The mathematical portion of the definition is simple enough, but it clearly tells us nothing causal. If the formula just provided exhausted the meaning of "attributable," then we could just as easily calculate the risk of measles attributable to spots as the risk of spots attributable to measles. But while there is no mathematical prohibition against conducting that calculation, it would be grossly misleading to represent the result as an attributable risk, and no responsible epidemiology journal would permit that terminology in publishing it.

Greenland argues that attributable risks should be split into two measures: excess fraction and etiologic fraction. The excess fraction can be calculated as above. The etiologic fraction, on the other hand, cannot be calculated directly. It may be inferred, but there is no direct measure of the etiologic fraction. Greenland's distinction is useful, but it is too pessimistic about the possibility of measuring etiologic fraction. Where a causal inference is warranted, it will sometimes be the case that we really can be confident—as confident as we are of the causal inference in the first place—that the excess measured by the calculation earlier is due to the exposure. This is because, as we shall see later, it is often the case that causal inferences proceed by ruling out other potential explanations for the association. When we are confident that other explanations are ruled out, we make the causal inference; but to say that we are confident that nothing else other than our exposure explains the association is just to say that we are confident that at least the whole excess fraction is caused by the exposure.

However, Greenland is right to insist that we cannot infer that at most the excess fraction is caused in this way. It is possible that an exposure may be a causal factor even among the cases which would have occurred anyway—those cases with counterparts in the unexposed group. For example, even if we can infer that 0.05 percent of smokers would have got lung cancer anyway, we cannot infer that smoking was causal in only the remaining 0.095 percent making up the total 10 percent risk among smokers. It is very possible that smoking was a causal factor in all smokers who develop lung cancer, whether or not they would have developed it as nonsmokers. Elsewhere I have drawn an analogy with porters in the Himalayas. Carrying heavy loads all day might cause them to suffer from bad backs more frequently than their peers in different occupations. But some of them no doubt would have suffered a bad back anyway, due to some innate weakness in the back. It is quite possible that carrying heavy loads is a causal factor in these porters' bad backs too—not the only one, but a causal factor nonetheless—despite the fact that they would have suffered a bad back anyway (Broadbent, 2011a, p. 256).

My own preferred solution to the causal interpretation problem is to see measures of causal strength as asserting that the exposure explains the net difference between two populations, as that net difference is expressed by the measure of association (Broadbent, 2013, pp. 50–54). This allows Greenland's point that it may be causal in more cases than are enumerated in the net difference, but also allows what Greenland is more doubtful about, that a direct causal interpretation can be given to these measures of association in some circumstances. However, my preferred solution leaves a number of further questions about exactly what the explanation in question amounts to.

Causal Inference in Epidemiology

Causal inference is a persistent topic in methodological reflections of epidemiologists. The rise of the modern discipline in response to the growing evidence of a causal link between smoking and lung cancer involved a great deal of reflection on the circumstances in which one may or may not be warranted in making a causal inference. Even if we set aside the complex and interesting issues about making practical recommendations in a situation of incomplete information, the nature of good causal inference remains a hotly contested topic among contemporary epidemiologists, long after the debates about smoking and lung cancer have been settled.

The starting point for discussions of causal inference in epidemiology is Austin Bradford Hill's 1965 discussion of the topic. In a presidential address to the Section of Occupational Medicine of the Royal Society of Medicine, Bradford Hill (1965, p. 11) identified nine "viewpoints" from which an association might be assessed for causality: strength, consistency, specificity, temporality, biological gradient, plausibility, coherence, experiment, and analogy.

> None of my nine viewpoints can bring indisputable evidence for or against the cause-and-effect hypothesis and none can be required as a sine qua non. What they can do, with greater or less strength, is to help us to make up our minds on the fundamental question—is there any other way of explaining the set of facts before us, is there any other answer equally, or more, likely than cause and effect?

Although he stressed that none of these could be taken as a sine qua non, his list is often referred to as "the Bradford Hill criteria." Similar lists have been developed in other places, but they mostly omit what was arguably his most important insight, or at least his central point, which was the all-things-considered judgment as to whether there is "any other way" of explaining the association.

The approach is a nice example of what philosophers of science now call inference to the best explanation (Lipton, 2004). In Hill's piece, and in other opinion-forming pieces of the time, the central characteristics of causal inference are the all-things-considered judgement of a number of potentially diverse pieces of evidence, the resistance to taking any one piece of evidence as decisive, and a resistance to judging the significance of evidence solely by the kind of evidence that it is or the methods that produced it. Thus one of the seminal papers in the debate on smoking and lung cancer, as well as the seminal surgeon general's report, drew evidence from a very wide array of sources. Since an association between smoking and lung cancer was widely accepted, the method was to address the various competitor explanations for this hypothesis. Depending on which competitor hypothesis was being addressed, different pieces of evidence would be appealed to. Some of these would, out of context, have been incredibly weak evidence for smoking causing lung cancer, as the previous discussion of time trend data illustrates.

There was general suspicion of any attempt to formalize causal inference, even though the leaders of the day were also pioneers in formal statistical methods and in epidemiological study design. Thus, Hill regrets the tendency of some journals to require statistical significance reports for all values reported. Hill also doubts that any single method should be given general priority over others, even though he was one of key figures in the development of the randomized controlled trial, which is sometimes considered the "gold standard" of evidence. This is ironic because it is not clear that Hill would have been comfortable with the whole idea of attaching special significance to a particular study type, or of "better" kinds of evidence trumping "worse" kinds, given his adherence to the idea of trying to find the best explanation of all the evidence.

In recent years, a different trend has emerged. There has been development in both study design and formal statistical methods, naturally enough, but in addition there is a conceptual shift concerning the place of these methods in causal inference. The EBM movement discussed in Howick's chapter 5 of this volume is one manifestation of this trend. EBM seeks to rank evidence according to the kind of study that produced it, with randomized controlled trials coming at the top (of primary research), cohort studies further down, case-control studies below them, and expert opinion in joint bottom place with evidence from laboratory sciences. The difficulties with evidence hierarchies of this kind are well known, but less widely discussed among philosophers is the corresponding development in the conceptual framework for thinking about causal inference in epidemiology.

This framework is characterized by a counterfactual view of causation, and more particularly, a contrastive view. That is, causes are thought of as things such that, had they been absent, the effect would have been absent; and moreover, the way in which the causes are absent—the value of the variable representing the cause—needs to be specified for a causal assertion or question to make sense. An even stronger requirement is that for an exposure to be a cause, it must be "manipulable," where that term refers to the possibility to intervene and manipulate the exposure.

This view has remarkable consequences. It has given rise to a debate about whether sex, race, and obesity can be meaningfully thought of as causes. This is quite revolutionary in a discipline that has developed measures of attributability, such as the one discussed in the previous section, which are very commonly used and perhaps even designed to enable us to express and quantify causal claims about this kind of exposure.

One of the most influential justifications for this very tight restriction on what counts as a cause is by Miguel Hernán and Sarah Taubman (2008). They tell a fictitious story about a king who wants to know how much excess mortality is attributable to obesity. He orders three enormous randomized trials to test the effect of diet, exercise, and a combination of the two on mortality among obese people. Their interventions are equally effective in reducing obesity, but result in different reductions in obesity. This means that the king does not get a straight answer to his question, because the way in which obesity is reduced has an effect on mortality, meaning that "the" excess attributable to obesity does not have an unequivocal value.

In a neighboring country, a president, unable to order such trials because of the constitution, employs an analyst to review historical health records to answer the same question. Hernán and Taubman (2008) point out that the analyst would be able to answer the question, enjoying an apparent advantage over the trial investigators in the neighboring kingdom. However, the real advantage lies with the investigators, since they can tell the king what to do to reduce obesity-related mortality: he should institute the policy corresponding to the intervention that reduced mortality the most. The analyst, on the other hand, cannot tell the president what policy to implement, other than "reduce obesity."

Hernán and Taubman (2008) are concerned about the usefulness of knowledge that, on the face of it, tells us about causes of outcomes of interest, and yet leaves us in the dark about how to act to bring about a desired change in that outcome. Although they do not draw the link themselves, there is a connection with an older dissatisfaction with "risk factor epidemiology"—research that tells us that certain exposures increase the risk of certain outcomes, and which are apparently causal, and yet whose importance for population health is questionable. The reason is that, while it may be that (for example) paracetamol is causal in some cases of asthma (quite doubtful, but let us suppose for the sake of argument), it does not follow that if one restricts paracetamol usage, one will reduce asthma prevalence. Fever and alternative drugs (nonsteroidal anti-inflammatories such as ibuprofen) might also cause asthma. Thus, the putative knowledge, even if it is truly causal (which, again, is doubtful), is useless until we know more about what would happen if we were to intervene upon it. This relates to the discussion of the previous section, since multifactorial thinking encourages research to simply catalogue causal risk factors, without seeking any more general and potentially useful explanation of the contrast between diseased and nondiseased people (Broadbent, 2013, pp. 155–57).

There is something extremely appealing about Hernan and Taubman's point, and also something quite strange about it. They are surely right to warn against too-easy claims about "the effect of obesity on mortality," when there are multiple ways to reduce obesity, each with different effects on mortality, and perhaps no ethically acceptable way to bring about a sudden change in body mass index from say 30 to 22 (Hernán and Taubman, 2008). To this extent, their insistence on assessing causal claims as contrasts to well-defined interventions is useful.

On the other hand, they imply some conclusions that are harder to accept. Hernán and Taubman (2008) suggest, for example, that observational studies are inherently more likely to suffer from this sort of difficulty, and that experimental studies (randomized controlled trials) will ensure that interventions are well-specified. They express their point using the technical term "consistency . . . can be thought of as the condition that the causal contrast involves two or more well-defined interventions (S10). Hernán and Taubman go on:

> [C]onsistency is a trivial condition in randomized experiments. For example, consider a subject who was assigned to the intervention group…in your randomized trial. By definition, it is true that, had he been assigned to the intervention, his counterfactual outcome would have been equal to his observed outcome. But the condition is not so obvious in observational studies. (p. S11)

This is a non-sequitur, however, unless we appeal to a background assumption that an intervention—something that an actual human investigator actually does—is necessarily well-defined. Without this assumption, there is nothing to underwrite the claim that "by definition," if a subject actually assigned to the intervention had been assigned to the intervention, he would have had the outcome that he actually did have.

Take, for example, the intervention of one hour of strenuous exercise a day, which Hernán and Taubman use in their article. "Strenuous exercise" is not a well-defined intervention. Weightlifting? Karate? Swimming? The assumption behind their paper seems to be that if an investigator "does" an intervention, it is necessarily well-defined; but on reflection this is obviously not true. An investigator needs to have some knowledge of which features of the intervention might affect the outcome (such as what kind of exercise one performs), and thus need to be controlled, and which do not (such as how far west of Beijing one lives). Even randomization will not protect against confounding arising from preference for a certain type of exercise (perhaps because people with healthy hearts are predisposed both to choose running and to live longer, for example), unless one knows to randomize the assignment of exercise-types and not to leave it to the subjects' choice.

This is exactly the same kind of difficulty that Hernan and Taubman (2008) press against observational studies. So the contrast they wish to draw, between "trivial" consistency in randomized trials and much more problematic situation in observational studies, is a mirage. Both can suffer from failure to define interventions.

Another hard-to-swallow conclusion also concerns the link between human actions and causes, but in the other direction. As well as apparently supposing that human action is sufficient for well-defined intervention, they also seem to suppose that it is necessary, and thus that we cannot meaningfully—or at least usefully—talk about causes that are not humanly manipulable. This consequence might seem absurd to philosophers; indeed it is a "stock objection" to interventionist and agency accounts that they make causes co-extensive with humanly manipulable things (Menzies and Price, 1993). But the question of how to understand nonmanipulable has recently attracted a number of high-profile discussions in epidemiology (VanderWeele and Hernán, 2012; VanderWeele and Robinson, 2014; cf. Glymour and Glymour, 2014). Very complex treatments of race and gender are offered, whereby potentially manipulable socioeconomic mediators are devised and offered for substitution in place of these variables in future research. But there is no good reason to think that something we cannot do thereby fails to be a well-defined intervention. The effect of drought on GDP compared to average annual rainfall, for example, appears to be a reasonably well-defined contrast, but not one upon which we can realistically intervene. This example also shows that the restriction to humanly manipulable causes is not well-motivated by considerations of usefulness, since it is clearly useful to be able to estimate (quantitatively) the effect of a drought on GDP, even if one cannot do anything about the drought itself.

A final and perhaps most troubling aspect of this whole way of thinking about causal inference is its tendency to focus on the mechanics of a single study, when real-life causal inference in the history of epidemiology has always been a complex, multifaceted exercise involving a range of different kinds of evidence. The model of inference to the best explanation remains much truer to seminal historical episodes in epidemiology. Yet there is a real tension between thinking of causal inference in this way, and thinking of it as a technical, formalized, and indeed mathematical exercise. It is as if there is an intellectual battle being joined between the ideas of Judea Pearl and those of Peter Lipton, and epidemiology is one of the main theatres of action.

Separating out the insights and confusions of this new way of thinking about causal inference is probably the most pressing philosophical issue in contemporary epidemiology. There clearly does seem to be an important insight in the admonition to think clearly about causal contrasts when framing causal questions and claims. Yet the allure of a neat technical apparatus is not a reason to revise our conceptual framework for thinking about causal inference, and causality itself, merely to ensure that the apparatus is universally applicable. Empirical realities have a way of intruding.

Additional Topics

I have surveyed some of the main philosophical issues in epidemiology, restricting my attention to those connected fairly directly with causation. There are additional topics, and plenty of papers waiting to be written. I can indicate those I am aware of, but there must be others that I do not know about, and I would invite the interested reader to try to locate some.

One interesting question is whether ethical as well as methodological factors play a role in epidemiological research, especially in situations where a precautionary action is contemplated. In 2012, a well-known pediatrician reasoned that the evidence of an association between paracetamol use and asthma was insufficient to infer a causal link, but sufficient to ground a recommendation that children at risk of asthma should not be prescribed paracetamol, when combined with the ethical principle of nonmaleficence. I have argued elsewhere that his reasoning was flawed (Broadbent, 2013, p. 83), but the point here is that in some situations, a weighing up of the costs of action against inaction might lead either to a blurring of distinctions between practical and scientific decisions, or else to distance between what is scientifically accepted and what is done in practice.

Another recent example concerns the effect of being slightly overweight (not obese) on mortality, which some research shows is negligible once various other factors (diabetes, blood pressure, etc.) are controlled for. Although there is a respectable body of evidence for this view, it is vigorously resisted by some epidemiologists, who fear that it clouds the public health message, and that it remains the case that the majority of overweight (and obese) people would benefit from taking the steps required to lose weight.

Another interesting topic that I have not discussed here is what is known as risk relativism. Relativism is the tendency to express risks in particular as relative measures, which are often said to be more useful for causal inference than absolute measures, and it is supposed to be more useful for public health policy (Northridge, 1995). Understanding the absolute/relative distinction is a challenge in itself, apart from evaluating the claims about the relative usefulness of these different measures (Poole, 2010; Greenland, 2012). I have suggested that there is a degree of "physics envy" at work when epidemiologists use relative measures, and that there is an attempt to devise universal laws—an attempt which, in my view, must fail (Broadbent, 2013, pp. 129–44; 2015). But the topic is certainly not one on which the last word has been spoken.

Another area ripe for philosophical investigation is the relation between epidemiology and law. The use of epidemiological evidence to prove causation presents interesting difficulties of a philosophical character. Since epidemiology is often a pioneer science, identifying causes before we fully understand how those causes operate, it may sometimes be the only scientific evidence available to establish that some exposure—arising from a defendant's wrongful act—caused some harm to a claimant. Yet the courts traditionally take a dim view of statistical evidence, as do jurisprudential theorists (notably: Cohen, 1977; Wright, 1988, 2008). My own view is that courts are irrational to exclude epidemiological evidence, but that view is not shared by many actual courts (for further discussion, see Broadbent, 2011a; 2013, pp. 162–81).

Yet another set of issues concerns social determinants of health. Epidemiological research on socioeconomic factors such as income and education level suggests that there is a causal connection between many of these factors and health (Marmot, 2006a, b). The causal claim remains contested, and there is tension between the disciplines of epidemiology and economics in this regard, since economists have provided some of the most stringent skepticism about the rigor of the claims made by epidemiologists working on the social determinants of health (Deaton, 2003, 2006). Aside from the causal question, there are questions about what we should do if the associations are indeed causal (Venkatapuram and Marmot, 2009; Wolff, 2011). A related topic in this area concerns the correct response to "neglected diseases" (Reiss and Kitcher, 2009; Broadbent, 2011b).

Finally, there is a slew of questions yet to be broached anywhere, to my knowledge, concerning the status of epidemiology as a natural or social science, and the status of epidemiology vis-à-vis the established debates about scientific realism.

Notes

1. A fuller account of the Semmelweis episode is given in Broadbent (2013, pp. 17–20).
2. The details of the Snow episode are more complex, of course. In particular, the events following the removal of the handle of the pump are taken by some to constitute evidence in favor of Snow's view (and removing the handle was an intervention). However, others argue that the incidence of cholera was already declining. In any case, the evidence that convinced the authorities to remove the handle in the first place was observational.
3. I am grateful to Jan Vandenbroucke for this point and the example of time trend data.
4. I am in the minority in thinking that causation is fundamentally selective (Broadbent, 2008, 2009b, 2012). For other nondismissive discussions of the topic, see Schaffer (2005, 2007) and Menzies (2007).
5. Nancy Cartwright (2010) gives a real-life example of a failed projection of this kind, where an infant nutrition program that worked in Tamil Nadu failed in Bangladesh. The project turned on educating mothers about what to feed their children. The projection from Tamil Nadu to Bangladesh failed because mothers in Bangladesh are considerably less empowered regarding what their children eat than they are in Tamil Nadu.

References

Broadbent, A. 2008. The difference between cause and condition. *Proceedings of the Aristotelian Society* 108: 355–64.

Broadbent, A. 2009a. Causation and models of disease in epidemiology. *Studies in History and Philosophy of Biological and Biomedical Sciences* 40: 302–11.

Broadbent, A. 2009b. Fact and law in the causal inquiry. *Legal Theory* 15: 173–91.

Broadbent, A. 2011a. Epidemiological evidence in proof of specific causation. *Legal Theory* 17: 237–78.

Broadbent, A. 2011b. Defining neglected disease. *BioSocieties* 6(1): 51–70. doi:10.1057/biosoc.2010.41.

Broadbent, A. 2012. Causes of causes. *Philosophical Studies* 158(3): 457–76. doi:10.1007/s11098-010-9683-0.

Broadbent, A. 2013. *Philosophy of Epidemiology: New Directions in the Philosophy of Science*. London and New York: Palgrave Macmillan.

Broadbent, A. 2015. Risk relativism and physical law. *Journal of Epidemiology and Community Health* 69(1): 92–94.

Cartwright, N. 2010. Will This Policy Work for You? Predicting Effectiveness Better: How Philosophy Helps. In PSA Presidential Address.

Cohen, L. J. 1977. *The Probable and the Provable*. Oxford: Clarendon Press.

Deaton, A. 2003. Health, inequality, and economic development. *Journal of Economic Literature* 41(1): 113–58.

Deaton, A. 2006. The determinants of mortality. *Journal of Economic Perspectives* 20(3): 97–120.

Evans, A. S. 1993. *Causation and Disease: A Chronological Journey*. New York, NY: Plenum Publishing Corporation.

Glymour, C., and Glymour, M. R. 2014. Race and sex are causes. *Epidemiology* 25(4): 488–90.

Greenland, S. 2012. Cornfield, risk relativism, and research synthesis. *Statistics in Medicine* 31: 2773–77.

Hernán, M. A., and Taubman, S. L. 2008. Does obesity shorten life? The importance of well-defined interventions to answer causal questions. *International Journal of Obesity* 32: S8–S14.

Hill, A. B. 1965. The environment and disease: Association or causation? *Proceedings of the Royal Society of Medicine* 58: 259–300.

Koch, R. 1876. *Verfrahen Sur Untersuchung Zur Conserviren Und Photographie Der Bakterien, Beitrag Der Pflanzen*. Breslow: Cohn's Bier.

Lipton, P. 2004. *Inference to the Best Explanation*, 2nd edition. London and New York: Routledge.

Mackie, J. 1974. *The Cement of the Universe*. Oxford: Oxford University Press.

MacMahon, B., and Pugh, T. F. 1960. *Epidemiologic Methods*. Boston, MA: Little, Brown.

MacMahon, B., and Trichopoulos, D. 1996. *Epidemiology: Principles and Methods*, 2nd edition. Boston: Little, Brown and Company.

Marmot, M. 2006a. Introduction. In *Social Determinants of Health*, eds. Michael Marmot and Richard Wilkinson, Second. Oxford: Oxford University Press, pp. 1–5.

Marmot, M. 2006b. Health in an unequal world: Social circumstances, biology, and disease. *Clinical Medicine* 6(6): 559–72.

Menzies, P. 2007. Causation in context. In *Russell's Republic Revisited: Causation, Physics, and the Constitution of Reality*, eds. Huw Price and Richard Corry. Oxford: Oxford University Press, pp. 191–223.

Menzies, P, and Price, H. 1993. Causation as a secondary quality. *British Journal for the Philosophy of Science* 44(2): 187–203.

Northridge, M. 1995. Attributable risk as a link between causality and public health action. *American Journal of Public Health* 85(9): 1202–204.

Poole, C. 2010. On the origin of risk relativism. *Epidemiology* 21(1): 3–9. doi:10.1097/EDE.0b013e3181c30eba.

Reiss, J., and Kitcher, P. 2009. Biomedical research, neglected diseases, and well-ordered science. *Theoria* 66: 263–82.

Rothman, K. J. 1976. Causes. *American Journal of Epidemiology* 104(6): 587–92.

Rothman, K. J., Greenland, S., and Lash, T. L. 2008. *Modern Epidemiology*, 3rd edition. Philadelphia: Lippincott Williams & Wilkins.

Schaffer, J. 2005. Contrastive causation. *Philosophical Review* 114(3): 297–328.

Schaffer, J. 2007. The metaphysics of causation. *Stanford Encyclopedia of Philosophy*. http://plato.stanford.edu/entries/causation-metaphysics/.

VanderWeele, T. J., and Hernán, M. A. 2012. Causal effects and natural laws: Towards a conceptualization of causal counterfactuals for nonmanipulable exposures, with application to the effects of race and sex. In *Causality: Statistical Perspectives and Applications*, eds. Carlo Berzuini, Philip Dawid, and Luisa Bernardinelli. Chichester: John Wiley and Sons, pp. 101–13.

VanderWeele, T. J., and Robinson, W. R. 2014. On the causal interpretation of race in regressions adjusting for confounding and mediating variables. *Epidemiology* 25(4): 473–84.

Venkatapuram, S., and Marmot, M. 2009. Epidemiology and social justice in light of social determinants of health research. *Bioethics* 23(2): 79–89.

Wolff, J. 2011. How should governments respond to the social determinants of health? *Preventive Medicine* 53: 253–55.

Wright, R. 1988. Causation, responsibility, risk, probability, naked statistics, and proof: Pruning the bramble bush by clarifying the concepts. *Iowa Law Review* 73: 1001–77.

Wright, R. 2008. Liability for possible wrongs: Causation, statistical probability, and the burden of proof. *Loyola of Los Angeles Law Review* 41: 1295–344.

5 Justification of Evidence-Based Medicine Epistemology

Jeremy Howick

Introduction

The Genesis of Evidence-based Medicine

The one-hundred-year period between 1885 and 1985 brought amazing medical discoveries. The rabies vaccine put an end to the fear of rabid dogs, the discovery of penicillin suggested that infectious disease would soon be altogether eradicated, and cure for most childhood cancer was a promising sign that all cancers could soon disappear. Open heart surgery, hip replacements, and kidney transplants indicated that we could dramatically extend our life span by replacing our "used" parts, and in vitro fertilization put an end to the misery caused by infertility (LeFanu, 2000). Infant mortality in the United States and Europe dropped from 140 to 5 in a thousand, and life expectancy rose from under 50 to almost 80 years. It was not unreasonable to suppose, in the middle of the twentieth century, that medicine would continue to advance at a furious pace and that quite soon most human suffering might all but disappear. Indeed, when Lord Horder (1949, p. 557) asked, "Whither medicine?" in 1949, he gave the only sensible answer he could at the time: "Whither else than straight ahead."

Eventually, however, reality set in. Infectious diseases proved more resistant than was initially envisaged, many cancers are proving to be formidable opponents, and a host of ailments such as obesity, diabetes, cardiovascular disease, and depression have replaced the traditional infectious diseases as major killers. At the same time the thalidomide scandal reduced the public's trust in medicine, and Thomas McKeown (1976) argued forcefully that increases in life span and decreases in infant mortality had more to do with economic improvements than with medical treatments. From out in left field, Ivan Illich (1977) contended that medicine did more harm than good (Daly, 2005). One thing was certain: the cost of healthcare continued (and continues) to rise each year, while improvements in healthcare (measured in life expectancy and infant mortality) have tapered off.

Against this background, many thoughtful clinicians began to question the value of the treatments they prescribed. Several best-selling autobiographies would be required to tell their interesting stories, so I will restrict myself to a particularly salient one.[1] Sir Iain Chalmers, who cofounded the Cochrane Collaboration, tells the following story that reflects the growing concern with failure to consider empirical observations adequately:

> It was while working for a couple of years in a Palestinian refugee camp in the Gaza Strip 30 years ago that I first became aware of just how devastating a disease measles can be. We had an immunization program, supervised by the World Health Organization (WHO) staff, but measles was nonetheless common among refugee children, many of whom were malnourished and in poor health in other ways, and complications were common.
>
> It had been drummed into me at medical school [based on mechanistic reasoning] in the early 1960s that antibiotics should never be prescribed for someone with a viral infection unless there was unambiguous evidence of bacterial superinfection. Accordingly, when a child was brought to me with early measles and I had convinced myself that there was no evidence of superinfection, I conserved our limited supply of antibiotics ... Distressingly often, my child patients had died a few days after I had seen them.
>
> My Palestinian medical colleague was seeing a very similar spectrum of patients with measles, but he seemed not to have a comparable experience. Toward the end of my first year working in the refugee camp, it was gently pointed out to me that this might be because he gave prophylactic antibiotics to children with measles, because, in his experience, rapid bacterial superinfection was very common in these vulnerable children. Having been convinced to change my practice, and doing exactly what I had been advised at medical school never to do, I had the impression that my child patients were less likely to die.
>
> This clinical impression was very sobering. It made me wonder whether what I had been taught at medical school might have been lethally wrong, at least in the circumstances in which I was working, and precipitated a now incurable "scepticemia" about authoritarian therapeutic prescriptions and prescriptions unsupported by trustworthy empirical evidence. (Chalmers, 2002, pp. 312–13)

What Is Evidence-based Medicine?

Evidence-based medicine (EBM) was introduced in the early 1990s with a rhetorical tour de force (Eddy, 1990; Evidence Based Medicine Working Group, 1992; Guyatt, 1991). The title of the paper that announced EBM to the wider community was: "Evidence-Based Medicine: A *New* Approach to Teaching the Practice of Medicine" (Evidence Based Medicine Working Group, 1992; emphasis added). The very first sentence of the paper reads: "A *new* paradigm for medical practice is emerging" (emphasis added).

The question of whether EBM is truly new is a historical one (Bernard, 1957; Celsus and Collier, 1831; Louis, 1836), and a comprehensive historical analysis of the origins and genesis of EBM lies beyond the scope of this work.[2] Similarly, the question of whether EBM is truly a new (Kuhnian) paradigm would involve an analysis of whether Kuhnian paradigms are applicable to methodological innovations in medicine, which would take us too far afield (Gillies, 1998, 2005). Moreover, both questions—whether EBM is new, and whether EBM is a new Kuhnian paradigm—require that we establish what EBM actually *is*. This is no straightforward task given the evolving definitions of the movement (Dawes et al., 2005; Guyatt et al., 2004; Sackett et al., 1996; Straus, 2004).

EBM was initially defined as follows: "Evidence-based medicine de-emphasizes intuition, unsystematic clinical experience, and pathophysiological rationale as sufficient grounds for clinical decision making and stresses the examination of evidence from clinical research" (Evidence Based Medicine Working Group, 1992, p. 2420). Yet given that "evidence" simply means "grounds for belief," medicine has always been evidence-based.[3] Barring cases of deliberate deception, even physicians deemed to be "quacks" have had grounds to believe that their therapies worked. If EBM is something new, as its proponents insist it is, then it must be a specific view of what counts as (good) evidence.

The terms "clinical experience," "pathophysiologic rationale," and "clinical research" require some clarification. By clinical experience, EBM proponents mean expert opinion that is *not* based explicitly on available empirical evidence. While this may be surprising, pre-EBM methods often failed to require that existing evidence be considered when making recommendations about the effects of medical therapies. A National Institute of Health report in 1990 in the United States, for example, praised the expert consensus method.

> Group judgment methods are perhaps the most widely used means of assessment of medical technologies in many countries. The consensus development conference is a relatively inexpensive and rapid mechanism

for the consideration and evaluation of different attributes of a medical technology including, for example, safety, efficacy, and efficiency, among many others. (Goodman and Baratz, 1990, p. 1)

Besides the United States, official representatives from Canada (Battista, 1990), Denmark (Jørgensen, 1990), Finland (Kauppila, 1990), The Netherlands (Kazinga et al., 1990), Norway (Backe, 1990), Sweden (Håkansoon and Eckerlund, 1990), and United Kingdom (Spilby, 1990) supported the report.

To be sure, the experts on the consensus panel were supposed to review the available evidence. However, the connection between the consensus statement and the best available evidence was often spurious. For example, Antman et al. (1992, p. 240) found that even textbook recommendations (written by experts) for treatments intended for heart attack routinely

failed to mention important advances or exhibited delays in recommending effective preventive measures. In some cases, treatments that have no effect on mortality or are potentially harmful continued to be recommended by several clinical experts.

By pathophysiologic rationale (mechanistic reasoning), EBM proponents mean inferences from (supposed) facts about the underlying pathological and physiological mechanisms of health and disease to conclusions that a treatment will or will not have effects. For example, the belief that antiarrhythmic drugs would reduce mortality was based on (supposed) facts about the causes of mortality (arrhythmias) and antiarrhythmic drugs' mechanism of action.

Unlike mechanistic reasoning, clinical research (I use the term "comparative clinical study") does not rely on evidence about *how* the intervention might produce an outcome, and instead involves directly observing the putative outcome relative to the putative outcome produced by a control treatment. A famous example of a comparative clinical study is the Cardiac Arrhythmia Suppression Trial (CAST), which began in 1987. The trial was designed to test whether antiarrhythmic drugs would reduce mortality in patients who had suffered from myocardial infarction (heart attack). In the study, twenty-seven clinical centers randomized 1,455 patients to receive encainide, flecainide, or placebo, while 272 were randomized to receive moricizine or placebo. The encainide, flecainide, placebo arm of the study was discontinued because of excess mortality in the experimental groups. Of 730 patients, 33 (4.5 percent) taking either encainide or flecainide had died after an average of 10 months of follow-up, while only 9 of 725 (1.2 percent) of patients taking placebo had died from arrhythmia and nonfatal cardiac arrest over the same time period (Investigators TCASTC, 1989). The experimental drugs also accounted for higher total mortality (56 of 730, or 7.7 percent in the treatment group versus 22 of 725 or 3.0 percent in the "placebo" group). Similar negative results were soon found for moricizine (Trial, CAS & II Investigators, 1992). Based on prevalence data, it was estimated that antiarrhythmic drugs had killed more people every year than died in action during the whole of the Vietnam War (Evans et al., 2006, p. 8).

The CAST study did not rely on any underlying facts about pathological and physiological mechanisms. In fact the randomized trial results *contradicted* the purported mechanisms. EBM proponents, however, do not view all comparative clinical studies as equal: randomized trials are deemed to provide the best evidence for therapeutic effects (Evidence Based Medicine Working Group, 1992, p. 2423).

Another central aspect of the EBM system of evidence that is not explicit in the definitions is the belief that *all* the relevant evidence must be considered before making a decision. This is supported by the principle of total evidence because, in principle, they aim to include all *relevant* studies. The justification for what counts as relevant is, of course, subject to legitimate questioning. However, because the volume of research in all fields—including philosophy—is growing, evidence synthesis of some sort is necessary for progress. This does not justify whether the methods currently used in EBM to systematically review the literature are justified, but rather points out that since all disciplines synthesize evidence, to criticize EBM for making their methods explicit is not even handed.

What is the Philosophy of EBM?

The EBM philosophy of evidence, which is the focus of this chapter, is best expressed in the EBM hierarchies of evidence (Canadian Task Force, 1979; Guyatt et al., 2008; Harbour, 2008; Phillips et al., 2001; Sackett, 1986, 1989). The idea behind the many different hierarchies can be summed up quite simply with three central claims (Figure 5.1):

1. Randomized trials (RCTs), or systematic reviews of many randomized trials, generally offer stronger evidential support than observational studies.
2. Comparative clinical studies in general (including both RCTs and observational studies) offer stronger evidential support than mechanistic reasoning (pathophysiologic rationale) from the basic sciences.
3. Comparative clinical studies in general (including both RCTs and observational studies) offer stronger evidential support than expert clinical judgment.

Early EBM proponents showed that many widely used therapies that had been adopted based on "lower" forms of evidence proved to be useless or harmful when subjected to randomized trials as the aforementioned antiarrhythmic drug trial exemplified.

In spite of the compelling rationale, the EBM hierarchy leads to several paradoxes. The first is that many of the treatments in whose effectiveness we have the most confidence—that we consider most strongly supported by evidence—have never been supported by randomized trials of any description. These treatments include automatic external defibrillation to start a stopped heart, tracheostomy to open a blocked air passage, the Heimlich maneuver to dislodge an obstruction in the breathing passage, rabies vaccines, penicillin for the treatment of pneumonia, and epinephrine injections to treat severe anaphylactic shock. Meanwhile we often lack confidence in some treatments that are supported by evidence from higher up in the hierarchy. The antidepressant Prozac, for instance, has proven superior to placebo in some double-blind RCTs, yet the effects of Prozac (over and above placebo effects) are hotly disputed (Healy, 2004, 2006; Kirsch and Sapirstein, 1998; Kirsch and Moore, 2002; Moncrieff and Kirsch, 2005). Strictly speaking this critique is unfair since the EBM movement has always acknowledged that treatments with dramatic effects do not require support from randomized trials (Glasziou et al., 2007; Sackett et al., 1997, p. 94; Sackett, 2000, p. 108; Straus et al., 2005, p. 119). Yet with one recent exception (Guyatt et al., 2008) current hierarchies have ignored this paradox: randomized trials still feature at the pinnacle of the EBM hierarchies.

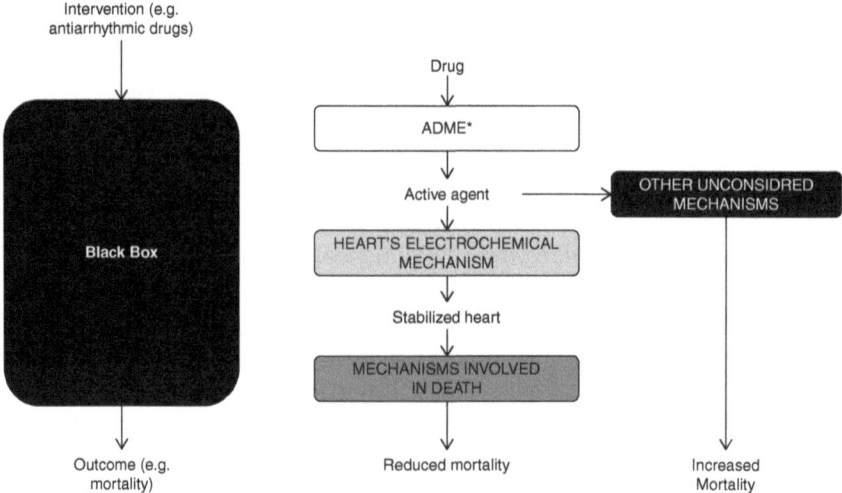

Figure 5.1 Black boxes and mechanisms.

The EBM rationale for the view that comparative clinical studies provide stronger evidential support to mechanistic reasoning and clinical expertise and that randomized trials usually provide better evidence than observational studies also demands further analysis. While EBM proponents have always acknowledged that mechanistic reasoning is important for generalizing, and that expertise should be integrated with external evidence, the view that comparative clinical studies provide stronger evidence than mechanistic reasoning or clinical expertise is unsupported by a defensible rationale. A stubborn objector could always claim that the conclusions from mechanistic reasoning and expert judgment were more reliable than the admittedly different conclusions from randomized trials. This leads to the paradox that the EBM hierarchy itself appears to be supported by weak (according to EBM) evidence, namely, the opinion of EBM experts!

What Is to Come?

In this chapter, I provide a concise overview of current philosophical controversies in the philosophy of EBM, with a focus on the EBM epistemology.[4] I focus on current *actual* philosophical controversies that surround the claims that systematic reviews of randomized trials usually provide better evidence than observational studies and mechanistic reasoning. Other philosophical controversies about the methodology of diagnostic reasoning, prognostic markers, expertise, and systematic reviews are emerging but not enough has been written about them to warrant being included here.[5] I also assume—for simplicity and due to the scope of this chapter—that the evidential role of expert judgment is (at least partly) parasitic upon how familiar experts are with the evidence. Hence I will not discuss the evidential role of expert judgment separately here.

Philosophical Controversies in EBM: Are Observational Studies as Good as Randomized Trials as Evidence?

Most EBM "hierarchies" of evidence rank randomized trials *categorically* above observational studies (Canadian Task Force, 1979; Harbour, 2008; Phillips et al., 2001; Sackett, 1986, 1989; La Caze, 2009). Yet strict adherence to this ranking view leads to the paradox that what we take to be our most effective therapies, ranging from the Heimlich maneuver to unblock an airway to eating to reverse the effects of starvation, have never been tested in randomized trials. Taking the EBM hierarchy at face value (which, as I argue later, might be a misrepresentation), it seems to follow that our most effective therapies are not supported by best (randomized) evidence. Exploiting this irony, Gordon Smith and Jill Pell (2003), wrote a spoof article entitled "Parachute use to prevent death and major trauma related to gravitational challenge: a systematic review of randomized controlled trials." They concluded that:

> Advocates of evidence-based medicine have criticised the adoption of interventions evaluated by using only observational [i.e. not from RCTs] data. We think that everyone might benefit if the most radical protagonists of evidence based medicine organized and participated in a double blind, randomised, placebo controlled, crossover trial of the parachute. (p. 1459)

While this parachute example is a spoof, it represents a real paradox in the EBM epistemology. The most dramatically effective treatments, ranging from the Heimlich maneuver to dislodge an airway obstruction, adrenaline to cure ana-phylactic shock, and external defibrillation to regulate heart rhythms, are not supported by evidence from randomized trials. If randomized trials provide "best" evidence, then it would seem that these treatments are not supported by "best" evidence. Since we believe these dramatically effective treatments to be effective, this is paradoxical.

No doubt partly motivated by these critiques, many have criticized the EBM view that randomized trials offer the best evidence (La Caze, 2009; Borgerson, 2009; Cartwright et al., 2007; Tonelli, 1998; Upshur, 2005; Worrall, 2002, 2007a, 2010a, 2010b). Here I argue that while most critiques of randomized trials are straw men, the EBM view must be modified to avoid the straw men attacks and to overcome the paradox of effectiveness. More specifically, I contend that categorical hierarchies of evidence that place randomized trials above obser-vational studies can be replaced with the view that *comparative clinical studies provide good evidence when the effect size outweighs the combined effect of plausible confounding factors*. The most recent EBM hierarchy (Guyatt et al., 2008), and other developments in the EBM system (Glasziou et al., 2007; Howick et al., 2009) with a few minor modifications, can be viewed as an operational expres-sion of the view I propose.

To anticipate, I begin by describing observational studies and randomized tri-als. While the concept of a randomized trial is rather simple, many philosophers and medical professionals misunderstand its essential features. Randomized trials differ from observational studies in that they are randomized, and that they can (but do not have to) employ double masking and "placebo" controls. Since randomization rules out allocation bias, while double masking and "pla-cebo" controls rule out performance bias, it seems to follow that randomized trials provide better evidence. Next, I review common critiques of the EBM position. Some, including Howson, Urbach, and Worrall, have argued that randomization does not add (much) methodological benefit. Others, including Cartwright and Mant, note that randomized trials lack external validity. I argue that both critiques are straw men against the EBM view.

Observational Studies: Definition and Problems

The most common observational designs are case studies, case series, case–control studies, cohort studies, and historically controlled studies. A detailed description of all these study designs would take us far afield. It suffices to note the essential features of observational studies that are *not* shared by randomized trials. In controlled observational studies (case studies and case series do not involve direct comparisons and I ignore them here), investigators compare people who take an intervention with those who do not. The investigators neither allocate patients to receive the intervention not administer the intervention. Instead, they compare records of patients who had taken an intervention and been treated in routine practice with similar patients who had not taken the intervention. The main problems with observational studies is that they suffer from (a) self-selection bias (sometimes called patient preference bias), (b) allocation bias, and (c) performance bias.

In one typical observational study, Petitti et al. (1987) compared the records of 2,656 women who took hormone (estrogen) replacement therapy (HRT) with those of 3,437 who did not and followed them for 10 or more years to measure rates of coronary heart disease (CHD) and overall mortality. They found that HRT users were only half as likely to die as HRT non-users. Stampfer and Colditz (1991) conducted a systematic review of all the available studies of the effects of HRT to prevent coronary heart disease (all but one were observational), and found that women taking HRT appeared to be, on average, half as likely to die as women who did not take HRT. They concluded that: "The preponderance of evidence from the epidemiologic studies strongly supports the view that postmenopausal estrogen therapy can substantially reduce the risk for coronary heart disease (p. 61). Based on these observational studies millions of women, including my mother, were prescribed and took HRT to protect (allegedly) against CHD and premature mortality.

However the observational studies of the effects of HRT, like all observational studies, suffered from the problem that people who choose to take (or are chosen by their doctors to take) HRT are likely to be very different in many ways from people who choose not to take (or are not chosen by their doctors to take) HRT. Those who choose to take HRT might be healthier, wealthier, have better medical care, eat fewer vegetables, live in less polluted neighborhoods, or differ in any number of other ways from people who choose not to take HRT. These differences are all potential confounders because they could all affect how likely people are to contract disease *independent* of whether or not they take HRT. Collectively, confounding differences between people in the experimental and control groups at the outset of a study and before the treatment is administered (the baseline) are often referred to as selection bias. Selection bias arising from the fact that patients choose to take a therapy (they select it) is referred to as self-selection bias.

To be sure, researchers are well-aware of self-selection bias. Petitti et al. (1987), for example, adjusted for age, smoking, body mass index, alcohol intake, hypertension, marital status, and education, and Stampfer and Colditz (1991) were careful to rank the studies in their review according to whether investigators had controlled for age, smoking, and types of menopause. After considering the effects of these potential confounders, they concluded that the apparent protective effect of HRT is "unlikely to be explained by confounding factors or selection" (p. 61).

Careful adjusting reduces confounding and therefore undoubtedly increases the quality of observational studies. Indeed many high quality observational studies produce the same results as randomized trials. At the same time, some differences inevitably prove difficult to adjust for. How, for example, would we control for the possibility that women who chose HRT had richer husbands, ate more vegetables, took public transportation, were more optimistic, or had a more extensive social network? These factors could all influence the risk of CHD but are, to say the least, not easy to measure, and hence to control for.

The following example suggests that even subtle differences between people who choose to take a treatment can have important effects. In one interesting study researchers found that there was no difference in mortality between men treated with clofibrate and those in the control group (who were treated with "placebo"): the mortality was 20 percent in both groups. Investigators then found that patients who adhered to the treatment regimen more strictly had a lower mortality (15 percent) than those who did not (25 percent) (Canner, 1980). The adherers had better outcomes whether they had the experimental or placebo treatments. This study has been replicated with consistent results that have recently been summarized in a systematic review (Simpson et al., 2006). These studies suggest that something to do with a patient's personality (whether or not they adhere to the treatment regime) can affect the outcome. Presumably, there are a disproportionate number of adherers among those who chose to take a treatment compared with those who do not in an observational study. After all, the choice to take a treatment is to adhere at least at the outset to a treatment regime. Here we have a confounding difference between the two groups in an observational study—a disproportionate number of adherers—that would be difficult if not impossible to control for in an observational study.

Similar biases arise when caregivers are in charge of deciding whether or not to prescribe a treatment. Caregivers could systematically favor the healthier (or less healthy), richer, or younger. They are certainly more likely to prescribe treatments to people who bother showing up to their appointments than those who do not. These differences could also confound the observational study and lead to what is often referred to as allocation bias.

Things get worse. Other potentially confounding factors can arise *after* the treatment regime has begun could further confound any comparison between people who take HRT and those who do not. Once people begin taking HRT, they could receive more attention from their doctors, reinforce their social network, or view themselves as victims and worry more. Potential confounding factors that enter after the intervention (HRT) has been chosen are often referred to as forms of performance bias because they arise during the performance phase of the trial.

A final problem with observational studies is that they do not rule out common causes. We might find a very strong correlation between possession of ashtrays and lung cancer; however, it does not follow that ashtrays increase the incidence of lung cancer. The common cause of possessing ashtrays and a higher risk of lung cancer is smoking.

Randomized Trials to the Rescue

Randomized trials differ from most observational studies in that they involve random allocation and experimental administration of treatments. Unlike in an observational study where patients choose to take the intervention themselves, participants in a randomized trial are *randomly* allocated to receive either an experimental intervention (such as HRT) or a control. *Simple* random allocation is a process whereby all participants have the same chance of being assigned to one of the study groups (Jadad, 1998, p. 2). Restricted randomization involves employing various strategies to ensure that the number of participants and various characteristics such as sex are similarly distributed between groups. A fair coin, random number tables, or (pseudo-)random generators on a computer can achieve this. For example, we might flip a coin and assign the next participant in the queue to receive the experimental intervention if the coin lands heads up, and the control if the coin lands tails up. In practice, of course, coin tosses are rare. Instead, investigators might have a pile of envelopes with instructions inside about which group to assign the next patient to.

Randomization, when adhered to, rules out self-selection bias and allocation bias. When a random allocation method is used to allocate people to receive the experimental or control treatment, neither participants nor caregivers can influence who receives the experimental intervention. However, unless the allocation sequence is *concealed*, randomization can be, and is commonly, subverted. Concealing allocation involves hiding the knowledge of which group receives the experimental intervention from the investigators and participants. For instance, the envelopes containing the allocation schedule could contain the letters "A" and "B" instead of experimental and control. Then, whether "A" refers to the experimental therapy or control therapy could be kept secret.

Allocation is particularly easy to decipher (and subvert) when the sequence is pseudo-random, involving alternation or allocation according to date of birth. While these pseudo-random methods rule out self-selection and allocation bias if strictly adhered to, the sequence can be easily deciphered. Real random allocation sequences are also detectable. For example, investigators have opened envelopes containing the sequence or holding them up to translucent lightbulbs reveals the assignment sequence. Kenneth Schulz (1995, p. 1457) conducted a workshop where investigators anonymously revealed the methods they used to decipher the allocation scheme, and heard many stories similar to the following rather amusing one.

> Still another workshop participant had attempted to decipher a numbered container scheme but had given up after her attempts bore no success. One evening she noticed a light on in the principal investigator's office and dropped in to say hello. Instead of finding the principal investigator, she found an attending physician who also was involved in the same trial. He unabashedly announced that he was rifling the files for the assignment sequence because he had not been able to decipher it any other way. What materialized almost as curious was her response. She admitted being impressed with his diligence and proceeded to help in rifling the files.

Knowledge of the allocation sequence is not dangerous provided that it is not subsequently tampered with. The problem is that once caregivers and participants know what treatment they are allocated to, allocation and self-selection bias become worrisome again. For example, a particularly ill patient might enter a caregiver's office to be randomly allocated to one of the treatment arms. A caregiver who was aware of the allocation sequence might not want the very ill patient to receive the risky experimental intervention and suggest that the patient exercise their right to withdraw from the trial, tell the patient to return in a few days to try again, or even reach for another envelope in the pile until the right allocation for that patient is selected. If a caregiver does this systematically, a disproportionate number if ill patients may end up in the control group. As a result, the experimental therapy could appear effective simply because those in the experimental group are healthier. The bias could work in the other direction as well. The clinician might believe that the experimental therapy is the next miracle drug, and make sure that the most ill patients are assigned to the experimental group. Violations of the assignment scheme are particularly dangerous when the investigator has a personal or financial interest in the new therapy appearing to be effective.

Participants' knowledge of the group to which they are assigned can corrupt the randomization schedule in an analogous way. Participants might have learned about the potential benefits of the new drug from the internet and drop out unless they are assigned to the experimental group. Others might fear potential unknown side effects of the new drug and drop out unless they are assigned to the control group. A good early example of concealed random allocation involved the now famous 1948 Streptomycin trial:

> Determination of whether a patient would be treated by streptomycin and bed-rest (S case) or by bed-rest alone (C case) was made by reference to a statistical series based on random sampling numbers drawn up for each sex at each centre by Professor Bradford Hill; the details of the series were unknown to any of the investigators or to the co-ordinator and were contained in a set of sealed envelopes, each bearing on the outside only the name of the hospital and a number. After acceptance of a patient by the panel, and before admission to the streptomycin centre, the appropriate numbered envelope was opened at the central office; the card inside told if the patient was to be an S or a C case, and this information was then given to the medical officer of the centre. (Medical Research Council Streptomycin in Tuberculosis Trials Committee, 1948)

In short, the distinguishing feature of a *randomized* trial is that it involves random allocation to experimental and control groups. To preserve the random nature of the allocation, concealment is generally required. The benefit of random allocation is that it acts to reduce the potentially confounding effects of dispenser attitudes (allocation bias) and patient preference (self-selection bias).

Since all *randomized* trials are controlled by definition, it is redundant to include the "C" in RCT. Randomized trials all involve comparing the experimental therapy with a control therapy. Although there can, in principle, be more than one test group and more than one control group, I limit my discussion to the simple case where there is a single experimental and a single control group. The control group can either receive another treatment, a placebo, or no treatment. A placebo is a treatment capable of making people believe it is, or could be, the experimental treatment when in fact it is not. A sugar pill that is indistinguishable to the senses from vitamin C could be a placebo. No-treatment controls are difficult to construct in practice. Either participants in the no-treatment groups are more or less left alone, in which case the investigators lose control over whether they choose to treat themselves with some other treatment of their own accord. Or, they are closely monitored in which case the effects of being monitored could, indeed has been known to, play a role (Cocco, 2009; McCarney et al., 2007).

A medical study is a trial—an experiment—when the investigators are in control of allocating participants to receive the experimental or control intervention(s), *and* they (or other investigators) are in charge of administering the experimental intervention (Jadad, 1998, p. 2; Bland, 2000, p. 5; Armitage et al., 2002, p. 6). Mill (1973), drawing what might be a more accurate distinction, distinguished "artificial" from natural experiments. In observational studies, investigators neither allocate participants to test or control groups nor administer the experimental intervention but rather examine records of patients who have been treated in routine practice.

In theory randomization is not required for experimental allocation. Investigators could allocate people experimentally by alternation, rotation, or date of birth. Such allocation would not be randomized, but since investigators perform the allocation, it would be experimental. A practical advantage of random allocation over other experimental methods for allocation is that it is more difficult to decipher and subsequently subvert.

Experimental administration of test and control treatments provides randomized trials with two further *potential* advantageous features over observational studies. Briefly, randomized trials, but not observational studies, can employ double masking and placebo controls.

To rule out the potentially confounding factors arising from caregiver and participant expectations and beliefs, we can blind or mask the participants and caregivers in charge of administering the intervention. Masking, like concealment, involves hiding the knowledge of who receives the experimental intervention. A double-blind or double-masked study is a study in which neither the participants who receive the intervention nor caregivers who administer the intervention are aware of who gets the experimental intervention. For example, in a double-blind randomized trial of HRT versus placebo, neither the participants nor the caregivers know whether the particular pill they take (or administer) is real HRT. Not knowing whether they are in the experimental or control group, the participants' expectations, and any effects of these expectations, is not confounded by the knowledge that they are taking a particular treatment. Similarly, if the physicians who administer the intervention do not know which participants are in the experimental or control groups, their treatment of participants is not different because of their knowledge of who is taking the experimental treatment.

Because they involve observations of what happens in routine practice, it is practically impossible for observational studies to be conducted in double-masked conditions. Unless something has gone wrong, caregivers know what interventions they are administering, and (one hopes) they tell their patients.

Exceptions include cases where the healthcare practitioner prescribes something by accident, or if the patient is unconscious.

Thus, double masking then can reduce the potentially confounding influence of several confounding factors that arise from knowledge of who receives the experimental treatment. For example, if a patient knows they are receiving the latest and best therapy, they might improve because of their beliefs and expectations and not because of the experimental therapy itself. In fact people can recover, even quite dramatically, from various ailments simply because they believe they are taking a powerful treatment (or *report* that they are recovering more quickly, which is all that is at issue when the outcome is subjective). Depressed patients, for instance, seem to recover more quickly (or report they recovered more dramatically) when they *know* they are receiving a "real" antidepressant drug than they do if they are not sure whether they are taking a real antidepressant drug (Moncrieff and Wessely, 1998; Moncrieff, 2003; Moncrieff et al., 2004; Tuteur, 1958). Similarly, investigator attitudes have been known to influence interpretation of rat (Rosenthal and Lawson, 1964) and human (Eisenach and Lindner, 2004) behavior, and also more objective measures such as blood cell counts (Berkson et al., 1939). Besides confounding influences of expectations and beliefs, participant and caregiver knowledge can lead to other confounders including differential drop-out rates and concomitant medication.

Second, placebo controls are often required to achieve double masking. In order to deceive trial participants into believing that they *might* be taking the experimental intervention, it must be possible to disguise the control intervention as the experimental intervention. Often the easiest way to achieve this is by designing an intervention that looks superficially like the experimental treatment but does not contain its characteristic features. For example, we might design a pill that looks like a HRT tablet but that contains no actual estrogen. Like double masking, placebo controls are practically impossible to employ in observational studies. In routine practice, treatments already have (supposedly) proven effects. To be sure, some treatments prescribed in routine practice are, for all intents and purposes, placebos. For example, doctors sometimes knowingly prescribe antibiotics for viral infections when the patient demands that something be done, or when the doctor herself would like to appear as though she is doing something. One might argue on this basis that we *could* conduct observational studies with placebo controls. These studies would compare, for example, antibiotics prescribed as placebos in routine practice with antibiotics prescribed for bacterial infections in routine practice. However, this would be practically impossible because it would be difficult to identify a control group that had been treated with placebo antibiotics in routine practice. Doctors are unlikely to freely admit they did this. And even if we could it would not help in studies involving other types of treatments.

To summarize this section, the essential feature of a randomized trial is that it involves random allocation to treatment groups. Randomization, provided it were adhered to (which is often impossible unless the allocation is concealed), helps to reduce baseline confounders. The experimental nature of randomized trials permits them to employ two features that are generally unavailable to observational studies designs, namely, double masking and placebo controls. These further, potential features of randomized trials allow them to reduce potential *performance bias* introduced by participant and caregiver knowledge of who receives the experimental intervention. In spite of their theoretical appeal, the benefits of randomized trials have been difficult to detect empirically (Odgaard-Jensen et al., 2011; Anglemyer et al., 2014), and philosophers therefore legitimately criticize the special place for randomized trials within the EBM system. However, when the effect is dramatic, as it is in the case of parachutes to prevent death, the Heimlich maneuver, and other dramatically effective treatments, observational evidence can be as strong as evidence from randomized trials. Current EBM "hierarchies" acknowledge this and thus avoid the paradox presented by highly effective therapies that are not supported by randomized trials.

Philosophical Controversies in EBM: The Role of Mechanistic Reasoning

Mechanisms are all the rage in current philosophical work on causality, where relatively strong ontological claims are made on their behalf (Bechtel and Abrahamsen, 2005; Glennan, 1996; Machamer et al., 2000). Mechanisms are allegedly responsible for generating causal regularities, if not all causal regularities, at least a good number of causal regularities of central interest in science. Expressing this view, Glennan (1996, p. 64) states that "a mechanical theory of causation suggests that two events are causally connected when and only when there is a mechanism connecting them." If mechanisms allegedly play such essential roles in underwriting causal regularities in the life sciences, it seems reasonable to expect that evidence about mechanisms should play a central role in supporting claims about the effectiveness of medical interventions, since these are just causal regularity claims with medical interventions as inputs and change in patient-relevant outcomes as outputs. Russo and Williamson (2007, p. 159), in a recent and interesting paper, insist on just this: "To establish causal claims, scientists need the mutual support of mechanisms and dependencies."

In stark contrast EBM proponents do not highly rate mechanistic reasoning. Far from being required, mechanistic reasoning does not even appear in the most recent, and arguably dominant, evidence-ranking scheme (Guyatt et al., 2008). Is this reasonable?

Here I argue that we do not require both evidence from mechanisms and evidence from comparative clinical studies to establish that interventions produce their effects. Moreover, there are a number of overlooked problems that beset the use of mechanistic reasoning. My overall conclusion, however, is not in support of the view popular in EBM that mechanistic reasoning is not evidence at all. Instead, I shall argue that where problems with our relevant knowledge of mechanisms can be overcome, mechanistic reasoning can and should be used to support claims that medical interventions have their putative patient-relevant effects. I begin by disambiguating *mechanisms* from *mechanistic reasoning*, and argue that only the latter is evidence (at least evidence relevant to clinical decision-making).

Terminology: Patient-relevant Effects, Comparative Clinical Studies, Mechanisms, and Mechanistic Reasoning

I am concerned here with evidence that a medical intervention produces a patient-relevant outcome. A patient-relevant outcome is, in brief, one that makes people feel better or live longer, as opposed to evidence about whether certain molecules latch on to rat cell receptors. Unless otherwise specified, I henceforth use the term "evidence" as shorthand for "evidence that a medical intervention has a patient-relevant outcome."

Different types of evidence support claims that interventions are effective. The idea behind Mill's (1973) methods, the numerical method (Louis, 1836), the statistical method (Bernard, 1957), and difference-making evidence (Russo and Williamson, 2007) is similar, and I refer to them collectively as comparative clinical studies. In these studies, some (experimental) groups receive the experimental intervention while other (control) groups do not. Then, outcomes in the groups are compared. If the outcomes differ significantly, the study counts as evidence that the intervention had some effect. In these studies the mechanism for *how* the intervention caused the outcome is generally a "black box" (Figure 5.1, left side). Randomized trials and controlled observational studies are examples of controlled clinical studies.

For example, in the antiarrhythmic example cited earlier, not only were the mechanisms explaining how the drugs might increase mortality unknown, but the prevailing mechanistic knowledge suggested that the drugs would *reduce* mortality.

There are various problems with evidence from comparative clinical studies that have been discussed elsewhere (Worrall, 2007b; Howick, 2011). It is beyond the scope of this chapter to evaluate these problems. Although effort has been spent over the past several decades researching the methodology of comparative clinical studies, the methodology of mechanistic reasoning has been altogether ignored.

Besides comparative clinical studies, evidence can be inferred from mechanistic knowledge, or "evidence of a mechanism." A problem with exploring just how mechanisms provide evidence is that mechanism has recently been characterized in several ways:

- Mechanisms are entities and activities organized such that they are productive of regular changes from start or set-up to finish or termination conditions (Machamer et al., 2000, p. 3).
- A mechanism underlying a behavior is a complex system that produces that behavior by the interaction of a number of parts according to direct causal laws (Glennan, 1996, p. 52).
- A nomological machine is a stable enough arrangement of components whose features acting in consort give rise to (relatively) stable input/output relations (Cartwright, 2009a, p. 8).

For present purposes these definitions are sufficiently similar. The heart (as a pump), the brain (as a control center), and the liver (as a detoxifying agent) are all mechanisms in the senses described here.

A central point of this chapter is that evidence of a mechanism by itself—even if good evidence—does not count as evidence that a treatment will have a clinical benefit. To see why, consider the mechanistic reasoning that led to the widespread adoption of antiarrhythmic drugs once again. Evidence of the heart and other mechanisms—although correct—did not amount to evidence that antiarrhythmic drugs reduce mortality. Instead, an implicit chain of reasoning is required to infer from evidence of mechanism(s) to the claim that a treatment will have a clinical benefit (Figure 5.1, middle). I refer to the inference from evidence of a mechanism to the claim that a treatment has a clinically relevant benefit as "mechanistic reasoning." The mechanisms involved in getting an orally administered drug to its pharmacological targets on a cell are relatively well understood and referred to as ADME (mechanisms for absorption, distribution, metabolism, and excretion). Once the drug reaches its cellular target, it reduces the frequency of ventricular extra beats (VEBs) by modifying the heart's electrochemical mechanism. (Myocardial infarction often damages the muscle and electrical system in the heart, leaving it susceptible to arrhythmias such as VEBs.) VEBs can cause the heart to pump insufficient blood. Without treatment, VEBs can degenerate into ventricular fibrillation followed by sudden death in the absence of electric shock. Based on this mechanistic knowledge, several antiarrhythmic drugs were developed and found to be successful for regulating VEBs (Moore, 1995, p. 44). Next, a reduction in VEBs (allegedly) reduces the risk of sudden death, presumably by reducing the risks associated with insufficient blood flow to vital organs. Finally, taking death as sustained lack of electrical activity in the brain, any reduction in mortality is related to brain mechanism(s).

As illustrated in Figure 5.1, descriptions of a single mechanism (such as the heart mechanism) rarely suffice to provide evidence for a link between an intervention and a patient-relevant outcome. Instead, we require identification and descriptions of *all* relevant mechanisms linking the intervention with the patient-relevant outcome *and* knowledge of what happens to each mechanism under intervention. With that in mind, "mechanistic reasoning" can be defined as follows: Mechanistic reasoning involves an inferential chain (or web) linking the intervention (such as anti-arrhythmic drugs) with a patient-relevant outcome, via relevant mechanisms. We can usually redescribe mechanisms in terms of lower-level mechanisms. For example, we might have included some of the heart's cellular mechanisms in our account of mechanistic reasoning for antiarrhythmic drug effects. But even in this case, the main feature of mechanistic reasoning—that it involves an inference from (alleged) knowledge of relevant mechanisms—remains.

Why the View that Mechanistic Reasoning is Necessary to Establish Causal Claims is Mistaken

Russo and Williamson (2007) support their view that mechanistic reasoning is required alongside comparative clinical studies with historical and theoretical arguments. The historical argument is based on three anecdotes. First, Semmelweis had strong evidence from comparative clinical studies, but his antiseptic procedures were rejected (arguably) because the Germ Theory of Disease was not available to explain *why* the procedure might work. Second, Doll and Hill's studies linking smoking and lung cancer were not fully accepted until the mechanism was established. Third, Warren and Marshall's claim that *Helicobacter pylori* caused peptic ulcers was practically laughed at until the mechanism was established.

However, in these anecdotes, the demand for mechanistic reasoning before causation was supposedly established delayed the adoption of life-saving interventions. Countless mothers and babies would have been saved had Semmelweis's intervention been adopted after the comparative clinical study, and life expectancy in many countries would have risen decades earlier if government strictures on smoking had been introduced before the mechanism linking smoking and lung was established. Hence Gillies (2005, p. 180) uses the very same examples to argue that it is unwise to require mechanistic reasoning alongside *strong* evidence from comparative clinical studies.

Russo and Williamson's (2007, 159) theoretical argument supporting the view that evidence of a mechanism is required to support causation is "if there is no plausible mechanism from C to E, then any correlation is likely to be spurious." It is true that comparative clinical studies sometimes support spurious relationships (although tightly controlled randomized trials are far less prone to spurious correlations than observational studies, and Russo and Williamson do not distinguish between the two different categories of comparative clinical study). But the requirement to include evidence of a mechanism as support for claims about therapeutic effectiveness does not play the theoretical role Russo and Williamson ascribe to it. Bloodletting was adopted on the basis of both mechanistic reasoning (derived from the humoral theory) and comparative clinical studies (observations of patients recovering after being bled, mostly due to placebo effects), yet it is safe to say that bloodletting was useless or harmful in most cases. The example of bloodletting may be unfair because we now know that the evidence supporting its efficacy was weak. But more recent examples, including the antiarrhythmic drug example, show that even apparently stronger evidence of a mechanism is insufficient for predicting clinical effectiveness.

Are Mechanisms Required to Justify External Validity?

Average study results may not apply to individuals or subgroups *within a study*, and target populations could be relevantly different from study populations. This problem is commonly discussed in the context of randomized trials, but it also applies to controlled observational studies and, as I shall point out later, studies that investigate underlying mechanisms. It is a problem whether the studies are analyzed using frequentist or Bayesian methods (Teira, 2010).

Consider the following imaginary example. If half the participants in a trial experienced 100 percent recovery, and the other half experienced no effect, the average outcome (50 percent recovery) would not describe what happened to any individual in the study. In a real example taken from Rothwell (1995), investigators conducting the European Carotid Surgery Trial (ECST) found that carotid endarterectomy appeared to carry an obvious risk of a ~0.5 percent increase in mortality (European Carotid Surgery Trialists' Collaborative Group, 1998; Ferro et al., 1991). However, when Rothwell (1995) restricted the analysis to patients with severe carotid stenosis, the intervention was found to be beneficial. This is not a problem with implementing the study results to populations outside the trial; hence, the term "external validity" is misleading. Unless there is no variation, average study results do not even apply to individuals *within* the trial.

But even if there is no variation within the subjects in a trial, target populations can be different from study populations. Up to 90 percent of potentially eligible participants are sometimes excluded from trials according to often poorly reported and even haphazard criteria (Mant, 1999; Penston, 2003; Travers et al., 2007; Zimmerman et al., 2002a, b; Zetin and Hoepner, 2007). For example, even the most effective antidepressants in adults have doubtful effects in children (Bylund and Reed, 2007; Deupree et al., 2007). In another example taken from Worrall (2007b), the drug benoxaprofen (Oraflex™ in the United States and Opren™ in Europe) proved effective in trials in 18- to 65-year-olds, but killed a significant number of elderly patients when it was introduced into routine practice. The problem that average results do not apply to individuals or subgroups within a trial is exacerbated by the fact that people can change over time. Result from a study that were applicable at time T_1 might not apply at a different time T_2.

Besides differences between study and target populations, study and target contexts can differ. In a Presidential Address to the Philosophy of Science Association, Cartwright (2010) illustrated this aspect of the problem with the example of the Tamil Nadu Integrated Nutrition Programs (TINP I and TINP II). These programs aimed to improve the nutritional status of preschool children (6–36 months old) and pregnant and nursing women. To achieve the aim, investigators provided a package of services that included nutrition education, primary healthcare, supplementary on-site feeding of children, education for diarrhea management, vitamin A, deworming, supplementary feeding of women, and growth monitoring through monthly weighing of all children aged 6–36 months.

TINP success was measured by comparing changes within TINP districts with changes in non-TINP districts. Independent surveys showed that severe malnutrition declined by at least 33 percent among children aged 6–24 months, and by 50 percent among those aged 6–60 months (Chidambaram, 1989; World Bank, 1990). TINP II was similarly successful, with a more conservative independent estimate of a 44 percent decline in severe malnutrition over 5 years (Nutrition NIo, 1998; World Bank, 1998).

Inspired by the TINP successes, a similar project was implemented in Bangladesh. Unsurprisingly, the project was called Bangladesh Integrated Nutrition Project (BINP). Unfortunately, BINP enjoyed little success: independent agencies reviewed the evidence and found little reason to believe that the project had had any impact (Federation StC, 2003; Karim et al., 2003). While the relevant biological traits of the study participants in Tamil Nadu and Bangladesh are unlikely to have been very different, the social contexts in Bangladesh were dissimilar in important ways. The first main difference appeared to be leakage: the food supplied by the project in Bangladesh was often used as substitutes for other family members rather than supplements for mothers and children. Other related reasons were the mother-in-law factor, and the man-shopper factor:

The program targeted the mothers of young children. But mothers are frequently not the decision makers . . . with respect to the health and nutrition of their children. For a start, women do not go to market in rural Bangladesh; it is men who do the shopping. And for women in joint households—meaning they live with their mother-in-law—as a sizeable minority do, then the mother-in-law heads the women's domain. (White, 2009, p. 6)

To recap, the problem of implementation is the problem of justifying claims that average study results apply to target populations. For present purposes, we take target populations to be individuals or subgroups within a study, or populations that were not, and perhaps would not have been, included in a study.

There are at least five (nonexclusive) potential solutions to the problem of implementation, including simple induction (Petticrew and Chalmers, 2011), n-of-1 trials (Guyatt et al., 1990), or pragmatic trials (Della, Gruppo Italiano Per Lo Studio, 1986), or clinical expertise. None of these are adequate (see Howick et al. (2013) and Howick (2011) for discussion). The solution preferred by most philosophical critics of EBM is the appeal to alleged knowledge of mechanisms. In a growing body of literature that began with discussions of the applicability of results from animal studies to humans, philosophers of science have argued that knowledge of mechanisms can justify implementing average study results to target populations by *analogy* (Cartwright, 2010; Lafollette and Shanks, 1995; Guala, 2005, 2010; Steel, 2008, 2010; Thagard, 1999). On this view, implementation is justified insofar as the relevant mechanisms—and hence the mechanistic reasoning linking the intervention and outcome—are shared in the study and target populations.

Dan Steel (2008, 2010) correctly points out that this simple mechanistic solution to the problem of implementation fails because of the "extrapolator's circle." In order to determine whether the mechanism in the target is sufficiently similar to the mechanism in the study population to justify extrapolation, we must know how relevant mechanisms in the target behave. But, Steel argues, if we had knowledge of mechanisms in the target population, then we would have strong mechanistic reasoning supporting the claim that the intervention caused the outcome in the target population. This would make the initial study (i.e., in the model) redundant. In Steel's (2008, p. 78) words, "[I]t needs to be explained how we could know that the model and the target are similar in causally relevant respects without already knowing the causal relationship in the target."

To escape from this circle, Steel (2008) offers a more sophisticated account of how mechanistic knowledge might help us justify implementing study results, namely, *comparative process tracing*. Comparative process tracing involves two steps: "First, learn the mechanism in the model organism, by means of process tracing or other experimental means[6] . . . Second, compare stages of the mechanism in the model organism with that of the target organism in which the two are most likely to differ significantly" (p. 89). A key feature of Steel's account is that we need not know everything about the mechanisms in the target, but only the relevant parts of the mechanism. Often, the needed points of comparison can be limited to stages of the mechanism close to the endpoint—the reasoning being that differences upstream matter only if they generate differences further downstream. This significantly reduces the number of points in the mechanism that we need to compare. Hence, we need not know everything about the mechanism in the target in advance, and the extrapolator's circle is allegedly avoided.

Some influential proponents of EBM have a position that could be interpreted as supporting the view that mechanistic reasoning can help solve the problem of implementation. They state, for example:

> A sound understanding of pathophysiology is necessary to interpret and apply the results of clinical research. For instance, most patients to whom we would like to generalize the results of randomized trials would, for one reason or another, not have been enrolled in the most relevant study. The patient may be too old, be too sick, have other underlying illnesses, or be uncooperative. Understanding the underlying pathophysiology allows the clinician to better judge whether the results are applicable to the patient at hand. (Evidence Based Medicine Working Group, 1992, p. 2423)

This advice continues in three editions of an EBM textbook (Sackett et al., 1997; Sackett, 2000; Straus et al., 2005). Interestingly, critics of EBM share this view (Tonelli, 2006). To be sure, the term used by some EBM proponents (pathophysiologic rationale) appears to be different from our mechanistic reasoning. At the same time, pathophysiology involves the study of how bodily processes behave in normal and abnormal circumstances, and rationale is a synonym of reasoning. Hence we take pathophysiologic rationale to mean (roughly) the same as mechanistic reasoning.

By way of support for the EBM view, Gordon Guyatt and Paul Glasziou (in conversation) have offered the following illustration. A trial might exclude everyone over the age of 60. They claim that mechanistic considerations support the view that the intervention is likely to work for a 61-year-old but may not work for a 90-year-old. Presumably they take it that the success of the intervention depends on the operation of pathophysiologic mechanisms that change only slowly beyond 60 and so would not have changed substantially in most 61-year-olds but would be highly likely to have changed by 90.

In spite of its intuitive appeal, mechanistic reasoning, even in Steel's more sophisticated account, is plagued by several problems that make it unsuitable as a robust solution to the problem of implementation. First, suppose mechanistic knowledge is useful only insofar as we correctly identify relevant mechanisms. But as we saw earlier, correct identification of all relevant mechanisms in any population is far more difficult than is often presumed. For example, a plausible (but incorrect) mechanism for blood creation led to various erroneous diagnoses and treatments such as bloodletting. Even if we correctly identify some mechanisms, we often fail to identify all the relevant links in the mechanistic web or chain linking the intervention with the outcome. This can lead to mistaken predictions about efficacy, as we saw in the CAST example earlier.

Even in areas that are very well understood, such as the cholesterol pathway, drugs can activate unexpected mechanisms, with harmful and very costly consequences (Joy and Hegele, 2008). Indeed, there are dozens of cases in which incomplete or mistaken knowledge of underlying mechanisms has led to the adoption of (sometimes fatally) harmful or useless therapies (Howick, 2011).

Another problem with using mechanistic reasoning to extrapolate from a study to a target population is that functioning of most mechanisms is discovered in tightly controlled laboratory experiments that expressly exclude as many potentially interfering variables as possible. Why would functions discovered in tightly controlled laboratory circumstances generalize more readily than effects discovered in controlled clinical studies? If they do not, then any knowledge about the mechanisms gained in these controlled settings is less likely to be shared by real-world populations. For example, St. John's wart has been shown in laboratory settings to induce the activity of cytochrome P450 (CYP) isoenzymes, which are extensively involved in metabolizing about 50 percent of known drugs (Markowitz et al., 2003), including many steroids. However, a clinical study suggested St. John's wart did not reduce the concentrations of androgenic steroids (Donovan et al., 2005). In this example the behavior of a mechanism in the laboratory was not reproducible in a real clinical setting.

Second, evidence of mechanisms do not guarantee that input/output relationships are regular. Claude Bernard (1957, p. 214), perhaps the grandfather of contemporary mechanistic reasoning in medicine, believed that mechanisms were productive of stable deterministic laws that precluded the need for any further empirical evidence (e.g., from controlled studies):

Now that the cause of the itch is known and experimentally determined, it has all become scientific, and empiricism has disappeared. We know the tick, and by it we explain the transmission of the itch, the skin changes and the cure, which is only the tick's death through appropriate application of toxic agents ... We cure it *always* without any exception, when we place ourselves in the known experimental conditions for reaching this goal. (Emphasis added)

While few today believe that more than a handful of diseases (if any!) are cured "always and without exception" (Broadbent, 2009)—and indeed Claude

Bernard himself advocated clinical trials when mechanisms were unknown (Morabia, 2006)—the belief that mechanisms produce stable relationships is widely held among mechanist philosophers of science. Consider other excerpts from the recent literature. Mechanisms are (supposedly):

> entities and activities organized such that they are productive of *regular* changes from start or set-up to finish or termination conditions. (Machamer et al., 2000, p. 3; emphasis added)

And:

> the existence of a mechanism provides evidence of the *stability* of a causal relationship. If we can single out a plausible mechanism, then that mechanism is likely to occur in a range of individuals, making the causal relation stable over a variety of populations. (Russo and Williamson, 2007, p. 159; emphasis added)

Furthermore:

> Nomological machines [mechanisms] generate causal laws between inputs and *predictable* outputs. (Cartwright, 2009b, p. 156; emphasis added)

The belief that mechanisms are productive of stable relationships might be borrowed from mechanics, where, if we ignore the quantum level, there *are* many mechanisms productive of stable input–output relationships. For instance, Cartwright (2009a) cites the example of a toaster's mechanism. But mechanisms in the human body and social world, especially those that are pertinent to clinically relevant outcomes, are generally far more complex than toasters. Besides epistemological problems with discovering assumed regularity (extreme sensitivity to initial conditions, complex interactions), mechanisms themselves might not behave regularly (Desautels, 2011).

Mechanisms' irregular behavior is perhaps best exemplified by paradoxical reactions, and many drugs that sometimes worsen the condition for which they are indicated (Hauben and Aronson, 2006). To name a few, antiepileptic drugs can both prevent and cause seizures (King et al., 2005; Lai et al., 2001), antidepressants can both ameliorate and worsen depressive symptoms (Saperia et al., 2006; Damluji and Ferguson, 1988), and antiarrhythmic drugs can cause arrhythmias (Winkle et al., 1981). Even the same molecule can initiate different mechanisms depending on its environment within the body. Most genes, at least, do many things. Manipulating one gene can therefore have unexpected and sometimes paradoxical consequences. One might object that the irregularity of mechanisms was due to ignorance of some other mechanism, which, if known, would be able to explain the irregularity by appealing to the regularity of presently unknown mechanisms. This is possible, but given that counterexamples to the claim that mechanisms behave in regular ways are unlikely to disappear, this objection risks becoming a metaphysical rather than evidence-based view.

Are Mechanisms Required to Generate Hypotheses?

Roughly 70 percent of biomedical funding is devoted to basic (animal, in vitro) science studies investigating the mechanisms of health and disease. The justification for this generous resource allocation appears to be that the basic mechanism research eventually leads to treatments that benefit humans. Philosophers of science discuss some widely celebrated historical cases where discovering a mechanism did just that. For example, Clarke et al. (2014) correctly note that Pasteur's understanding of the mechanism linking bacteria with disease was required to develop anthrax and rabies vaccines. Perhaps the most dramatic of Pasteur's tests was the case of young Joseph Meister, a 9-year-old boy who had been bitten by a rabid dog before the rabies vaccine had been tested in humans. Meister was vaccinated and subsequently survived, establishing the usefulness of rabies vaccinations.

However, it does not follow from the fact that some useful treatments are discovered on the back of basic mechanism research that mechanism research is *required* for treatment discovery. Empirical observations are also very useful for this purpose. Many of our most commonly used and beneficial treatments, ranging from analgesics and anesthesia for treating pain to digitalis for treating atrial fibrillation, were discovered by empirical trial and error, often by lay people. I am also willing to wager that at least 50 percent of the readers of this chapter have tried one of the following treatments: chicken soup for the cold or flu, gargling salt water for a sore throat, or pouring water (sometimes with salt) into the nostril to treat a blocked nose. All these treatments have been used for centuries if not millennia and anecdotal evidence suggests they are effective. Reports of chicken soup as a cure for the flu date back to at least Babylonian times (Ohry and Tsafrir, 1999). However none of these treatments have been evaluated in clinical trials.

There are two reasons why the usefulness of mechanism research for treatment has been exaggerated. First, the theoretical and empirical problems with mechanistic reasoning are serious but have been all but ignored by philosophical proponents of mechanisms. Mechanisms and theories in physics—the ones that philosophers of science often appeal to when propounding the importance of mechanisms (Cartwright and Hardie, 2012)—are exceptionally successful at making practical predictions. The fact that proponents of mechanisms choose the 150-year-old example of Pasteur to illustrate the benefits of mechanisms is telling more because it is an exception in the sense that it illustrates mechanism- and theory-driven discoveries. Even Pasteur's discoveries, have empirical roots that are rarely discussed. To name just one such root, many centuries before Pasteur discovered the germ theory, St. Hildegard of Bingen discussed scabies in her treatise, *Physika*, naming the itch mite "snebelza." She treated scabies using sulfur ointment, a treatment that is still used to treat scabies mites. At the time it was not known that microorganisms caused scabies, and physicians (due to prevalence of Galen's ideas) did not believe her.[7]

Second, empirical studies suggest that when it comes to methods for treatment discovery, mechanism research is not the only—or, as I shall argue, most efficient—game in town. The best estimate for the proportion of beneficial treatments that were discovered by conducting basic research are between 2 and 21 percent (Chalmers et al., 2014). This evidence needs to be taken into account when allocating public funds to research.

It is worthwhile clarifying that neither the views in this chapter nor the views of actual medical researchers (whether or not they subscribe to EBM) are antimechanism. Anyone who has done a clinical trial or a Cochrane Review knows that plausible mechanisms are considered and valued. I have defended the use of (evidence-based) mechanisms in several previous papers. Rather the argument I put forth here, like the arguments I put forth in my previous papers, is that the importance of mechanisms has been wildly exaggerated and that other methods are superior.

Conclusion

I have argued that the EBM epistemology is, on the whole, justified because systematic reviews of randomized trials are more likely to provide good evidence than observational studies, and mechanistic reasoning. At the same time, the view that systematic reviews of randomized trials provide the best evidence leads to the paradox that our most effective treatments are not supported by "best" evidence. This paradox can be overcome by taking the effect size of a treatment into account when evaluating strength of evidence, as more recent EBM hierarchies do. The diminished role of mechanistic reasoning within the EBM system is also viewed as controversial by many philosophers of science. I argue that while mechanistic reasoning can be useful for establishing treatment effects, it is not required, and that empirical evidence supports the view that randomized trials provide better evidence than mechanistic reasoning.

Notes

1. See Daly (2005) for a great overview.
2. See Tröhler (2001) for a good review of the recent historical roots of EBM.
3. See *Oxford English Dictionary*, online version. 2nd edition: Oxford University Press, 1989.
4. See Fulford et al. (2012) for an interesting discussion. One might argue that values are required to *know* what the best treatment is, and hence that a discussion of values is required also for the epistemology of EBM. I have great sympathy for this view. However, there remains a sense in which the effectiveness of a medical intervention are not value-dependent. Hence I exclude a discussion of the role of values in EBM epistemology to another work.
5. See Howick et al. (2015) for a brief discussion of these controversies.
6. In broad terms, "process tracing" involves a step-by-step reconstruction of the path connecting an end-point (an initial cause or a final effect) with other elements of the mechanism via intermediate nodes.
7. This is one of many examples, consistently ignored by proponents of mechanisms, where appeal to mechanisms prevented useful treatments from benefiting patients. To name just a few examples, a placebo controlled trial of antiarrhythmic drugs was deemed unethical by those who believed the drugs to work based on apparent knowledge of mechanisms, Fisher did his best to prevent antismoking regulations based on an alleged genetic mechanism causing both people to smoke and lung cancer, and Warren and Marshall's claim that *Helicobacter pylori* caused peptic ulcers was not believed because it was believed that bacteria could not live in the hostile stomach wall's hostile environment.

References

Anglemyer, A., Horvath, H. T., and Bero, L. (2014). Healthcare outcomes assessed with observational study designs compared with those assessed in randomized trials. *Cochrane Database Syst Rev* 4: MR000034.

Antman, E. M., Lau, J., Kupelnick, B., Mosteller, F., and Chalmers, T. C. (1992). A comparison of results of meta-analyses of randomized control trials and recommendations of clinical experts. Treatments for myocardial infarction. *JAMA* 268(2): 240–48.

Armitage, P., Berry, G., and Matthews, J. N. S. (2002). Statistical Methods in Medical Research, 4th edition, P. Armitage, G. Berry, J. N. S. Matthews, eds. Oxford: Blackwell Science.

Backe, B. (1990). Profile of a consensus development program in Norway: The Norwegian Institute for Hospital Research and the National Research Council. In *Improving Consensus Development for Health Technology Assessment: An International Perspective*, eds. C. Goodman and S. R. Baratz. Washington, DC: National Academy Press, pp. 118–24.

Battista, R. N. (1990). Profile of a consensus development program in Canada: The Canadian Task Force on the Periodic Health Examination. In *Improving Consensus Development for Health Technology Assessment: An International Perspective*, eds. C. Goodman and S. R. Baratz. Washington, DC: National Academy Press, pp. 87–92.

Bechtel, W., Abrahamsen, A. (2005). Explanation: A mechanist alternative. *Studies in the History and Philosophy of Biological and Biomedical Sciences* 36: 421–41.

Berkson, J., Magath, T., and Hurn, M. (1939). The error of estimate of the blood cell count as made with the hmocytometer. *Am J Physiol* 128: 309–23.

Bernard, C. (1957). *An Introduction to the Study of Experimental Medicine*. New York: Dover Publications, Inc.

Bland, M. (2000). *An Introduction to Medical Statistics*, 3rd edition. Oxford: Oxford University Press.

Borgerson, K. (2009). Valuing evidence: Bias and the evidence hierarchy of evidence-based medicine. *Perspect Biol Med* 52(2): 218–33.

Broadbent, A. (2009). Causation and models of disease in epidemiology. *Studies in History and Philosophy of Science Part C: Studies in History and Philosophy of Biological and Biomedical Sciences* 40(4): 302–11.

Bylund, D. B., and Reed, A. L. (2007). Childhood and adolescent depression: Why do children and adults respond differently to antidepressant drugs? *Neurochem Int* 51(5): 246–53.

Canadian Task Force on the Periodic Health Examination. (1979). The periodic health examination. *Can Med Assoc J* 121(9): 1193–254.

Canner, P. L. (1980). Influence of adherence to treatment and response of cholesterol on mortality in the coronary drug project. *N Engl J Med* 303(18): 1038–41.

Cartwright, N. (2009a). How to do things with causes. *APA Proceedings and Addresses* 83(2).

Cartwright, N. (2009b). Causal laws, policy predictions, and the need for genuine powers. In *Dispositions and Causes*, ed. T. Handfield. Oxford: Oxford University Press.

Cartwright, N. (2010). Will this policy work for you? Predicting effectiveness better: How philosophy helps (Presidential Address). *Philosophy of Science Association*.

Cartwright, N., Goldfinch, A., and Howick, J. (2007). Evidence-based policy: Where is out theory of evidence? *Graduate Conference of the Graduate School for Social Sciences*, Milan.

Cartwright, N., and Hardie, J. (2012). Evidence-Based Policy: A Practical Guide to Doing It Better. Oxford; New York: Oxford University Press.

Celsus, A. C., and Collier, G. F. (1831). *A Translation of the Eight Books of Aul. Corn. Celsus on Medicine*. London: Simpkin and Marshall.

Chalmers, I. (2002). Why we need to know whether prophylactic antibiotics can reduce measles-related morbidity. *Pediatrics* 109(2): 312–15.

Chalmers, I., Bracken, M. B., Djulbegovic, B., Garattini, S., Grant, J., Gülmezoglu, A. M., Howells, D. W., Ioannidis, J. P. A., and Oliver, S. (2014). How to increase value and reduce waste when research priorities are set. *Lancet* 383(9912): 156–65.

Chidambaram, G. (1989). *Tamil Nadu Integrated Nutrition Project—Terminal Evaluation*. Madras: Directorate of Evaluation and Applied Research, State Planning Commission.

Clarke, B., Gillies, D., Illari, P., Russo, F., and Williamson, J. (2014). Mechanisms and the evidence hierarchy. *Topoi* 33(2): 339–60.

Cocco, G. (2009). Erectile dysfunction after therapy with metoprolol: The Hawthorne effect. *Cardiology* 112(3): 174–77.

Daly, J. (2005). *Evidence-Based Medicine and the Search for a Science of Clinical Care*. Berkeley, CA; London: University of California Press.

Damluji, N. F., and Ferguson, J. M. (1988). Paradoxical worsening of depressive symptomatology caused by antidepressants. *J Clin Psychopharmacol* 8(5): 347–49.

Dawes, M., Summerskill, W., Glasziou, P., Cartabollotta, A., Martin, J., Hopayian, K., Porzsolt, F., Burls, A., and Osborne, J. (2005). Sicily statement on evidence-based practice. *BMC Med Educ* 5(1): 1.

Della, Gruppo Italiano Per Lo Studio. (1986). Effectiveness of intravenous thrombolytic treatment in acute myocardial infarction. *Lancet* 1(8478): 397–402.

Desautels, L. (2011). Against regular and irregular characterizations of mechanisms. *Philosophy of Science*, 78(5): 914–25.

Deupree, J. D., Reed, A. L., and Bylund, D. B. (2007). Differential effects of the tricyclic antidepressant desipramine on the density of adrenergic receptors in juvenile and adult rats. *J Pharmacol Exp Ther* 321(2): 770–76.

Donovan, J. L., DeVane, C. L., Lewis, J. G., Wang, J. S., Ruan, Y., Chavin, K., and Markowitz, J. S. (2005). Effects of St John's wort (Hypericum perforatum L.) extract on plasma androgen concentrations in healthy men and women: A pilot study. *Phytother Res* 19(10): 901–906.

Eddy, D. M. (1990). Practice policies: Where do they come from? *JAMA* 263(9): 1265, 9, 72 passim.

Eisenach, J. C., and Lindner, M. D. (2004). Did experimenter bias conceal the efficacy of spinal opioids in previous studies with the spinal nerve ligation model of neuropathic pain? *Anesthesiology* 100(4): 765–67.

European Carotid Surgery Trialists' Collaborative Group. (1998). Randomised trial of endarterectomy for recently symptomatic carotid stenosis: Final results of the MRC European Carotid Surgery Trial (ECST). *Lancet* 351(9113): 1379–87.

Evans, I., Thornton, H., and Chalmers, I. (2006). *Testing Treatments: Better Research for Better Healthcare*. London: British Library.

Evidence Based Medicine Working Group. (1992). Evidence-based medicine: A new approach to teaching the practice of medicine. *JAMA* 268: 2420–25.

Federation StC. (2003). *Thin on the Ground. Questioning the Evidence Behind World Bank-Funded Community Nutrition Projects in Bangladesh*. London: Save the Children Federation.

Ferro, J. M., Oliveira, V., Melo, T. P., Crespo, M., Lopes, J., Fernandes, J., Damiao, A., and Campos, J. G. (1991). [Role of endarterectomy in the secondary prevention of cerebrovascular accidents: results of the European Carotid Surgery Trial (ECST)]. *Acta Med Port* 4(4): 227–28.

Fulford, K. W. M., Peile, E., and Carroll, H. (2012). *Essential Values-Based Practice: Clinical Stories Linking Science with People*. Cambridge: Cambridge University Press.

Gillies, D. (1998). Debates on Bayesianism and the theory of Bayesian networks. *Theoria* 64(1): 1–22.

Gillies, D. (2005). Hempelian and Kuhnian approaches in the philosophy of medicine: The Semmelweis case. *Studies in History and Philosophy of Biological and Biomedical Sciences* 36(1): 159–81.

Glasziou, P., Chalmers, I., Rawlins, M., and McCulloch, P. (2007). When are randomised trials unnecessary? Picking signal from noise. *BMJ* 334(7589): 349–51.

Glennan, S. S. (1996). Mechanisms and the nature of causation. *Erkentnis* 44(1): 49–71.

Goodman, C., and Baratz, S. R. (1990). *Consensus Development at the NIH: Improving the Program*. Washington, DC: National Academy Press.

Guala, F. (2005). *The Methodology of Experimental Economics*. Cambridge: Cambridge University Press.

Guala, F. (2010). Extrapolation, analogy, and comparative process tracing. *Philosophy of Science* 77(5): 1070–82.

Guyatt, G. (1991). Evidence-based medicine. *American College of Physicians Journal Club* 114: A16.

Guyatt, G., Cook, D., and Haynes, B. (2004). Evidence based medicine has come a long way. *BMJ* 329(7473): 990–91.

Guyatt, G. H., Keller, J. L., Jaeschke, R., Rosenbloom, D., Adachi, J. D., and Newhouse, M. T. (1990). The n-of-1 randomized controlled trial: Clinical usefulness. Our three-year experience. *Ann Intern Med* 112(4): 293–99.

Guyatt, G. H., Oxman, A. D., Vist, G. E., Kunz, R., Falck-Ytter, Y., Alonso-Coello, P., and Schünemann, H. (2008). GRADE: An emerging consensus on rating quality of evidence and strength of recommendations. *BMJ* 336(7650): 924–26.

Håkansoon, S., and Eckerlund, I. (1990). Profile of a consensus development program in Sweden: The Swedish Medical Research Council and the Swedish Planning and Rationalization Institute for the Health and Social Services. In *Improving Consensus*

Development for Health Technology Assessment: An International Perspective, eds. C. Goodman and S. R. Baratz. Washington, DC: National Academy Press, pp. 125–30.

Harbour, R. T. (ed.) (2008). *SIGN 50: A Guideline Developer's Handbook*. Edinburgh: NHS Quality Improvement Scotland.

Hauben, M., and Aronson, J. K. (2006). Paradoxical reactions: Under-recognized adverse effects of drugs. *Drug Saf* 29(10): 970.

Healy, D. (2004). *Let Them Eat Prozac*. New York: New York University Press.

Healy, D. (2006). Did regulators fail over selective serotonin reuptake inhibitors? *BMJ* 333(7558): 92–95.

Horder, L. (1949). Whither medicine? *Br Med J* 1(4604): 557–60.

Howick, J. (2011). *The Philosophy of Evidence-Based Medicine*. Oxford: Wiley-Blackwell.

Howick, J., Glasziou, P., and Aronson, J. K. (2009). The evolution of evidence hierarchies: What can Bradford Hill's "guidelines for causation" contribute? *J R Soc Med* 102(5): 186–94.

Howick, J., Glasziou, P., and Aronson, J. K. (2013). Problems with using mechanisms to solve the problem of extrapolation. *Theor Med Bioeth* 34(4): 275–91.

Howick, J., Graham Kennedy, A., and Mebius, A. (2015). Philosophy of evidence-based medicine (2015). Oxford bibliographies. *Oxford Bibliographies*.

Illich, I. (1977). *Limits to Medicine: Medical Nemesis: The Expropriation of Health*, new edition. Harmondsworth: Penguin.

Investigators TCASTC. (1989). Preliminary report: Effect of encainide and flecainide on mortality in a randomized trial of arrhythmia suppression after myocardial infarction. *N Engl J Med* 321(6): 406–12.

Jadad, A. (1998). *Randomized Controlled Trials*. London: BMJ Books.

Jørgensen ,T. (1990). Profile of a consensus development program in Denmark: The Danish Medical Research Council and the Danish Hospital Institute. In *Improving Consensus Development for Health Technology Assessment: An International Perspective*, eds. C. Goodman and S. R. Baratz. Washington, DC: National Academy Press, pp. 96–101.

Joy, T. R., and Hegele, R. A. (2008). The failure of torcetrapib: What have we learned? *British Journal of Pharmacology* 154(7): 1379–81.

Karim, R., Lamstein, S. A., Akhtaruzzaman, M., Rahman, K. M., and Alam, N. (2003). *The Bangladesh Integrated Nutrition Project: Endline Evaluation of the Community Based Nutrition Component*. Boston; Dhaka: The Institute of Nutrition and Food Sciences, The Friedman School of Nutrition Science.

Kauppila, A.-L. (1990) Profile of a consensus development program in Finland: The Medical Research Council of the Academy of Finland. In *Improving Consensus Development for Health Technology Assessment: An International Perspective*, eds. C. Goodman and S. R. Baratz. Washington, DC: National Academy Press, pp. 102–109.

Kazinga, N. S., Casparie, A. F., and Everdingen, J. J. E. (1990). Profile of a consensus development program in Finland: National Organization for Quality Assurance in Hospitals. In *Improving Consensus Development for Health Technology Assessment: An International Perspective*, eds. C. Goodman and S. R. Baratz. Washington, DC: National Academy Press, pp. 110–17.

King, T., Ossipov, M. H., Vanderah, T. W., Porreca, F., and Lai, J. (2005). Is paradoxical pain induced by sustained opioid exposure an underlying mechanism of opioid antinociceptive tolerance? *Neurosignals* 14(4): 194–205.

Kirsch, I., and Moore, T. (2002). The emperor's new drugs: An analysis of antidepressant medication data submitted to the U.S. Food and Drug Administration. *Prevention & Treatment* 5.

Kirsch, I., and Sapirstein, G. (1998). Listening to prozac but hearing placebo: A meta-analysis of antidepressant medication. *Prevention & Treatment* I.

La Caze, A. (2009). Evidence-based medicine must be. *J Med Philos.*

Lafollette, H., and Shanks, N. (1995). Two models of models in biomedical research. *The Philosophical Quarterly* 45(179): 141–60.

Lai, J., Ossipov, M. H., Vanderah, T. W., Malan, T. P., Jr., and Porreca, F. (2001). Neuropathic pain: The paradox of dynorphin. *Mol Interv* 1(3): 160–67.

LeFanu, J. (2000). *The Rise and Fall of Modern Medicine.* London: Abacus.

Louis, P. C. A. (1836). *Researches on the Effects of Blood Letting in Some Inflammatory Diseases, and on the Influence of Tartarized Antimony and Vesication in Pneumonitis,* C. G. Putnam, trans., with preface and appendix by J. Jackson. Boston: Hillart, Gray.

Machamer, P., Darden, L., and Craver, C. F. (2000). Thinking about mechanisms. *Philos Sci* 67: 1–25.

Mant, D. (1999). Can randomised trials inform clinical decisions about individual patients? *Lancet* 353(9154): 743–46.

Markowitz, J. S., Donovan, J. L., DeVane, C. L., Taylor, R. M., Ruan, Y., Wang, J. S., and Chavin, K. D. (2003). Effect of St John's wort on drug metabolism by induction of cytochrome P450 3A4 enzyme. *JAMA* 290(11): 1500–504.

McCarney, R., Warner, J., Iliffe, S., van Haselen, R., Griffin, M., and Fisher, P. (2007). The Hawthorne Effect: A randomised, controlled trial. *BMC Med Res Methodol* 7: 30.

McKeown, T. (1976). *The Role of Medicine: Dream, Mirage or Nemesis?* London: Nuffield Provincial Hospitals Trust.

Medical Research Council Streptomycin in Tuberculosis Trials Committee. (1948). Streptomycin treatment for pulmonary tuberculosis. *BMJ* 2: 769–82.

Mill, J. S. (1973). *A System of Logic, Ratiocinative and Inductive: Being a Connected View of the Principles of Evidence and the Methods of Scientific Investigation.* Toronto: University of Toronto Press.

Moncrieff, J. (2003). A comparison of antidepressant trials using active and inert placebos. *Int J Methods Psychiatr Res* 12(3): 117–27.

Moncrieff, J., and Kirsch, I. (2005). Efficacy of antidepressants in adults. *BMJ* 331(7509): 155–57.

Moncrieff, J., and Wessely, S. (1998). Active placebos in antidepressant trials. *Br J Psychiatry* 173: 88.

Moncrieff, J., Wessely, S., and Hardy, R. (2004). Active placebos versus antidepressants for depression. *Cochrane Database Syst Rev* (1): CD003012.

Moore, T. J. (1995). *Deadly Medicine: Why Tens of Thousands of Heart Patients Died in America's Worst Drug Disaster.* New York; London: Simon & Schuster.

Morabia, A. (2006). Claude Bernard was a 19th century proponent of medicine based on evidence. *Journal of Clinical Epidemiology* 59(11): 1150–54.

Nutrition NIo. (1998). *Endline Evaluation of Tamil Nadu Integrated Nutrition Project II.* Hyderabad: Indian Council of Medical Research.

Odgaard-Jensen, J., Vist, G. E., Timmer, A. Kunz, R., Aki, E. A., Schünemann, H., Briel, M., Nordmann, A. J., Pregno, S., and Oxman, A. D. (2011). Randomisation to protect against selection bias in healthcare trials. *Cochrane database of systematic reviews* 13(4): MR000012.

Ohry, A., and Tsafrir, J. (1999). Is chicken soup an essential drug? *CMAJ* 161(12): 1532–33.

Penston, J. (2003). *Fact and Fiction in Medical Research: The Large-Scale Randomised Trial.* London: The London Press.

Petitti, D. B., Perlman, J. A., and Sidney, S. (1987). Noncontraceptive estrogens and mortality: Long-term follow-up of women in the Walnut Creek Study. *Obstet Gynecol* 70(3 Pt 1): 289–93.

Petticrew, M., and Chalmers, I. (2011). Use of research evidence in practice. *Lancet* 378(9804): 1696; author reply 967.

Phillips, B., Ball, C., Sackett, D., Badenoch, D., Straus, S., Haynes, B., and Dawes, M.. (2001). Oxford Centre for Evidence-based Medicine Levels of Evidence. http://www.cebm.net/?o=1021, accessed July 21, 2009.

Rosenthal, R., and Lawson, R. (1964). A longitudinal study of the effects of experimenter bias on the operant learning of laboratory rats. *J Psychiatr Res* 69: 61–72.

Rothwell, P. M. (1995). Can overall results of clinical trials be applied to all patients? *Lancet* 345(8965): 1616–19.

Russo, F., and Williamson, J. (2007). Interpreting causality in the health sciences. *International Studies in the Philosophy of Science* 21(2): 1157–70.

Sackett, D. L. (1986). Rules of evidence and clinical recommendations on the use of antithrombotic agents. *Chest* 89(2 Suppl): 2S–3S.

Sackett, D. L. (1989). Rules of evidence and clinical recommendations on the use of antithrombotic agents. *Chest* 95(2 Suppl): 2S–4S.

Sackett, D. L. (2000). *Evidence-Based Medicine: How to Practice and Teach EBM*, 2nd edition. Edinburgh: Churchill Livingstone.

Sackett, D. L., Richardson, W. S., Rosenberg, W., and Haynes, B. (1997). *Evidence-Based Medicine: How to Practice & Teach EBM*. London: Churchill Livingstone.

Sackett, D. L., Rosenberg, W. M., Gray, J. A., Haynes, R. B., and Richardson, W. S. (1996). Evidence based medicine: What it is and what it isn't. *BMJ* 312(7023): 71–72.

Saperia, J., Ashby, D., and Gunnell, D. (2006). Suicidal behaviour and SSRIs: Updated meta-analysis. *BMJ* 332(7555): 1453.

Schulz, K. F. (1995). Subverting randomization in controlled trials. *JAMA* 274(18): 1456–58.

Simpson, S. H., Eurich, D. T., Majumdar, S. R., Padwal, R.S., Tsuyuki, R.T., Varney, J. and Johnson, J.A. (2006). A meta-analysis of the association between adherence to drug therapy and mortality. *BMJ* 333(7557): 15.

Smith, G. C., and Pell, J. P. (2003). Parachute use to prevent death and major trauma related to gravitational challenge: Systematic review of randomised controlled trials. *BMJ* 327(7429): 1459–61.

Spilby, J. (1990). Profile of a consensus development program in the United Kingdom: The King's Fund Forum. In *Improving Consensus Development for Health Technology Assessment: An International Perspective*, eds. C. Goodman and S. R. Baratz. Washington, DC: National Academy Press, pp. 131–36.

Stampfer, M. J., and Colditz, G. A. (1991). Estrogen replacement therapy and coronary heart disease: A quantitative assessment of the epidemiologic evidence. *Prev Med* 20(1): 47–63.

Steel, D. (2008). *Across the Boundaries: Extrapolation in Biology and Social Science.* Oxford: Oxford University Press.

Steel, D. (2010). A new approach to argument by analogy: Extrapolation and chain graphs. *Philosophy of Science* 77(5): 1058–69.

Straus, S. E. (2004). What's the E for EBM? *BMJ* 328(7439): 535–36.

Straus, S. E., Richardson, W. S., Glasziou, P., and Haynes, R. B. (2005). *Evidence-Based Medicine: How to Practice and Teach EBM*, 3rd edition. London: Elsevier: Churchill Livingstone.

Teira, D. (2010). Frequentist versus Bayesian clinical trials. In *Philosophy of Medicine*, ed. F. Gifford. Amsterdam: Elsevier, pp. 255–97.

Thagard, P. (1999). *How Scientists Explain Disease*. Princeton, NJ; Chichester: Princeton University Press.

Tonelli, M. R. (1998). The philosophical limits of evidence-based medicine. *Acad Med* 73(12): 1234–40.

Tonelli, M. R. (2006). Integrating evidence into clinical practice: An alternative to evidence-based approaches. *J Eval Clin Pract* 12(3): 248–56.

Travers, J., Marsh, S., Williams, M., Weatherall, M., Caldwell, B., Shirtcliffe, P., Aldington, S., and Beasley, R. (2007). External validity of randomised controlled trials in asthma: To whom do the results of the trials apply? *Thorax* 62(3): 219–23.

Trial, CAS & II Investigators. (1992). Effect of the antiarrhythmic agent moricizine on survival after myocardial infarction. *N Engl J Med* 327(4), 227–33.

Tröhler, U. (2001). *To Improve the Evidence of Medicine: The 18th Century British Origins of a Critical Approach*. Royal College of Physicians of Edinburgh.

Tuteur, W. (1958). The double blind method: Its pitfalls and fallacies. *Am J Psychiatry* 114(10): 921–22.

Upshur, R. (2005). Looking for rules in a world of exceptions: Reflections on evidence-based practice. *Perspectives in Biology and Medicine* 48(4): 477–89.

White, H. (2009). *Theory-Based Impact Evaluation: Principles and Practice*. New Delhi: International Initiative for Impact Evaluation.

Winkle, R. A., Mason, J. W., Griffin, J. C., and Ross, D. (1981). Malignant ventricular tachyarrhythmias associated with the use of encainide. *Am Heart J* 102(5): 857–64.

World Bank. (1990). Project Completion Report. India. Tamil Nadu Integrated Nutrition Project. Washington: World Bank, Operations Evaluation Department. Internal Report.

World Bank. (1998). Implementation Completion Report. India. Second Tamil Nadu Integrated Nutrition Project. Washington: World Bank, Operations Evaluation Department.

Worrall, J. (2002). What evidence in evidence-based medicine? *Philosophy of Science* 69(Supplement): S316–S30.

Worrall, J. (2007a). Why there's no cause to randomize. *British Journal for the Philosophy of Science* 58(3): 451–88.

Worrall, J. (2007b). Evidence in medicine. *Compass* 2(6): 981–1022.

Worrall, J. (2010a). Evidence: Philosophy of science meets medicine. *Journal of Evaluation in Clinical Practice* 116: 356–62.

Worrall, J. (2010b). Do we need some large, simple randomized trials in medicine? In *EPSA Philosophical Issues in the Sciences*, eds. M. Suarez, M. Dorato, and M. Redei. Dordrecht: Springer, pp. 978–90.

Zetin, M., and Hoepner, C. T. (2007). Relevance of exclusion criteria in antidepressant clinical trials: A replication study. *J Clin Psychopharmacol* 27(3): 295–301.

Zimmerman, M., Mattia, J. I., and Posternak, M. A. (2002b). Are subjects in pharmacological treatment trials of depression representative of patients in routine clinical practice? *Am J Psychiatry* 159(3): 469–73.

Zimmerman, M., Posternak, M. A., and Chelminski, I. (2002b). Symptom severity and exclusion from antidepressant efficacy trials. *J Clin Psychopharmacol* 22(6): 610–14.

6 Evolutionary Medicine: Philosophical Aspects

Michael Ruse

Why so Long a Wait for Evolutionary Medicine?

When Charles Darwin published his *Origin of Species* in 1859, things (in Britain) were just starting to change dramatically in the area of medical education. Increasingly, it was realized that something had to be done about the quality of training of doctors and related healthcare workers. The Crimean War had shown dramatically how inadequate was the state of British medicine, for more soldiers died off the battlefield than on it. Had Florence Nightingale and her devoted followers not been there, things would have been even worse.

One of the people most involved in the reforming of Victorian Britain in general and medical training in particular was Darwin's great supporter, his "bulldog," Thomas Henry Huxley (Desmond, 1997). He was by the 1860s, especially through the new science university (now Imperial College) being built on profits from the Great Exhibition of 1851, much involved in the reform of science education, and realized that a key component was going to be finding jobs for his students and reciprocally support for his teachers (Ruse, 1996). As a biologist, he saw two major possibilities—school education and medicine. Let us train teachers in basic biology and then they in turn can pass on this knowledge to their pupils, something of far greater use to them in the modern world than older subjects like classics. Let us train would-be doctors in basic biology and then pass them over for clinical training in the great teaching hospitals. They will build on a far better foundation than medics of the past.

Huxley was successful in both of these aims. He himself sat on the London School Board and was influential in getting biological science into the curriculum. (One of his own students and later a schoolteacher in his own right was H. G. Wells, the novelist.) The medical profession loved what he proposed and supported him enthusiastically, snapping up his now properly trained graduates. However, our story starts to get really interesting when we delve into what exactly Huxley was teaching his students. You might think that, as Darwin's greatest booster, his students would get a firm training in evolutionary theory. After all, was not Theodosius Dobzhansky (1973) to say that

147

nothing in biology makes sense except in the light of evolution? Not so at all! Evolution was virtually nonexistent in Huxley's courses. A lecture program of 165 sessions covered anatomy and embryology in great detail. Evolution would get half a lecture at most and Darwin's mechanism of natural selection a mere 10 minutes.

Why this, something remarked on by his own students? Father Hahn (S.J.), who studied under him in 1876, writes:

> One day when I was talking to him, our conversation turned upon evolution. "There is one thing about you I cannot understand," I said, "and I should like a word in explanation. For several months now I have been attending your course, and I have never heard you mention evolution, while in your public lectures everywhere you openly proclaim yourself an evolutionist." (Huxley, 1900, p. 2428)

Basically Huxley's response, to Father Hahn and to the world at large, was that embryology and anatomy—and physiology, a subject that Huxley got trained assistants to teach—were serious parts of professional science, whereas evolution had a different role. It was more a world picture, a kind of secular religion if you like, that made sense of existence and of our place in it, but that did not belong in the teaching classroom. Or putting the matter another way, Huxley could not see how evolution could cure a pain in the belly, and it was to that end that his biological teaching was directed.

So evolutionary theory got excluded from medical training, and that was the way that things went for a hundred or more years (Ruse, 2012). There were some cracks in the wall. Obviously with the rise of eugenics there was interest in health and disease and biological factors involved. This brought up some evolutionary speculating. More pertinently, in the 1950s as with the incorporation of genetics into the evolutionary world picture, and the recognition that Darwinian selection is the main cause of evolutionary change, every now and then medical issues started to emerge. Best known probably was the work on sickle-cell anemia, where it was shown that it is a function of a certain gene in the population, where one dose of the gene (heterozygote) meant that the bearer had a natural immunity to malaria, whereas two doses of the gene (homozygote) meant that the bearer died in childhood of anemia (Alison, 1954a, b). It was shown also that the reason why the sickle-cell gene persists is that the protection offered for the heterozygotes balances the cost of the deaths of the homozygotes. Evolution—natural selection—was at the center of this understanding, as it also was in related work done particularly at the University of Liverpool by students of the British ecological geneticist E. B. Ford. He got money from the Nuffield Foundation—a charity founded on the fortune of the British equivalent of the American automobile magnate Henry Ford—to show how the work of his group on evolution in the Lepidoptera (butterflies and moths) is a good model for human diseases.

But these were isolated instances, and it was not really until the 1990s, when the mega-phenomenon of the Human Genome Project was inaugurated, that serious interest started to arise in evolutionary questions pertaining to medicine. Nothing however compared to the influence of the jointly authored book, by physician Randolph Nesse and evolutionary biologist George C. Williams, *Why We Get Sick: The New Science of Evolutionary Medicine*, published in 1994. With this major call to arms, the modern field of evolutionary medicine was launched. I will leave it to others to talk about its successes, and the extent that it has or has not made inroads into the conservative area of medical school education. Here I want to focus on what I think is a matter of some considerable interest, the philosophical aspects and implications of Darwinian medicine. What does philosophy have to say about the subject? Can it help at all? Does it have existing resources? Does Darwinian medicine point to areas that need further philosophical development? As my guide, I will rely on the superb textbook *Principles of Evolutionary Medicine* (2009), by the eminent New Zealand medical scientist Sir Peter Gluckman and his associates (Alan Beedle and Mark Hanson). He offers an eightfold classification of the ways in which evolution can have relevance for medicine; so let us start there.

Evolution and Medicine

First, there is the obvious (although perhaps overlooked) but crucial factor of our environment outstripping our evolved nature. For obvious reasons, having a sweet tooth might be of great evolutionary advantage. If food supplies are scarce, being prepared to go that extra mile for (let us say) honey could be of great advantage, given the quick and important boost a foodstuff like this can offer. So having the biological motivation could be a major factor in biological success. But today, with agriculture and easy access to valuable foodstuffs, the advantages of a sweet tooth are much less obvious, and clearly, given the obesity problem in modern advanced society, it can be counterproductive.

Somewhat more subtle is something like lactose tolerance and intolerance. Humans used to be intolerant of milk stuffs—at least after childhood. Why would they need to be otherwise? But then with the domestication of cattle in particular an easy-to-obtain-but-valuable source of protein became available. So there seems to have been strong selection in this direction—at least strong selection of populations for whom milk was available. This does mean obviously that some peoples are going to be intolerant even today, and with easy transport and the possibility of living elsewhere one needs to be sensitive to these points. Students from China, for instance, may well be intolerant. And there will be people in our own society for whom selection has not done the needed job. There is some suggestion that Charles Darwin may have been lactose intolerant and that this accounts for his ongoing adult illnesses (Dixon and Radick, 2009). It is noteworthy that when he went off for cures at spas and the like, his health improved. Perhaps it had little to do with a regime of cold baths and much with the Spartan diet to which he was subjected. When he returned home to the heavily cream-laden meals his wife prepared, he once again fell sick.

Second, there are life-history factors. Today, again speaking of advanced countries, we tend to live very much longer than we did hitherto. Selection will be indifferent to this fact. In biologically unsuspected old age, things could break down because selection has not worked on human bodies in this state. Selection is interested in a functioning prostate at 20 not at 70. In fact, of course, selection might even work against old age if it benefits youth. It is thought that stem cells in tissues might be a case in point. They promote healthy tissue in youth but can misfire and bring on cancers in old age.

Third come defense mechanisms out of control. Morning sickness might well be a good adaptation because it is a sensitivity toward certain food stuffs in early pregnancy. The fetuses of women with morning sickness could well be better off than the fetuses of women without morning sickness. For obvious reasons, with information like this, one might well want to modify the treatment offered. It does not follow that no treatment should be offered, but if one thought one was working with someone particularly sensitive to certain food-stuffs and the like, one might aim for avoidance in the first place rather than covering up after the problem starts. The same is true of fever when sick. There is evidence that this is an adaptation used in fighting infection. Simply bringing down a fever might be counterproductive.

The fourth factor centers on "evolutionary arms races." Going back to Darwin himself, it is a well-documented fact that lines of organisms compete against each other. (More strictly the individuals in lines of organisms compete against each other.) The prey gets faster and so the predator gets faster. The boring apparatus gets more efficient. The shell gets thicker (Dawkins and Krebs, 1979). In the health world, such races are practically the norm rather than the exception. A new drug to fight bacteria is introduced. Within months, the bacteria have developed a natural immunity to the drug. Penicillin is the classic case. Introduced in 1942, by the end of the war resistant strains were starting to appear. Moreover methods of resistance can vary, so no one simply modifying solution may be possible.

Fifth comes the matter of design or constraints (Amundson, 1994). Childbirth tends to be difficult for human beings. A major reason is the size of the child's head. Likewise, humans are prone to lower back pain simply because our design is that of two-legged animals on a four-legged frame. The wonder is that we do not suffer more than we do. Obviously realizing what is going on here does not necessarily solve problems, but if nothing else one might get away from some of the nonsense talk about being "natural" and not doing things that go against nature. If nature could not do the job properly—and there is no a priori reason why it always should and, given the nature of natural selection, many reasons why sometimes it does not—then there is hardly objection to our trying to improve on things. If an episiotomy prevents vaginal tears, then go for it.

Sixth is the case we have discussed already, where selection balances good effects against bad. Sickle-cell anemia is the textbook case. It is thought possibly that cystic fibrosis may be another, with protections for those with just one gene against typhoid and tuberculosis. The tragedy of course is that as we develop ways of preventing things like malaria—perhaps simply by moving to a part of the world where there is no malaria—we do not thereby remove the dangerous genes. Unfortunately even if selection now swings into action against these genes, it will be many generations before they are reduced in number appreciably.

The seventh factor centers on Darwin's secondary mechanism, sexual selection (Darwin, 1871). At the least, this can obviously lead to societally disruptive behavior, particularly by young males. Of course, and here we can see how philosophical issues lurk, a major issue is going to revolve around how we distinguish responsibility from genuine disorder calling for medical understanding. When does a compulsion about sex move from fun to irritating to positively unhealthy?

Finally, number eight, there are issues to do with history. If one belongs to a small group that may possibly have gone through a bottleneck where the population numbers were very much reduced, one may well be more liable to certain diseases than members of the general public. One thinks, for instance, of the high prevalence of Tay Sachs disease among Ashkenazi Jews. There is nothing in the Jewish way of life as such that makes one liable to Tay Sachs disease—circumcision or avoidance of pork—rather it is that mutations occurred in their group and have persisted because (until fairly recently) there was not significant breeding outside the group.

The Science

Starting to veer toward the more philosophical end of the spectrum, one has first questions about the nature of the science being presupposed in evolutionary medicine. Generally speaking, and this is going to apply particularly to any discipline where George Williams (1966) was a major influence, evolutionary understanding today is going to make natural selection the chief underlying causal factor. No one, for instance, is going to give much credence to any approach depending on Lamarckian factors—the inheritance of acquired characteristics. Evolutionary medicine is going in this sense to be Darwinian. However, making selection important does not preclude a number of other issues raising questions of some interest. There are two big factors that need discussion.

First, to what extent is selection going to be considered all-powerful and all-inclusive? Already we can see that no one—and this includes the most ardent of Darwinians—is going to say that selection has produced perfection in every respect on every occasion (Gould and Lewontin, 1979; Ruse, 2006). The whole point about natural selection is that it is a comparative matter. It is not a question of being perfect but of being better than the competition. In the land of the blind, the man with one eye is king. Or to use the old joke: when you are running from a bear in the forest, it is not a matter of breaking world records but of running faster than the other chap. George Williams (1966) himself makes this point strongly, pointing out that the male urogenital tract is about as badly designed as it possibly could be, with tubes wandering all around the lower body rather than going directly to get on with the job.

This is not to say that there may not be differences and disputes about whether or not something is under the control of selection, and if so to what end. To take a classic case of dispute from outside the medical realm, it is well known that many plants exhibit what is known as phyllotaxis—a rather stylized pattern of parts. Sunflowers show this in the packing of the seeds in the flower; so also do pinecones; even cauliflowers are subject to the same rules. There has been much discussion about the reason for phyllotaxis, with early Darwinians claiming that it provided a triumph of selective explanation, for the patterns had clear utility, for instance, in helping seeds to get distributed (Gray, 1879). More recently, critics have argued that phyllotaxis has no selective advantages and is simply a function of mathematics and the purely contingent matter of the order in which plant parts are produced (Goodwin, 2001). Nevertheless, Darwinians argue that while mathematics is indeed involved, natural selection picks up and works with and on top of all of this (Niklas, 1988). One can see how there might be all sorts of related types of questions in medicine. Fever is a good example. The body clearly has its own natural defenses against disease, but is fever one of them? If it is, then in what way is it defending the body? Is it killing alien attackers directly or is it stimulating the production of other factors that then kill or repel the attackers? Or is fever just an unfortunate by-product of the body defending itself or even just a result of the attack? How one answers these questions is clearly going to be pertinent to proposed treatments. Even if fever itself has no value, if one reduces it, will one thereby be reducing the associated factors that do have value?

The second question is about the nature of selection itself. As is well known, for 50 years now there has been intense debate about the level at which natural selection works—although in fact this is a debate that goes back to the codis-coverers of natural selection, Charles Darwin and Alfred Russel Wallace (Ruse, 1980; Dawkins, 1976; Sober and Wilson, 1997). Does selection always work for the individual, perhaps even at the level of the gene—"selfish genes"—or can selection work for the group perhaps even the species? Often this does not make much difference. If let us say every individual in a species of cat is doing well, then in a sense one can say that the species is doing well. Although of course this does not necessarily follow. The cats individually may be doing well, but compared to another species of cat the species as a whole might be falling behind. More particularly, within a species organisms may be compet-ing, and what is good for one organism is certainly not good for others, or perhaps in the end for the species as a whole. In sexual selection, for instance, a feature might be very effective in attracting mates but then might get so accen-tuated and bizarre that in the end the individuals collapse in on themselves and the species goes extinct. Some have thought that the exaggerated antlers of the Irish elk might be a case in point.

Mother–offspring Conflict

Where the debate about whether selection works for the individual always or can work for the group starts to have real bite is where the interests are clearly in opposition. This happens most obviously in the case of social organisms. Can it ever be the case that an individual can give to others—show "altruism"—at its own expense? Can selection work against the individual and in favor of the group? Most Darwinians think that although this is logically possible, it is very unlikely to happen in practice (West and Gardner, 2013). Altruism of this nature can never be stable and will always been wiped out quickly. If we have two individuals, one of whom is giving and other taking without return, then it is the second who will be favored by selection and soon the former and its kind will go extinct. This is not to say that we might not get altruism of a more mod-erate kind, where although an individual may not benefit directly its relatives will benefit and so (since they are sharers of the same genes) the individual benefits biologically indirectly. A mother feeding her baby, for instance. The mother gets no direct reward, but through the baby her line goes on (Hamilton, 1964; Smith, 1982).

Harvard biologist David Haig (2008) argues that a particularly striking example of individual selection, where an organism has an adaptation that seems almost counterintuitive, occurs in the case of preeclampsia—a danger-ous ailment in pregnancy that involves high blood pressure and carries a severe risk of stroke and possible death. Intuitively it seems obvious that the biologi-cal interests of the unborn child and its mother are identical. After all, having babies is what Darwinian evolution is all about. But in fact their interests do not necessarily coincide. Suppose a mother has a couple of children and that if unattended both will die but that if one is killed the other will survive. It is in the mother's interests to kill off one of her children, although it is hardly in the interests of that child to be killed. Conversely, if there are limited resources it might be in the child's interests to see the mother go, even though it will now have to do without the help that mother can give. Haig suggests that we might have just such a case here. The child needs the benefits from the mother's blood and high blood pressure in the mother increases those benefits. So the risk of death of both mother and infant might be worth it. Haigh notes that, interestingly, preeclampsia more often occurs in cases of twin births, where there might well be stronger competition for nutrients from the mother.

Multilevel Selection

But isn't there something to be said for different levels of selection, a kind of "multilevel" selection as one might say? Consider a fairly recent discussion (by Carl T. Bergstrom and Michael Feldgarden, 2008) of ways in which one might apply insights from evolution to the creation of new barriers to invasive organisms. The dangers posed by bacteria are often not from the individual bacteria as such, but come when they are in groups and start acting together. When we have, what the authors call, a "quorum." Could it be that a solution might lie in tricking the bacteria into thinking that such a quorum does not exist? And could it be that, when the bacteria social behavior is disrupted, it might not rebound as quickly as one might suppose. In their words:

> Where bacterial cooperation occurs, it is not an unavoidable consequence of direct individual selection as antibiotic resistance usually is, but rather a finely balanced consequence of multilevel selection. Thus if bacterial cooperation is disrupted, it may not return as readily as individually selected traits. To see how this might work, imagine a population of bacteria in which social behavior has been halted by disrupting quorum sensing. Whereas with conventional antibiotics the first antibiotic-resistant mutant has a substantial growth advantage, with quorum-sensing disrupters the first resistant mutant has a growth disadvantage. It provides a public good by producing constitutively, but it receives no benefits from the other members of the population who are not producing due to the quorum sensing disrupter. Moreover, because these behaviors are selected at the population level, if resistance does evolve it is likely to do so on the time scale of populations, rather than on the time scale of individuals. While a bacterium may reproduce in a matter of hours, populations often turn over on scales of

weeks to months and thus resistance to quorum sensing disruptors is likely to evolve much more slowly than does resistance to conventional antibiotics. (pp. 134–35)

Prima facie it seems that group selection is at work—"behaviors are selected at a population level." However a careful reading shows that no such mechanism is really being proposed. The behaviors occur at the population level, but because they do not at first serve the interests of individuals—"it receives no benefits from the other members of the population"—they do not spread quickly. Indeed, the question is why they spread at all. "Multilevel selection" is not a term being used to bring in group selection. It is rather to acknowledge that individual selection can have group effects that are going to be important to the individual.

Health and Disease

Let us move now from the more epistemological side of things—what kind of theory are we dealing with and why—to the more ethical, or at least value-laden, side of things. For some years now, there has been a steady literature on the key medical notions of health and sickness or disease. How do these play out against the background of evolutionary medicine? Health in a way is the fundamental notion; it is certainly the state to which medicine aspires (although somewhat paradoxically medicine exists only because aspirations fail); but it is also in a way the more difficult to capture. Turn first therefore to the idea of sickness, brought on by disease. There are two ways to regard disease—one is to regard it as a natural phenomenon (Peter has chicken pox), and the other is to see it as normative from the start (the philosophy graduate student did much better after he had had treatment for his sexual addictions). The well-known philosopher Philip Kitcher puts matters in terms of objectivity and subjectivity.

Some scholars, objectivists about disease, think that there are facts about the human body on which the notion of disease is founded, and that those with a clear grasp of those facts would have no trouble drawing lines, even in the challenging cases. Their opponents, constructivists about disease, maintain that this is an illusion, which the disputed cases reveal how the values of different social groups conflict, rather than exposing any ignorance of facts, and that agreement is sometimes even produced because of universal acceptance of a system of values (Kitcher, 1997, pp. 208–209).

Start with the naturalistic or objective treatment of disease. The standard treatment comes from Christopher Boorse (1975, also 1977, 1987). He specifies: "On our view, disease judgments are value neutral . . . their recognition is a matter of natural science, not evaluative decision" (Boorse, 1977, p. 543). But how does one cash out the reference to natural science? In some sense, it has to be a matter of what is normal or natural for the species. "There is a definite standard of normality inherent in the structure and effective functioning of each species or organism ... Human beings are to be considered normal if they possess the full number of ... capacities natural to the human race, and if these ... are so balanced and inter-related that they function together effectively and harmoniously" (p. 554). But how now are we to understand the "definite standard of normality"? It cannot be—or surely should not be—just a matter of counting. Homosexuals are in a minority, but that as such neither makes them sick nor healthy. Sickle-cell anemia sufferers are in a minority, but we do not say that they are diseased because of this. Rather it is because having sickle-cell anemia means that you are in pain, you are unhappy, you are not functioning well.

Now, if you are determined to push the naturalist position, you might seize on the last of these criteria and try to work from there—"not functioning well." Surely if one is functioning well or not is an objective matter, because the sense of "well" here is not a normative one in the sense of good or bad, but rather an evaluative one in the sense of keeping up to a standard properly. One might say, for instance, that the electric chair is a good method of execution, without in any sense believing that execution is ever a good thing. A Mormon with five wives and thirty kids may be functioning well biologically, even though you disapprove strongly of his lifestyle. But that is the problem here. Is someone with sickle-cell anemia not functioning well? At a personal level, presumably not. However the whole system is promoted by natural selection, because the heterozygotes are doing super-well. So the system as a whole is functioning nicely.[1] And yet one surely wants to say that sickle-cell anemia is an illness in some sense.

Part of the problem here, as Randolph Nesse is always stressing, is that selection does not care about how you feel, whether you are happy or sad, but only about whether you are surviving and reproducing (Nesse and Williams, 1994). This has led some, Kenneth Schaffner (1993), for instance, to argue that we should always take ultimate ends—like survival and reproduction—out of the discussion, and focus just on the immediate ends and issues.

Schaffner (1993) has argued very convincingly that although medicine might use teleological talk in its attempts to develop a mechanistic picture of how humans work, the teleology is just heuristic. It can be completely dispensed with when the mechanistic explanation of a given organ or process is complete. Schaffner argues that as we learn more about the causal role a structure plays in the overall functioning of the organism, the need for teleological talk of any kind drops out and is superseded by the vocabulary of mechanistic explanation, and that evolutionary functional ascriptions are merely heuristic; they focus our attention on "entities that satisfy the secondary [i.e., mechanistic] sense of function and that it is important for us to know more about" (p. 390; see also Murphy, 2008).

We have to be careful here when we are talking about "just heuristic." My suspicion is that many (and I would include myself here) would be very uncomfortable with the claim that the teleology in evolutionary biology could ever, even in theory, be eliminated (Ruse, 2003). Evolutionary biology is infused with the design metaphor, seeing organisms as if designed by a conscious intelligence. Evolutionary biologists today do not think that they necessarily were designed by such an intelligence—although presumably there are those today who would follow Darwin in thinking that there was such an intelligence at work, but at a distance. But it is hard to see how evolutionary biology could function without the assumption of design. Without the assumption one would not ask questions like: "What is the function of the plates on the back of the Stegosaurus?" Nor would one get answers like: "They exist in order to control the bodily temperature of that particular kind of dinosaur" (Kant, in his *Third Critique—The Critique of Judgement* (1790), although no evolutionist is very good on this point).

But perhaps this is not really Schaffner's main point. Perhaps his real worry is that we spend our time thinking through the biology when we should be focusing on the immediate issues and specifically the things worrying people right here and now—this calls for a material explanation, that is, one in terms of efficient causes rather than final causes (to use an Aristotelian mode of understanding).[2] At one level, I doubt the evolutionary medicine supporter is going to disagree. While we need to know the objective or natural causes of an illness or disease, ultimately it is hard not to agree that value considerations do enter into the judgment. One is ill if one is feeling bad or if one has something with the potential to make one feel bad—this latter would, I take it, cover something like high blood pressure or an unfelt lump on the prostate or such things. Tristram Engelhardt Jr. (1976, p. 259) is the point person here: "We identify illnesses by virtue of our experience of them as physically or psychologically disagreeable, distasteful, unpleasant, deforming." Obviously, this is not enough. I am not ill if I am unjustly condemned to death. At once the normativists start moving over toward the naturalist side. We identify them "by virtue of some form of suffering or pathos due to the malfunctioning of our bodies or our minds. We identify disease states as constellations of observables related through a disease explanation of a state of being ill" (p. 259).

At another level though, I suspect that the supporter of evolutionary medicine would argue that someone like Schaffner is missing something very important. Suppose you have a high fever and this makes you feel wretched. It is hard to deny that you are sick or that this is something brought on by a disease. However, if you then learnt that the high fever was an adaptation put in place by natural selection to fight diseases, then while you might still think of the person as sick, you might modify your response.

Health and Well-being

What finally about health and well-being? Usually, as illness and disease seem to call for normative judgments, so health and well-being are taken to call for such judgments also. The philosopher Hans-Georg Gadamer (1996) defined "health" as "a condition of being involved, of being in the world, of being together with one's fellow human beings, of active and rewarding engagement in one's everyday tasks." In a like fashion, the World Health Organization (WHO, 1946) defines "health" as "a state of complete physical, mental and social well-being and not merely the absence of disease or infirmity."

Clearly if you do think of health somewhat along these lines, biology is going to play into the discussion, but it is going to be far from definitive. One is not going to define health purely in terms of survival and reproduction. Having a sense of fulfillment and being worthwhile is part of being healthy, and obsession with numbers of children is surely odd to the point of imbalance somewhere. Nevertheless, having children may be a very important part of what one considers full and healthy living. It is true that today there are voices (especially in the Western world) who argue that children are an option and not necessarily the best or right option. Most people however do not think this way and (although they may hesitate to say it too loudly) rather think of people who voluntarily forego having children as if not sick then sadly truncated as human beings. Moreover unless you are essentially free from disease and handicap, you are probably less likely to have total fulfillment and thus less likely to be judged totally healthy. So biology surely does come in somewhere, and the pertinence of the evolutionary approach is not to be denied totally or even in large part.

Epilogue

Evolutionary medicine is still young and growing. I hope that I have convinced you that it raises questions of great philosophical interest and that in return it offers rewards to those prepared to understand and engage.

Notes

1. This is not group selection. There is no suggestion that selection is benefiting the group. What is happening is that selection is promoting the good of some organisms at the expense of others. One could well imagine that the costs of caring for the afflicted could be so great that as a group all suffer. Better that the group be completely less than super-fit individuals, but able to manage, and go from there.

2. An efficient cause is one that brings things about—the hammer hit the nail and the nail penetrated further into the wooden board. A final cause is one that gives the reason why things happen—the carpenter drove the nail into the board in order to hang pictures from it. Although the efficient cause works from the past to the present whereas the final cause works from the future to the present, they are not strictly symmetrical. If there is an effect, the efficient cause has occurred. If the nail is in the wood, the efficient cause occurred. It may well be that the final cause never occurs. The nail is in the wood, but no one bothers to hang pictures from it.

References

Allison, A. C. (1954a). Protection by the sickle-cell trait against subtertian malarial infection. *British Medical Journal* 1: 290.

Allison, A. C. (1954b). The distribution of the sickle-cell trait in East Africa and elsewhere and its apparent relationship to the incidence of subtertian malaria. *Transactions of the Royal Society of Tropical Medical Hygiene* 48: 312.

Amundson, R. (1994). Two concepts of constraint: Adaptationism and the challenge from developmental biology. *Philosophy of Science* 61: 556–78.

Bergstrom, C. T., and M. Feldgarden. (2008). The ecology and evolution of antibiotic-resistant bacteria. In *Evolution in Health and Disease,* 2nd edition, eds. S. C. Sterns and J. C. Koella. Oxford: Oxford University Press, pp. 125–37.

Boorse, C. (1975). On the distinction between disease and illness. *Philosophy and Public Affairs* 5: 49–68.

Boorse, C. (1977). Health as a theoretical concept. *Philosophy of Science* 44: 542–73.

Boorse, C. (1987). Concepts of health. *Health Care Ethics* 359–93. Philadelphia: Temple University Press.

Darwin, C. (1859). *On the Origin of Species by Means of Natural Selection, or the Preservation of Favoured Races in the Struggle for Life.* London: John Murray.

Darwin, C. (1871). *The Descent of Man, and Selection in Relation to Sex.* London: John Murray.

Dawkins, R. (1976). *The Selfish Gene.* Oxford: Oxford University Press.

Dawkins, R., and Krebs, J. R. (1979). Arms races between and within species. *Proceedings of the Royal Society of London B* 205: 489–511.

Desmond, A. (1997). *Huxley: From Devil's Disciple to Evolution's High Priest.* New York: Basic Books.

Dixon, M., and Radick, G. (2009). *Darwin in Ilkley.* Stroud, UK: History Press.

Dobzhansky, T. (1973). Nothing in biology makes sense except in the light of evolution. *American Biology Teacher* 35: 125–29.

Engelhardt, H. T. (1976). Ideology and etiology. *Journal of Medicine and Philosophy* 1: 256–68.

Gadamer, H.-G. (1996). *The Enigma of Health.* Stanford: Stanford University Press.

Gluckman, P., Beedle, A., and Hanson, M. (2009). *Principles of Evolutionary Medicine.* Oxford: Oxford University Press.

Goodwin, B. (2001). *How the Leopard Changed Its Spots,* 2nd edition. Princeton: Princeton University Press.

Gould, S. J., and Lewontin, R. C. (1979). The spandrels of San Marco and the Panglossian paradigm: A critique of the adaptationist programme. *Proceedings of the Royal Society of London, Series B: Biological Sciences* 205: 581–98.

Gray, A. (1879). *Structural Botany.* New York and Chicago: Ivison, Blakeman, Taylor.

Haig, D. (2008). Intimate relations: Evolutionary conflicts of pregnancy and childhood. In *Evolution in Health and Disease*, 2nd. edition, eds. S. C. Sterns and J. C. Koella. Oxford: Oxford University Press, pp. 65–76.

Hamilton, W. D. (1964). The genetical evolution of social behaviour. *Journal of Theoretical Biology* 7: 1–52.

Huxley, L. (1900). *The Life and Letters of Thomas Henry Huxley*. London: Macmillan.

Kant, I. [1790] (1951). *Critique of Judgement*. New York: Haffner.

Kitcher, P. (1997). *The Lives to Come: The Genetic Revolution and Human Possibilities*, 2nd edition. New York: Simon and Schuster.

Murphy, D. (2008). Concepts of health and disease. *The Stanford Encyclopedia of Philosophy*, E. N. Zalta, ed. http://plato.stanford.edu/entries/health-disease/.

Nesse, R. M., and Williams, G. C. (1994). *Why We Get Sick: The New Science of Darwinian Medicine*. New York: Times Books.

Niklas, K. J. (1988). The role of phyllotactic pattern as a "developmental constraint" on the interception of light by leaf surfaces. *Evolution* 42: 1–16.

Ruse, M. (1980). Charles Darwin and group selection. *Annals of Science* 37: 615–30.

Ruse, M. (1996). *Monad to Man: The Concept of Progress in Evolutionary Biology*. Cambridge, MA: Harvard University Press.

Ruse, M. (2003). *Darwin and Design: Does Evolution Have a Purpose?* Cambridge, MA: Harvard University Press.

Ruse, M. (2006). *Darwinism and Its Discontents*. Cambridge: Cambridge University Press.

Ruse, M. (2012). *The Philosophy of Human Evolution*. Cambridge: Cambridge University Press.

Schaffner, K. (1993). *Discovery and Explanation in Biology and Medicine*. Chicago: University of Chicago Press.

Smith, J. M. (1982). *Evolution and the Theory of Games*. Cambridge: Cambridge University Press.

Sober, E., and Wilson, D. S. (1997). *Unto Others: The Evolution of Altruism*. Cambridge, MA: Harvard University Press.

West, S. A., and Gardner, A. (2013). Adaptation and inclusive fitness. *Current Biology* 23: R577–R584.

Williams, G. C. (1966). *Adaptation and Natural Selection*. Princeton, NJ: Princeton University Press.

World Health Organization (WHO). (1946). WHO definition of Health. *Preamble to the Constitution of the World Health Organization as Adopted by the International Health Conference*.

7 Medical Humanism Part 1: Philosophical and Historical Underpinnings

Alfred I. Tauber

Introduction

The thought collective (or paradigm) governing clinical medicine for over a century centers on the scientific basis of defining disease and the therapeutic interventions based on that understanding. This preoccupation with the mastery of disease is, of course, the traditional mission of healthcare and as such dominates any philosophical comment on medical practice and the doctor–patient relationship. However, underlying this epistemological orientation rests an older humanist tradition attendant to deeper moral concerns, which grounds medicine in all of its manifestations: Traditional humanism embraces a logic or orientation that asserts the primacy of human dignity, tempered not so much by empathy, but rather an ethos directed toward fulfilling creative human potential, morally. Couple this orientation to Reason, which, in its broadest purview, promotes the attainment of human self-understanding, yields an ethical calculus that permits choice and self-responsibility based on rational deliberation. Thus the rich humanistic tradition regards humans as potentially self-willed and responsible for their fate, a sentiment perhaps best described by Giovanni Pico della Mirandola (1965, p. 5) in 1486:

> Thou, like a judge appointed for being honorable, art the molder and maker of thyself; thou mayest sculpt thyself into whatever shape thou dost prefer. Thou canst grow downward into the lower nature which are brutes. Thou canst again grow upward from thy soul's reason into the higher natures which are divine.

In the context of medical practice, which has repeatedly been accused of diluting its ethical concern for the person, humanism makes its claims for a reason that encompasses both the humane treatment with an appropriate balance between an austere objectivity (following the demands of a positivist science) and the rational measure of that power in the context of human suffering.

Critics repeatedly decry science's assumed authority that threatens its proper assessment and use, where the "scientific picture of the world *replaces* the common-sense picture" (Sellers, 1956, 1997, pp. 82–83; emphasis in the original), or what humanists would call the "measure of man." Despite the achievements of the scientific worldview, humanists rightly fear the unmitigated influence of a scientific reductionism accompanying the success of positivist medicine. They justly are troubled by the danger of misplaced applications and unbridled dominance over other forms of knowing. Scientism is imperialistic, assuming to apply its methods and logic in arenas where, because of its authority, caution is required. Humanists rightly are suspicious of claims that are by their very nature fallible and which history has repeatedly demonstrated are infected by pernicious cultural determinants. Couple intellectual arrogance to science's economic and political power, and the call of balancing scientism with a modifying humanism ground all appeals to a more humane approach to healthcare.

The history of this issue must be counted as one of the most perplexing chapters of the West's intellectual evolution. Modern science in many ways exemplifies the Age of Reason: Asserting a distinction between an understanding of reason that serves a predetermined goal (e.g., one defined by religious faith) as opposed to the use of enlightened reason that is unrestricted by prior dogma. Inquiry in this latter formulation has no *telos* other than the inquiry itself. In this sense, scientific knowledge is neutral; the process of study is putatively immune to bias and prejudice (at least in its theoretical prime state); fallibilism is assumed; objectivity is sought. This view of epistemic accomplishment is fundamental to liberal thought and thus binds science firmly to kindred liberal political and moral philosophies originating under the humanist banner. Each share the same critical values and, in many respects, the same methods of analysis and tireless questioning of the fruits of their respective studies. This kindred commitment places the call for a humanist-oriented medicine well within a historical trajectory, which justifies a renewed examination of those claims.

Specifically, from the humanist perspective, in the medical scenario how the science addresses the demands of the patient's needs as a *person* (as opposed to a disease-centered approach) claims dominance over any other concern. Accordingly, medicine becomes a humane-intended activity. This orientation puts medicine's science and technology in service to fulfilling human need along the entire spectrum spread from psychological and social concerns to the most effective applied technology for the treatment of disease (Pellegrino, 1979; Tauber, 1999). The tension between a scientific medicine oriented by the objectivist view and the humanistic demands of responding to the preservation of human dignity in the face of a patient's personal experience of illness finds its roots well before the advent of scientific medicine. The close linkage of science as "natural philosophy" and moral philosophy began to uncouple in the eighteenth century. That intellectual development frames our own imbroglio, for clinical medicine must adjudicate the rightful claims of each orientation. That history we now review.

The Enlightened Whole

"Natural philosophers" became "scientists" in the mid-nineteenth century, when practitioners, both natural and social scientists, distinguished their own technical and professional route from the more general concerns of humanists. The break, already evident at the end of the eighteenth century, clearly emerged when both poets and physicists recognized a seeming chasm opening between them. The issue focused on the character of "reason," which originally was conceived as undivided between these two domains.

The Enlightenment celebrated an unfettered reason; the relentless questioning of authority and doctrine; the promotion of individuality and free-choice; the centrality of autonomous selfhood and moral agency; the confidence in progress; and the sanctity of secularism. In this general view, "reason" spilled over into all endeavors of human thought and industry. Indeed, only with the growing appreciation that different kinds of reason coexisted in different domains did the "problem" of reason's unity arise. And as science increasingly demonstrated its own unique use and understanding of reason, it began to lose it tethers to other forms of reason from which it developed. After all, science became an expression of a form of rationality that had further developed the movement toward reasoned, open-ended inquiry that held the fallibility of knowledge as inviolate. This was an Enlightenment ideal, whose ancestry stretched into the Renaissance, when philosophers increasingly turned their attention to deciphering nature's secrets.

During the Enlightenment, those who pondered the nature of knowledge were struck by a growing separation of investigative methods employed by those who studied the natural world, on one hand, and those who commented on the social, spiritual, and psychological domains, on the other. Distinctions between opinion and knowledge, always a central concern of philosophy in one form or another, by the mid-eighteenth century had reached a critical crisis. David Hume drew these distinctions with particular sharpness. He presented Immanuel Kant with the challenge of refuting a skepticism that placed objective knowledge of the natural world in doubt. Indeed, on what basis could knowledge of the natural world or the moral universe be conceived as legitimate and well grounded? The place of reason, the role of emotions, the intuitions of the spiritual domain, and the ability to understand human psychology each required a model of the mind that would account for their respective claims to access these particular forms of knowledge.

Kant began by offering a schema of the mind that made the natural world intelligible, and thus susceptible to scientific investigation. He proposed a schema in which knowledge of the natural world and the moral domain required two different kinds of human cognition. He called these, respectively, "pure" and "practical" reason. "Pure" reason referred to the cognitive functions that humans apply to the natural world.[1] In contrast, "practical" reason dealt with the moral realm. In other words, Kant thought that humans possess one faculty for knowing the material world, best exemplified by scientific inquiry, and he held that a second universe, the moral–spiritual–personal, was, in terms of the first form of understanding, unknowable. People might believe in the freedom of the will, the immortality of the soul, and the divine, but the means by which humans might "know" such metaphysical claims was not discernable by the same means by which humans knew the natural world.[2]

The consequence of this division was, from Kant's perspective, a way to save Belief.[3] But what he in fact did (for those so inclined) was to legitimatize one way of knowing as "real" and the other as "less real." In short, science could claim a special legitimacy, albeit Kant's transcendental claims were immediately attacked and the philosophical basis of his theory of science led to unresolved debate (e.g., Brittan, 1978; Beiser, 1987; Friedman, 1992). In any case, science increasingly asserted its own agenda with more confidence, and some would say with arrogance. However, note, any commitment to this configuration of reason still required that some balance be sought between what Kant called the reason of the empirical domain and the reason of the moral. Specifically, where does scientific inquiry end and other modes of knowing take over? For instance, the hermeneutical (interpretive) disciplines employ a legitimate countervailing method of knowing. From this perspective, only an interpretative stance makes any sense when assessing a work of art or determining the meaning of behavior. Systems of justice, cultural practices, and human psychology cannot be reduced to strict objective inquiry, but rather rest on different kinds of assessment and interpretation. And when religious knowledge makes its claims, on what basis might a scientific attitude allow for the spiritual?[4]

These questions will not rest and, indeed, they frame the basic issues regarding the place of science in a world dominated by human-centered concerns and experience, of which clinical medicine holds a central place. When science is viewed circumspectly, it becomes only one of several modes of inquiry, albeit with its particular strengths, but also with limitations. The line separating objectivity from subjectivity remains highly dynamic, historically contingent, and continuously contested. Despite the obvious importance of making these distinctions, the history of science is marked by the controversy of defining those boundaries, and medicine is one of the crucial battlegrounds of this debate.

Defining Reality

In reaction to the contamination of subjective interpretation, a new objectivity developed in the nineteenth century. The "holistic scientist" was quickly replaced by a new kind of practitioner, a specialist employing a new positivist method. This shift in science's philosophical agenda required a new lexicon to distinguish practitioners of one sort from the other, and, in response, William Whewell (1840, p. cxiii) coined the term "scientist": "We need very much a name to describe a cultivator of science in general. I should incline to call him a *Scientist*." By the end of the nineteenth century, physicians were trained as scientists and aspired to a new ideal, the physician–scientist. Noteworthy is not this definition, but the late date of its birth. After all, the word "science" is ancient. The Latin *scientia* means "knowledge" as opposed to *sapientia*, wisdom. In other words, *scientia* is knowledge of, or cognition about, the world, as opposed to the more self-reflexive domain of *wisdom*. And *sciens*, "knowing," originally meant "to separate one thing from another, to distinguish," which also points to analysis of a particular kind. Certainly this etymology closely adheres to what we broadly understand to be what science seeks. In short, the word "science" has an ancient etymology, but the word "scientist" is distinctly modern.[5]

So, until the mid-nineteenth century, science was a category of philosophy, and philosophy sought to integrate epistemology and moral philosophy. Indeed, their separation was considered a problem, which required analysis and, ultimately, redress.[6] The examination of the natural world was part of what philosophers did, but that activity was in service to a humanist imperative of finding human's place *in* the world. Only as the methods of scientific inquiry became increasingly technical and a new objectivism took hold in its various disciplines did a "scientist" emerge as someone different from a philosopher. If one examines the Western intellectual world as late as the 1850s, the educated classes were comfortably conversant with the latest scientific findings, and many pursued what we would call amateur science (Tauber, 2001). Chemistry and physics began to separate a bit earlier, but certainly natural history remained the province of a wide audience. In short, until about 150 years ago, most scientists and philosophers shared the same intellectual bed (Postlethwaite, 1987).

However, advances in scientific techniques and methods of study required specialization and finally, professionalization.[7] The fruits of that labor resulted in new industries derived from scientific findings and their successful application to material culture. Since the Renaissance, science has been sold as a package deal: Invest in scientific inquiry and the discoveries will be converted into economic, military, and social power. Those promises have been delivered. We now have a huge medical–industrial complex that rivals the military. Most would concur that the investment has been true to its promise, and few could dispute that the triumphs of technology are inseparably linked to the success of the underlying science.[8]   And that achievement rests on the philosophical foundation of positivism, whose precepts were clearly articulate in the nineteenth century.

The Rise of Positivism and its Hegemony

Positivism carries several meanings and has been notoriously difficult to define, yet certain tenets may be identified, especially as espoused in its nineteenth century format (Simon, 1963; Kolakowski, 1968). Foremost, positivists championed a new form of objectivity, one that radically removed the personal report to one that was universally accessible. Thus knowledge, to be "true" and "real," must be attested to by a community of observers who shared common observation. This move from the private sphere of experience to a communal one had begun at the dawn of modern science, but in the mid-nineteenth century this ideal of truth became clearly enunciated as a scientific principle. Thus positivism sought a collection of rules and evaluative criteria by which to distinguish true knowledge.

Positivism contrasted with, indeed, was constructed in opposition to, the romantic view of the world by denying any cognitive importance to value judgments. Experience, positivists maintained, contains no such qualities of men or events as "noble," "good," "evil," or "beautiful." In radical reaction against the romantics, positivists sought instead to objectify nature, banishing human prejudice from scientific judgment. The total separation of observer from the object of observation—an epistemological ideal—reinforced the positivist disavowal of "value" as part of the process of observation. One might interpret, but such evaluative judgments had no scientific (i.e., objective) standing. Simply put, where the Romantics privileged human interpretation (exemplified by artistic imagination), the positivists championed mechanical objectivity (e.g., thermometer, voltmeter, chemical analysis). Indeed, the distinction of scientific "facts" and corrupting subjective "values" represents a crucial distinction in the development of modern science.

The positivists' position originated in the eighteenth century with Hume's famous proclamation that one cannot infer "ought" from "is" (i.e., a moral case cannot be deduced from a natural fact).[9] For Hume, the fact/value distinction originated in an argument against the illogical deduction of religious belief from natural facts and morality from similar constructions derived from natural law or other systems of supposed rational basis (Putnam, 2002). He argued instead that ethics is grounded in human emotions, needs, and caprices that are rationalized into moral justifications. His philosophy supported the scientific aspiration of objectivity, that is, facts divorced from contaminating personal values, which was then more fully developed in the nineteenth century by the positivists.

Cautionary voices were generally ignored. For instance, Goethe, at the end of the eighteenth century, resisting the allure of a radically objective science, appreciated that "facts" do not reside independent of a theory or hypothesis that must support them (a point well developed in twentieth-century philosophy of science) (Tauber, 1993). He contended that "everything factual is already theory" and thereby offered a warning about the epistemological complexity of some idealized notion of objective knowledge. He understood the potential danger of subjective contamination of scientific observation, and more to the point, the tenuous grounds of any objective "fact" that relied in any way on interpretation. ("Interpretation" stretches from inference to direct observation, for any perception must ultimately be processed to fit into a larger picture of nature and must cohere with previous experience.) Accordingly, the synthetic project of building a worldview begins by placing facts within their supporting theory, and continues with integrating that scientific picture with the broader and less obvious intellectual and cultural forces in which science itself is situated. Thus, facts as independent products of sensory experience are *always* processed—interpreted, placed into some overarching hypothesis or theory.

This epistemological critique argued that observations assume their meanings within a particular context, for facts are not just products of sensation or measurement as the positivists averred, but rather they reside within a conceptual framework, which places the fact into an intelligible picture of the world, which included an inescapable point of view (Nagel, 1985). Accordingly, each inviolate observer held a privileged vantage, and the vision so obtained was jealously protected (Tauber, 2001). In contrast, the world built from positivist principles appears essentially the same to all viewers, because facts for them have independent standing and universal accessibility, so that irrespective of individual knowers, facts constitute shared knowledge. From this orientation, the independence of the known "fact" rests on its correspondence to a reality, which any objective observer might know. This assumes both a universal perspective, that "view from nowhere" *and* a correspondence theory of reality. But as Hilary Putnam (1990) cogently argued, even the positivist standards or aspirations of natural science are values, which are developed historically and chosen in everyday practice. So, radical objectivity is compromised, and as stubborn as the positivists might have been in attempting to stamp out subjective influences, they only succeeded in making them seem disreputable (Daston and Galison, 2007). There is no escape from the constraints of an observer fixed by his individual perspective, contextualized in some observational setting, and committed to processing information through some interpretative (namely, subjective) schema. Such an observer cannot adhere to a rigid identification of "facts" based on an idealized separation of the knower and the known. Various kinds of values knit the factual world together into a more or less coherent worldview (Tauber, 2001, 2009).

Despite these caveats, the radical separation of the observing/knowing subject and his object of scrutiny is the single most important characteristic of positivist epistemology. Because of this understanding, positivists claimed that science should rest on a foundation of neutral and dispassionate observation. The more careful the design of the experimental conditions and the more precise the characterization of phenomena, the more likely subjective contaminants would be eliminated. Thus the strict positivist confined herself to phenomena and their ascertainable relationships through a vigorous mechanical objectivity. In the clinical scenario the patient has been displaced by her disease, whose investigation and treatment presumably requires little attention to the restraints imposed by the individual's psychological needs and expectations. In short, a tension divides medicine's scientific agenda from the moral concerns of patient care. That split results from an epistemology operating independently of a moral philosophy, just as the positivists had aspired!

In the life sciences, positivism exercised new standards in the study of physiology that applied the objective methodologies of chemistry and physics to organic processes. The research program found its explicit expression in a revised form of reductionism. Most would argue that the very success of biology and medicine has been in orienting the organic to a physical and genetic reductionism (Tauber and Sarkar, 1993), with the espousal of a strong positivism. This orientation began in the German physiology laboratories of the 1840s, which endeavored to rid biology of both vitalism and teleology as explanatory of life processes. That strategy to provide a comprehensive physico-chemical, and later genetic, explanation of the organic had profound epistemological and metaphysical consequences. The reductionists were initially a group of German physiologists, led by Hermann Helmholtz, who openly declared their manifesto of scientific inquiry (Galaty, 1974). They did not argue that certain organic phenomena were not unique, only that all causes must have certain elements in common. They connected biology and physics by equating the ultimate basis of the respective explanations. Reductionism, specifically physical reductionism as opposed to the later development of genetic reductionism, was also a reaction to romanticism's lingering attachment to vitalism, that is, the notion that life possessed a special "life force," and more generally to a holistic vision of biology. Romantic biology invoked a stratagem that combined vitalism and teleology. Logically independent of each other, they were to be generally viewed as interrelated. The eventual ascendancy of a reductionist science was achieved by mid-nineteenth century in the research program to reject vitalism, waged by the

German reductionist physiologists, and by a separate tributary, a materialistically based evolution invoked by Darwinism (Moulines, 1981; Lenoir, 1989). (Teleology has suffered a much slower expiration, and appears in new guises, but is largely irrelevant to modern discourses of scientific biology.)

This approach allowed newly adopted laboratory techniques to establish physiology as a new discipline and gave birth to biochemistry, whose central tenets held that the fundamental principles of organic and inorganic chemistries were identical, differing only inasmuch as the molecular constituents of living organisms were governed by complex constraints of metabolism. And, of course, this approach seeped into medicine as new standards of training and practice based in a scientific ethos took firm hold at the expense of older forms of humanistic medicine (Tauber, 1992, 2005a).[10]

Thus, positivism was intimately linked to the assumption that all of nature was of one piece, and the study of life was potentially no different in kind than the study of chemical reactions, the movement of heavenly bodies, or the evolution of mountains. Therefore, if all of nature was unified—constituted of the same elements and governed by the same fundamental laws—then the organic world was simply on a continuum with the inorganic. So, according to this philosophy, there was no essential difference between animate and inanimate physics and chemistry, and the organic world was therefore subject to the same kinds of study so successfully applied in physics. In the process, an insidious shift occurred. Man was displaced from his metaphysical perch and assumed a more naturalized standing. Accordingly, physicians were taught to treat the body essentially composed as a machine, governed by uniform chemistry, and thus susceptible to mechanical repair. The new problem became (1) how to reduce the organic to the inorganic, that is, to exhibit the continuity of substance and operation; and (2) concomitantly understand the distinct character of life processes. And as the science marched forward, the patient qua person was often lost in the enthusiasm of this invigorated scientism.[11]

Science from a Nineteenth-century Humanist Perspective

While the sciences were increasing their intellectual influence, more balanced views were clearly articulated and an equilibrium of sorts was still sought. Note how John Merz (1896, vol. 2, pp. 203–204), in his influential (and magisterial) review of nineteenth-century thought, summarized the situation at the end of the century:

> Clearly, besides the abstract sciences, which profess to introduce us to the general relations or laws which govern everything that is or can be real, there must be those sciences which study the actually existing forms as distinguished

from the possible ones, and "here" and "there," the "where" and "how," of things and processes, which look upon real things not as examples of the general and universal, but as alone possessed of that mysterious something which distinguishes the real and actual from the possible and artificial. These sciences are the truly descriptive sciences, in opposition to the abstract ones. They are indeed older than the abstract sciences, and they have, in the course of the period under review in this work, made quite as much progress as the purely abstract sciences. In a manner, though perhaps hardly as powerful in their influence on practical pursuits, they are more popular: they occupy a larger number of students; and inasmuch as they also comprise the study of man himself, they have a very profound influence on our latest opinions, interests, and beliefs—i.e., on our inner life.

Thus the broadest intellectual concerns of some leading scientists during the Victorian period attest to the humane character of their scientific endeavors and the falsity of dividing the intellectual world into simple proscience and antiscience groups. Nineteenth-century science was too multifarious an enterprise to be delineated so clearly, and more to the point, the deepest metaphysical aspirations of its practitioners arose from concerns shared with their poetic brethren.[12]

Humane scientists such as Darwin, Thomas Huxley, and John Tyndall, in promoting the power of scientific explanation, acknowledged the limits of the scientific dominion. With an appreciation that could only be developed from an education steeped in the humanistic tradition, they understood that science's values of objectivity were, indeed, *values.* Science is ultimately based on a belief in the values of objectivity, rationality, and order as construed within certain limits and prescriptions. These are chosen for particular purposes and undergo historical development. In this sense, scientific principles are themselves historically and culturally conditioned. To us, now, it may seem self-evident that the two discourses are governed by different rules of thought, that their respective rationalities possess different characteristics, and that their objects of study demand different methods of exploration. However, in the mid-nineteenth century a synthesis was still possible in the mind of the individual whose eclectic interests allowed diverse pursuits. The tensions and potential contradictions that resulted were widely appreciated (Tauber, 2001),[13] and spawned the rich twentieth century discussions discussed in the accompanying essay.

Binding Scientific Medicine to the Humanist Demand

The project of better aligning science with its humanistic origins, that is, science's deeper philosophical project, originates from the beginning of their schism. Not surprisingly, "humanism" was coined, like the word "scientist," in the nineteenth century to apply to the rediscovery of the classical tradition that had its rejuvenation in the medieval period. Humanists were originally concerned with a general education, which spans the classics to modern science. But humanists accorded particular importance to a liberal agenda: freedom of thought, tolerance, revision and correction of opinion, open communication, and a self-critical attitude. These underlying values tie together the central concerns of the humanities and science into a powerful alliance. In fact, one could argue that these values captured much of philosophy's ethos. Accordingly, the scientific worldview could make its claims based on a long history of coupling its particular concerns to this much larger agenda.

Recall that science also originated as a contributing member of the philosophy faculty, and on this broad view, science is part of a larger historical development of humanistic thought. Although we are usually struck by how science followed a naturalistic philosophy, even its empiricism is based on a rationality that had roots in philosophy, as discussed earlier. Scientific epistemology emerged directly from natural philosophy, which in turn was part of a larger intellectual orientation: through ruthless self-criticism, the frame of reference is always in doubt; the historical record reveals fallibility; the place of objective knowledge as opposed to subjective opinion is tested and contested. And when opinion is held, it is open to revision through free argument. These are the core values of science and the underlying philosophy guiding its methods and defining its aims. Science is sustained, indeed instantiated, by a self-critical philosophy, tested against the empirical investigations of nature. Nature devoid of human value and human caprices demanded plain answers to starkly posed questions. In short, although science and humanities pursue different objects of inquiry, they support each other in common purpose and the same critical attitude. And beyond this kinship we find other aspects that link them.

Subordinate the difference of science's object of study, the natural world, as well as differing methodologies (the empirical basis of scientific investigations), and we are left with an essentialist core—Science, like the humanities, is a human-centered focus of inquiry; "human-centered" in two senses: first, the standards of discourse are human-derived (as opposed to divinely inspired). Revelation has been displaced by a critical stance oriented by new standards of what is factual and what is not. What is knowledge and what is opinion? What is objective and what is subjective? The second component refers to knowledge directed at developing human industry. "Industry" does not refer here to material culture, but rather the more general understanding of industry as the systematic labor to create *value*. The study of nature is deeply committed to a personal comprehension of the world, a picture of reality that offers insight, and thereby an orientation, of Man in Nature. After all, science without its supporting self-critical foundations becomes instrumental, solely a tool for technology.[14]

Scientific findings alone are insufficient for determining significance, and thus interpretation is required (Tauber, 1996, 2009). Commentators from Goethe (Tauber, 1993) to Whewell (1840) to Michael Polanyi (1962) have understood that raw knowledge, a fact, is essentially meaningless. What is the significance of a scientific fact or larger theory unless it may be applied to human understanding? "Understanding" entails many layers of interpretation, and here the linkage to the humanistic disciplines becomes most evident. Science influences its supporting culture, the values that govern its use, and ultimately the sense of meaning and significance ascribed to the scientific portrait of the world. Polanyi called this final step "personal knowledge" when he wrote about the same time as Kuhn about the limits of positivism. Both recognized, as did an entire generation following them, that scientific knowledge was ultimately human-centered in the sense discussed here.[15] On this broad view, science is part of a larger historical development of humanism, and finds itself, ultimately, in its service.

Conclusion

Certain conclusions beckon: first, the "package deal" of *doing* science and *placing* science within its intellectual and social contexts argues that science and its study as a human activity cannot be separated. This interdisciplinary effort arises, because the boundaries of science cannot be circumscribed to the laboratory or technical discourse (Gieryn, 1995). The findings seep into applications, which affect our material culture, medicine, the military, and virtually all aspects of our society. Only an educated public can make appropriate use of the fruits of scientific labor, thus a close coordination between scientists and lay public is required to reap the greatest harvest from the investment made in research. In terms of our discussion, the prioritization of research initiatives, the allocation of resources, and the application of medical technologies are determined in a complex debate between policy makers, medical industrialists, heathcare providers, and the public. The net result of such deliberation reflects competing interests and the underlying cultural and social forces vying for control. So where does the humanistic approach to the patient appear in the vortex of what too often is a discussion based solely in economic terms? A full answer to that question falls beyond this essay, but it seems reasonable to assume that the legal context of medical ethics has become the most effective forum for addressing the broader needs of the patient (Tauber, 2005a, 2006b, 2007). Such protective measures fall well outside the more traditional discourse of humanist philosophies, but here the tossed ball of patient dignity has found its most hospitable home (Tauber, 2015).

Second, the critique of science is essential to its flourishing. Science gains its place at the table precisely because of its power to define a competing worldview.

The "naturalization" of humans, from the evolution of species to the biological character of the mental, testifies to how successfully scientific explanations have been translated into potent theories of Man and Society. However, notwithstanding the effective penetration of scientific theory into notions about the nature of our social and psychological existence, a careful scrutiny is required to apply the conceptual lessons appropriately. Closely linked to that application, the converse operation is also necessary, namely, a critical view of the truth claims made by scientists. With these critiques, philosophy and history of science find their most pressing calling.[16]

The mission of humanists is not only to interpret the development of science, and to assist efforts made from within the scientific establishment in its own self-critical evaluations, but in the setting of clinical medicine the mission is also to insist on, and explain why, misapplied scientistic approaches to clinical medicine are not only inadequate for the care of the patient, but harmful (Tauber, 2005b, 2006a, 2008). Identifying the special demands of caring for the ill fall within the traditional responsibilities of citizens to translate scientific discoveries and theories into wider conceptual and social contexts, where their significance is assessed and their impact enacted. After all, the application of science falls well beyond the laboratory and the bedside represents a notoriously difficult interface to integrate human need with the technological imperative (discussed in the accompanying essay).

Third, beyond the material fruits of scientific labor, the most profound effect is science's worldview, or, as Heidegger (1977) noted, that there *is* a worldview at all! The theories and methods that have demonstrated the worlds of molecular biology, biophysics, neurophysiology, and so on have markedly altered how we conceive the body and our very selfhood. Further, the human sciences, growing from the influence of contemporary biosciences, for better and for worse, have bestowed their own theories on human character and conduct. Indeed, the debate concerning the medicalization of complex behaviors (e.g., addictions, violence, sexual practices, and various sociopathies) has yet to find a resting place in the courts and in the wider world of social mores.

Such questions fall under the more general rubric of whether a scientific "consilience" will eventually replace humanism's own approach. This is an issue with a long intellectual pedigree. The crisis created by the ascendancy of a scientific material universe was aptly summarized by Schiller (1993, p. 121) at the beginning of the nineteenth century: "How are we to restore the unity of human nature" in a disenchanted world? Viewed from the secular perspective, science joined other cultural forces to offer alternative definitions of human identity and Man's relationship to the larger universe—cultural, natural, and supernatural. And today, our very self-consciousness provokes the problematic relationship of the Cartesian mind–body imbroglio in new ways as our corporality becomes more and more objectified.[17] Simply put, if humanism captures that constellation of values and meanings of human agency (selfhood), where does the scientific objectification of our heart, brain, and fingers leave human self-awareness (Flanagan, 2007)?

In conclusion, science's broadest philosophical agenda is historically aligned with the humanist tradition, which has too often been obscured by the hegemony of science's more parochial interests. In some sense, the irony of the seeming gulf between the dominance of scientific medicine and the humanistic demands of patient care may be perceived as a conflict of interests or an alienation, when, in fact, their combined efforts are actually complementary to their respective endeavors. The dichotomy is philosophically incongruous. Despite the obvious contrasts in their respective orientations, an abiding alliance between them is both natural and necessary. Natural, because they are linked by their shared histories and originally unified philosophies; necessary, because only their combined strength will offer a comprehensive approach to the suffering person.[18] On this account, the philosophical need to pursue a "unified reason" remains. But the call for a humanist medicine has other rationales as well, which are discussed in Part 2 of "Medical Humanism."

Acknowledgments

Tauber's essay has modified and excerpted previously published material appearing here with permission of the publishers: Tauber, A. I. "Science and reason, reason and faith: A Kantian perspective," in *Intelligent Design. Science or Religion? Critical Perspectives*, R. M. Baird and S. E. Rosenbaum (eds.), Amherst, NY: Prometheus Books, 2007, pp. 307–36. Republished in *Alhikma* 1:73–108, 2008. Originally published as the Herbert H. Reynolds Lectureship, Department of Philosophy, Baylor University, Waco, TX, 2006; and Tauber, A. I., *Henry David Thoreau and the Moral Agency of Knowing*, Los Angeles: University of California Press, 2001, pp. 127–30.

Notes

1. Such knowledge is derived from appearances—the cognitive product or the *phenomenon* that we perceive. The *noumenon*, the thing-in-itself we cannot know, and thus our ontology is of a "second-order." Kant (1787, 1998, p. 375 [B333]) was satisfied: "What the things may be in themselves I do not know, and also do not need to know."
2. As Kant (1787, 1998, p. 117 [Bxxx]) acknowledged: "Thus I had to deny *knowledge* in order to make room for *faith*" (emphasis in the original). Faith refers to metaphysics, by which Kant meant the possibility of going beyond the science of appearances to address moral pursuits. Thus, one kind of knowledge was differentiated from the other, and in fact, the argument followed a strong Christian tradition: "Faith is

the assurance of things hoped for, the conviction of things not seen" (Epistle to the Hebrews 11:1).

3. Beyond offering a model by which science and religion might coexist secure in their respective domains, Kant also offered a way of synthesizing scientific thinking with the aesthetic mode. He viewed aesthetic judgment as unlike either theoretical (i.e., cognitive) or practical (i.e., moral) judgment, in that it is effected entirely subjectively, that is, solely in reference to the knowing subject. This judgment nevertheless commands communal assent through the common ground of communal or shared subjectivity. Moreover, aesthetic judgment, according to Kant (1790), provides the essential focus for connecting the theoretical and practical aspects of human nature.

4. Indeed, Martin Heidegger's (2014) critique of Western philosophy rested on how logic, and science in particular, failed to address the question, "Why are there beings at all instead of nothing?" He called for a renewed attention to Being through poetry and a spiritual contemplation of Dasein's capacity to wonder, that is, to address the fundamental existential question. This "first" and deepest of all mysteries certainly have scientific explanations (e.g., universes created in the explosion of a particle/antiparticle collision in a quantum vacuum or a quantum fluctuation of a closed space–time sphere of zero radius), but *why* there is a universe (or universes) with particular physical laws, space–time, and the existence of energy-mass remains beyond scientific explanation (Holt, 2012).

5. Note, Charles Darwin, who wrote during the same period as Whewell, referred to himself as a "natural philosopher." Darwin was very careful with his language and as a gentleman he had good reason to prefer the older designation. The term "philosophical" was not explicitly defined, but generally stood for an approach to the study of the natural world (Rehbock, 1983, pp. 3–11), which included the search for laws in biology, a dissatisfaction with teleological arguments, a certain speculative or intuitive attitude in method (especially rampant among *Naturphilosophen*), and an idealist approach. In addition, "scientist" was too easily associated with commercial overtones of technical applications, and thus the designation carried a pejorative connotation of someone who was inclined to look for the economic benefits of discoveries, in contrast to the pristine search for knowledge. Not until the end of the nineteenth century could the term "scientist" assume its current neutrality.

6. For instance, the scientific fidelity to the truth of nature was seen by Thomas Huxley (1886, p. 146) as the basis of morality, believing that moral order might derive from natural order, for the same faith in, and search for, laws of cause and effect learned from nature might be applied to the understanding and the regulating of human conduct. This extrapolation was also sought by the American Transcendentalists (e.g., Ralph Waldo Emerson and Henry David Thoreau), albeit with different method (Tauber, 2001).

7. The techniques developed in the nineteenth century reflected a growing sophistication, both in terms of material investigations, as well as the mathematics supporting them. The field of "biology" was invented as its own discipline in the first decade of the nineteenth century and by the 1820s, Claude Bernard and other physiologists were reducing organic processes to physics and chemistry. Concurrently, physics and chemistry were employing new mathematics, primarily statistical in nature, which by the 1870s created statistical mechanics and all that it spawned. In short, focused attention to the rapid growth of technical knowledge became a prerequirement for active professional participation, and this demanded specialized training. Eventually this academic narrowing led to professional segregation. In short, by the 1870s, science was divided into various natural and social sciences, each of which assumed a high degree of technical competence and cognitive training (Smith, 1997).

8. As Aristotle observed, technology is *not* science, for they represent two distinct forms of knowledge, that is, technology is considered as the *application* of scientific knowledge for material innovation. However, while technology builds on scientific insight, technical advances may proceeed independently of new scientific findings and, more generally, no logically deductive method has been shown to account for technical progress (Staudenmaier, 1985; Vincenti, 1990).

9. The critique is sometimes referred to as Hume's Law and is introduced in his *A Treatise of Human Nature* (1739, 1978; Book III, Part 1, section I), where he is attacking the apparent rationality of various ethical or religious positions.

10. In the United States the establishment of the first research-based medical school (Johns Hopkins), the subordination of contenders to biomedicine through the 1910 Flexner Report, and the enthusiastic application and still unrealized expectations for the elimination of infectious diseases each date to this period (Tauber, 1992).

11. This general approach was not limited to the study of the natural world, for by the 1850s, positivism came to be understood as a philosophical belief that held that the methods of natural science offer the only viable way of thinking correctly about human affairs. And so were the human sciences born (Smith, 1997). Accordingly, empirical experience—processed with a self-conscious fear of subjective contamination—served as the basis of all knowledge. Facts, the products of sensory experience, and, by extrapolation, the data derived from machines and instruments built as extensions of that faculty, were first ascertained and then classified. "Hypothesis" was defined as the expectation of observing facts of a certain kind under certain conditions; and a scientific "law" could be defined as the proposition that under certain conditions of a certain kind, facts of a certain kind were uniformly observable. Any hypothesis or law that could not be defined in terms such as these would be written off as "pseudo-hypothesis" or "pseudo-law." And thus the sciences separated themselves from older traditions of inquiry.

12. Tess Cosslett (1982, pp. 11–30) has outlined the values of Victorian science in this humanistic context along the following lines: (1) Truth: the search for truth should reject the easy consolations of religion, for nature never lies and she provides a standard of veracity; (2) Law: science discerns laws of natural causation and thereby can perceive a deeper order in the universe than that expressed by poetic or religious imagination; (3) Kinship with nature: natural causation not only implies regularity but also confers an inherent unity with nature (Postlethwaite, 1984; Dale, 1989). So, while Darwinian evolution or Lyellian geology was metaphysically destabilizing in one sense, to be intelligible these theories still had to be coherent. Thus the interconvertibility of light and heat, the evolution of species, the rise and fall of mountains sounded the keynotes of unity and continuity. As a popularizer wrote in 1888, "[A]ll things are made of the same stuff differently mixed, bound by one force, stirred by one energy in divers forms" (Clodd, 1888, p. 231). On this view, "mechanism" has become "organism" and "matter" has been transmuted into "process." These formulations humanize nature into categories analogous to human agency and action; (4) Organic interrelation: each organic part is integral to the whole and each element has an essential effect on that whole. This view had deep aesthetic and moral implications, especially telling when human history and natural history were seen as one. Humanity from this vantage can be viewed as one perpetual, self-renewing, transgenerational organism. Regarded as of one piece, each constituent is responsible for, and to, the whole. In regard to the moral value of the present, each act, no matter how seemingly inconsequential or trivial, assumes a cosmic significance both in its own right and by its effects on subsequent human history; (5) Scientific imagination: while they rejected Romanticism's subjectivity, some Victorian scientists (e.g., John Tyndall) recognized that scientific creativity still rested on Imagination,

and they used the notion in the same way Coleridge did, albeit it must be regarded as a retained characteristic of Romanticism that did not readily find a compatible environment in a scientific culture increasingly dominated by a materialist positivism. The mystery and transcendental quality conferred by scientific insight fundamentally lies outside formal science praxis. Science has no voice to articulate its vision in terms that are subjective. So when the scientist faces the ultimate mysteries, he must step across the line dividing science from religion and poetry and acknowledge what Herbert Spencer called "The Unknowable." John Tyndall (1865, vol. 2, p. 52) eloquently attested:

> In one sense [science] knows, or is destined to know, everything. In another sense it knows nothing. Science understands much of this intermediate phase of things that we call nature, of which it is the product; but science knows nothing of the origin or destiny of nature. Who or what made the sun and gave his rays their alleged power? Who or what made and bestowed upon the ultimate particles of matter their wondrous power of varied interaction? Science does not know: the mystery, though pushed back, remains unaltered.

13. Positivism continued to garner strength into the twentieth century, and its program achieved its major influence from the 1920s into the 1950s under the guise of logical positivism (also called logical empiricism). This movement, often identified as the Vienna Circle, extended well beyond science into the social sciences and largely shaped analytic philosophy, whose principle concerns dealt with how sentences might be verified and thus determined as truthful or not (Kolakowski, 1968; Giere and Richardson, 1996). Putting aside the issues concerning the analytic basis of truth statements in ordinary language, logical empiricists, extrapolating from its key tenet that scientific method alone provides knowledge, regarded a statement as cognitively meaningful only if it was "scientific," that is, empirically veridical. In this context, propositions are meaningful only if they can be assessed by an appeal to some foundational form of sensory experience. Thus proponents of this Vienna Circle position espoused science as the gold standard of knowledge, because sense data—especially in the form of mechanical objectivity—were treated as worthy of foundational status; and, conversely, given such criteria for a basis for truth claims, these positivists judged religious, metaphysical, and ethical statements "meaningless." This strong empirical orientation has been justly challenged on many philosophical, historical, and sociological grounds. Most celebrated of those assailants was Thomas Kuhn, who, in *The Structure of Scientific Revolutions* (1970), argued that scientific evolution did not exclusively follow such precepts and that other social and aesthetic factors were important determinants of scientific truth. Coupled to historically based critiques, philosophers, led by Paul Feyerabend (1975), argued that there was no prescribed, orthodox scientific method and that science was better characterized as a plurality of philosophies and practices. Finally, sociologists firmly placed science among other social institutions and showed how scientific practice was influenced by a vast intellectual and cultural infrastructure (Hollis and Lukes, 1982; Jasanoff et al., 1995). In short, argued the critics, science was hardly the normative enterprise celebrated by the positivists, and because of an intricate matrix of philosophical, historical, and cultural contingencies, it could not possess a singular universal and prescribed method of discovery or verification, nor a transcendental, timeless norms of scientific practice and objectivity (Megill, 1994). Some further argued that as a result of these critiques, even science's cognitive content was open to new skepticism. And here we find the locus of contention. By the 1990s, critics and scientists were again

alienated from each other, not in C. P. Snow's original formula of mutual illiteracy, but because of aggressive polemics in which each side clearly understood what was being debated and what was at stake (Tauber, 2009).

14. Science's instrumentality has at least two dimensions: The first refers to science's intellectual activity, a mode of discovery and knowing, where the findings are used like a currency to buy different goods. The goods are findings or ideas, which are then placed into a conceptual context. The second meaning refers to how research is applied (perhaps, employed) to devise technologies. These might be put to constructive use (the usual case) or instead, employed as a tool for purposes quite at odds with the original intent of seeking knowledge for our social good. This instrumental quality of science (its technological power) holds one of its ironies: instead of maintaining its original philosophical credentials, science, more precisely its technological progeny, too often has become so divorced from those earlier concerns that the basic research has become a tool that may be applied independently of the primary intent of the investigation. Co-opted by those whose own agenda has nothing to do with promoting the Western values that spawned science in the first place, we have painfully learned how powerful technologies may be used as an instrument of power for sociopolitical ends at odds with our own. So molecular biology might be used to create a rogue virus, or Nazis might use the chemistry of poison gases to murder innocents. In these instances, the instrumental value of science is readily seen as a tool for technological applications radically divorced from the intent of those who either commissioned, or directly pursued, the investigations in the first place.

15. For instance, why should we preserve natural resources? When does a fetus become an individual? To what use should nuclear energy be applied? And when we consider the degree to which human behavior is determined by the genetic dimension, the discussion ranges from the evolutionary origins of morality to the conceptions of gender and sexuality; from the character of altruism to the very notion of "human nature" (Wright, 1995; Ridley, 1998; Wade, 2014).

16. Perhaps not surprisingly, as science assumed greater intellectual independence, the disciplines of history and philosophy of science matured. They filled a gaping hole. After all, as Thomas Kuhn (1970) noted almost 50 years ago, scientists were not interested in their own histories, much less the philosophy undergirding their discipline. In turn, the humanists lamented the scarcity of meaningful dialogue between themselves and their scientific colleagues. The sociologies of each group had radically diverged. But beyond this professional separation, the respective mode of discourse seemed foreign to the other and thus cross-fertilization had become increasingly barren.

17. The conflict is often traced to the unleashing of Descartes's mind–body dualism, which bequeaths a dilemma to both the subject and its world, i.e., to render whole that which is broken asunder. The Cartesian method imparts a tension, for in dissecting the world into parts it offers no means for those elements to become reintegrated. The holistic design is lost (Grosholz, 1991). Holism, as a philosophical construct, grew out of seventeenth-century debate over the metaphysical structure of Nature. In response to the dualistic construction of mind and body proposed by Descartes, Spinoza endeavored to unify the schism by transcending the alternative primacy of either mind or body with a new concept, substance: absolute, infinite, and unknowable. Spinozean pantheism was the direct antecedent to the Romantic notion of Nature's unity (McFarland, 1969), and to the extent that this holistic construct formed the metaphysical response to Descartes's mechanistic philosophy, it became associated with an antimechanical solution to the problem of life's unique property. Where, what, or how was the organic then to be defined?

18. This general discussion about the unity of reason follows Kant (Wein, 1961) and then developed by Whitehead (1925), Husserl (1935, 1970), and Gadamer (1976, 1981),

each of whom, despite the radical differences of their respective philosophies, profoundly understood that the bifurcation of reason bestowed a conundrum that could only be addressed by a synthesis of science and its supporting philosophical critique. In these terms, reason must "remain its own pupil" (Wein, 1961, p. 313).

References

Beiser, F. C. (1987). *The Fate of Reason*. Cambridge: Harvard University Press.

Brittan, G. G., Jr. (1978). *Kant's Theory of Science*. Princeton: Princeton University Press.

Clodd, E. (1888). *Story of Creation* London: Longmans.

Cosslett, T. (1982). *Science and Religion in the Nineteenth Century*. Cambridge: Cambridge University Press.

Dale, P. A. (1989). *In Pursuit of a Scientific Culture: Science, Art, and Society in the Victorian Age*. Madison: University of Wisconsin Press.

Daston, L., and Galison, P. (2007). *Objectivity* New York: Zone Books.

della Mirandola, G. P. (1965). *On the Dignity of Man and Other Works*, C. G. Wallis, trans. Indianapolis: Bobbs-Merrill.

Feyerabend, P. (1975). *Against Method*. London: Verso.

Flanagan, O. (2007). *The Really Hard Problem: Meaning in a Material World*. Cambridge: MIT Press.

Friedman, M. (1992). *Kant and the Exact Sciences*. Cambridge: Harvard University Press.

Gadamer, H.-G. (1976, 1981). *Reason in the Age of Science*, F. G. Lawrence, trans. Cambridge: The MIT Press.

Galaty, D. H. (1974). The philosophical basis for mid-nineteenth-century German reductionism. *Journal of the History of Medicine and Allied Sciences* 29: 295–316.

Giere, R. N., and Richardson, A. W. (eds.) (1996). *Origins of Logical Empiricism Minnesota Studies in Philosophy of Science, Vol. 16*. Minneapolis: University of Minnesota Press.

Gieryn, T. F. (1995). Boundaries of science. In *Handbook of Science and Technology Studies*, eds. S. Jasanoff, G. E. Markle, J. C. Petersen, and T. Pinch. Thousand Oaks, CA: Sage Publications, pp. 393–443.

Grosholz, E. R. (1991). *Cartesian Method and the Problem of Reduction*. Oxford: Clarendon Press.

Heidegger, M. (1977). The age of the world picture. In *The Question Concerning Technology and other Essays*, trans. W. Lovitt. New York: Harper Torchbooks, pp. 115–54.

Heidegger, M. (2014). *Introduction to Metaphysics*, 2nd edition, G. Fried and R. Polt, trans. New Haven: Yale University Press.

Hollis, M., and Lukes, S. (1982). *Rationality and Relativism*. Cambridge: The MIT Press.

Holt, J. (2012). *Why Does the World Exist? An Existential Detective Story*. New York: W.W. Norton.

Husserl, E. (1935, 1970). *The Crisis of European Science and Transcendental Phenomenology. An Introduction to Phenomenological Philosophy*, D. Carr, trans. Evanston, IL: Northwestern University Press.

Hume, D. (1739, 1978). *A Treatise of Human Nature*. Oxford: Clarendon Press.

Huxley, T. (1886). Science and morals. In *Collected Essays, Vol. 9, Evolution and Ethics*. London: Macmillan, 1893.

Jasanoff, S., Markle, G. E., Petersen, J. C., and Pinch, T. (eds.). (1995). *Handbook of Science and Technology Studies*. Thousand Oaks, CA: Sage Publications.

Kant, I. (1790, 1987). *Critique of Judgment*, W. S. Pluhar, trans. Indianapolis: Hackett Publishing Co.

Kant, I. (1787, 1998). *Critique of Pure Reason*, P. Guyer and A. W. Wood, trans. Cambridge: Cambridge University Press.

Kolakowski, L. (1968). *The Alienation of Reason. A History of Positivist Thought*, Norbert Guterman, trans. Garden City: Doubleday.

Kuhn, T. S. (1970). *The Structure of Scientific Revolutions*, 2nd edition. Chicago: University of Chicago Press.

Lenoir, T. (1989). *The Strategy of Life. Teleology and Mechanics in Nineteenth Century German Biology*. Chicago: University of Chicago Press. (Originally published, Dordrecht: D. Reidel Publ. Co., 1982).

McFarland, T. (1969). *Coleridge and the Pantheist Tradition*. Oxford: Clarendon Press.

Megill, A. (ed.) (1994). *Rethinking Objectivity*. Durham: Duke University Press.

Merz, J. T. (1896, 1965). A *History of European Thought in the Nineteenth Century*, Vol. 1–4. New York: Dover Publications Inc.

Moulines, C. U. (1981). Hermann von Helmholtz: A physiological theory of knowledge. In *Epistemological and Social Problems of the Sciences in the Early Nineteenth Century*, eds. H. N. Jahnke and M. Otte. Dordrecht: D. Reidel Publishing Co., pp. 65–73.

Nagel, T. (1985). *The View from Nowhere*. New York: Oxford University Press.

Pellegrino, E. D. (1979). *Humanism and the Physician*. Knoxville: University of Tennessee Press.

Polanyi, M. (1958, 1962). *Personal Knowledge: Towards a Post-critical Philosophy*, Corrected edition. Chicago: The University of Chicago Press.

Postlethwaite, D. (1984). *Making It Whole: A Victorian Circle and the Shape of Their World*. Columbus: Ohio State University Press.

Putnam, H. (1990). Why is a philosopher? In *Realism with a Human Face,* ed. J. Conant. Cambridge: Harvard University Press.

Putnam, H. (2002). *The Collapse of the Fact/Value Dichotomy and Other Essays*. Cambridge: Harvard University Press.

Rehbock, R. F. (1983). *The Philosophical Naturalists: Themes in Early Nineteenth Century British Biology*. Madison: The University of Wisconsin Press.

Ridley, M. (1998). *The Origins of Virtue: Human Instincts and the Evolution of Cooperation*. New York: Penguin.

Schiller, F. (1801, 1993). Letters on the Aesthetic Education of Man. In *Essays*, eds. W. Hinderer and D. O. Dahlstrom, trans. E. M. Wilkinson and L. A. Willoughby. New York, NY: Continuum Publishing, pp. 86–178.

Sellers, W. (1956, 1997). *Empiricism and the Philosophy of Mind*. Cambridge: Harvard University Press.

Simon, W. M. (1963). *European Positivism in the Nineteenth Century*. Ithaca, NY: Cornell University Press.

Smith, R. (1997). *The Norton History of the Human Sciences.* New York: W. W. Norton.

Staudenmaier, J. M. (1985). *Technology's Storytellers*. Cambridge, MA: MIT Press.

Tauber, A. I. (1992). The two faces of medical education/Flexner and Osler revisited. *Journal of the Royal Society of Med*icine 85: 598–602.

Tauber, A. I. (1993). Goethe's philosophy of science: Modern resonances. *Perspectives in Biology and Medicine* 36: 244–57.

Tauber, A. I. (ed.). (1996). *The Elusive Synthesis: Aesthetics and Science*. Dordrecht: Kluwer Academic Publishers.

Tauber, A. I. (1999). *Confessions of a Medicine Man: An Essay in Popular Philosophy*. Cambridge: MIT Press.

Tauber, A. I. (2001). *Henry David Thoreau and the Moral Agency of Knowing*. Berkeley: University of California Press.

Tauber, A. I. (2005a). *Patient Autonomy and the Ethics of Responsibility*. Cambridge: MIT Press.

Tauber, A. I. (2005b). Medicine and the call for a moral epistemology. *Perspectives in Biology and Medicine* 48: 42–53.

Tauber, A. I. (2006a). Medicine as a moral epistemology. In *Multidisciplinary Approaches to Theory in Medicine*. eds. R. Paton and L. McNamara. Amsterdam: Elsevier, pp. 63–88.

Tauber, A. I. (2006b). Seeking medicine's moral glue. *American Journal of Bioethics* 6: 41–44.

Tauber, A. I. (2007). Balancing medicine's moral ledger: Realigning trust and responsibility. In *Responsibility*, ed. Darling-Smith. Lanham: Lexington Books, pp. 129–48.

Tauber, A. I. (2008). Medicine and the call for a moral epistemology, Part II: Constructing a synthesis of values. *Perspectives in Biology and Medicine* 51: 450–63.

Tauber, A. I. (2009). *Science and the Quest for Meaning*. Waco, TX: Baylor University Press.

Tauber, A. I. (2015). Book review essay of *The Cambridge Handbook of Human Dignity. Interdisciplinary Perspectives*, eds. M. Düwell, J. Braarvig, R. Brownsword, and D. Mieth. Cambridge: Cambridge University Press, 2014. *Perspectives in Biology and Medicine*, 57: 560–68.

Tauber, A. I., and Sarkar, S. (1993). The ideological basis of the Human Genome Project. *Journal of the Royal Society of Medicine* 86: 537–40.

Tyndall, J. (1854). On the study of physics. In *Fragments of Science*, 7th edition. London: Longmans, 1889.

Tyndall, J. (1865). Vitality. In *Fragments of Science*, 7th edition. London: Longmans, 1889.

Vincenti, W.G. 1990. *What Engineers Know and How They Know It. Analytical Studies from Aeronautical History*. Baltimore, MD Johns Hopkins University press.

Wade, N. (2014). *A Troublesome Inheritance: Genes, Race and Human History*. New York: Penguin.

Wein, H. (1961). In defense of the humanism of science: Kant and Whitehead. In *The Relevance of Whitehead*, ed. I. Leclerc. London: George Allen & Unwin Ltd., pp. 289–315.

Whewell, W. (1840). *Philosophy of the Inductive Sciences*. London: J. W. Parker

Whitehead, A. (1925). *Science and the Modern World*. London: Macmillan.

Wright, R. (1995). *The Moral Animal: Why We Are the Way We Are: The Science of Evolutionary Psychology*. New York: Vintage.

7a Medical Humanism Part 2: Inspirations of the Twentieth Century

Lydie Fialová

Introduction

Medicine represents a very diverse and multifaceted social institution. It can be conceptualized as a space where the tradition of knowledge, grounded in the natural sciences and their technological applications, and the tradition of care for the ill intersect. Situated in the world of human relationships, yet making use of scientific knowledge, medicine is an endeavor with a strong ethical charge. Moreover, through its immediate relationship to life and death, health, illness, and suffering, medicine also provides unique insight into the cultural history and the history of philosophical ideas. The intertwined nature of life and death, the awareness of one's essential vulnerability and finitude, the attempt to transcend these limitations and to find meaning in the finitude of living, and the attempt to achieve some form of permanence or even perfection are constant characteristics of the human condition.

In the previous chapter, Alfred Tauber described the philosophical origins of humanism as well as the historical context of medicine's commitment to scientific objectivity, positivism, and reductionism. The understanding of medicine as a space where not only ethics and science intersect but where they also tend to create tension or even to clash in clinical care has been the point of departure for philosophy of medicine (Pellegrino, 1979; Pellegrino and Thomasma, 1981). In some ways this tension reflects the distinction between the realm of objectivity and subjectivity in medicine: the tendency to depersonalize the patient as an object of medical technology and bureaucratic practices contrasted with the inherently subjective experience of suffering. The attempts to rescue the humanistic dimension of medicine by attention to the experience of suffering have also guided many of the philosophical and social studies of medicine (Cassell, 2003; Kleinman, 1989; Frank, 1997). Drawing on these approaches and explorations this chapter will examine the landscape of medical humanism in the twentieth century.

During the twentieth century, hospitals in the Western world became places where most people were born and where they died. Medicine thus established itself as the institutional context for both the beginning and the end of human life. Moreover, the biomedical sciences established themselves as a "truth discourse" about the nature of human life understood in terms of its biology. Indeed, medicine has shaped our understanding of the beginnings of life and that of death in purely materialistic, biological terms. Images vividly depicting the earliest encounter between sperm and ovum, through various embryonic stages and fetal development have become part of the cultural imagination and understanding of the beginning of life. In the same way we rely on science and technology to define death: the flat EEG and absence of brain activity detected by imaging methods permit discontinuing life support and the harvesting of bodily organs.

Firmly grounded in the positivist tradition of the natural sciences, medicine exalts the objectivistic stance and transforms lived experience into an object of medical knowledge and intervention. Approaching pain and suffering, as well as procreation and death in a biological conceptual framework, transforms an existential condition into a medical one. This process, described as medicalization, tends to obscure the personal aspects of illness and suffering. As a result, medicine offers technological solutions even in situations where these might be inappropriate. The medicalization of life and death and the neutralization of the ethical space by the objectifying approach of applied science, as well as the institutionalization of medical care that becomes subordinated to the modern bureaucratic regimes, become therefore a target for critiquing medicine (e.g., Jaspers, 1989; Elias, 1986; Illich, 2000). Nevertheless, the encounter of patients with their caregivers and physicians still remains essentially ethical in nature (Tauber, 1999).

In this chapter, I explore the tendency of modern medicine to obscure this elemental ethical relationship between patients and their caregivers and physicians. First, considering medicine as a tradition of knowledge and applied science, I examine the tendency of medicine to depersonalize patients and transform them into a site of technological intervention. Unlike the natural sciences, which remain in a neutral descriptive mode, medicine is committed to the value of health, which it aims to restore and preserve. As such, it is a necessarily normative enterprise, and I examine the implications of this distinction. Second, I consider medicine as a tradition of care in which the primarily ethical act of compassion, responding to the suffering of another, became dominated by the institutional ethos of impersonal care. Finally, I suggest that these tendencies may be counteracted by retrieving the primacy of the ethical that reveals itself in solidarity with and as responsibility for the suffering Other. Medical humanism reflects the understanding that we all share the same human condition of vulnerability and finitude. I conclude by presenting the vision of the human condition as it was elaborated by phenomenological philosophy of existence with an emphasis on the temporal and interpersonal dimensions of human existence. The experience of illness, suffering, and death represents situations in which the essential fragility of human life is exposed. These limit situations also present a call for compassion with the suffering Other that grounds medicine as an ethical practice.

Medicine and its Objects

For centuries, the induction of students into medicine started with anatomical dissection. This practice is often considered as a rite of passage into the profession. The study of anatomy and pathology through dissection allows students to gain an understanding of the structure and function of the human body. However, the practice of dissection often plays also another role—perhaps not entirely deliberate yet very efficient—the depersonalization of the patient. The corpse, where all life is absent—the nameless body exposed in all its nakedness—is stripped of all meaning. The premortem identity is entirely irrelevant for the generalizable knowledge gained from such an exercise. This abstraction and depersonalization is necessary for physicians as a specific mode of thinking because it enables diagnostic and therapeutic considerations. This practice also offers some experiential explanation for the persistence of Cartesian dualism in medicine—when the life is gone, the only thing remaining is the material body. The focus on the structure of individual organs, bones, vessels, and nerves dissected apart contributes to the vision of human body as biological material functioning together as a complex machine. The task of medicine is to repair the damage caused by disease, thus transforming the body into an object of technical intervention.

Critics have long argued that the ideals of objectivity and rationality that characterize modern science lead to a narrowing of the focus of medicine to the physical signs of disease, many of which can be traced to the molecular level today (see Marianne Boenink's chapter 3 in this volume). As the human body is constituted as a separate entity, so are the organs, tissues, cells, and genes. The unprecedented success of the life sciences has been built on the possibility to identify, extract, isolate, and cultivate cells outside the body for the purposes of research (Landecker, 2010). This process of material abstraction then influences the way physicians think about these entities: altered organs, cells, and genes are conceived of as independent substances representing diseases and their causes. However, one can also argue that the human organism in its complexity is much more than the sum of its parts. However detailed the description, the unique life experience of each individual patient is not reducible to entities captured by medical categories (Canguilhem, 1991; Goldstein, 2000).

185

Such methodological reductionism easily becomes ontological reductionism, which in many respects proves inimical to humane care. The objectifying and generalizing approach that is perfectly effective and desirable in the realm of science thus does reach its limit when applied to patient care where, as a result, the disease then becomes the focus of intervention, and the patient disappears into the background of their pathology.

The impact of technology on the world of medicine has been enormous. Various technologies enhance human senses: in nineteenth-century medicine, the microscope expanded the possibilities of vision just as the stethoscope expands hearing. Modern technologies additionally allow for detection of phenomena undetected or unquantifiable by human senses—such as electrical impulses, magnetic fields, or sound waves. These technologies have transformed diagnostic and therapeutic possibilities in medicine: building on the knowledge gained by biomedical research, it allows for their application in the material world, making it possible to interfere with or manipulate physiological processes and create artifacts and imitations of biological substances. Technology thus represents an extension of both human senses and powers.

In his essays on technology, Hans Jonas examines the ways in which modern technology affects and transforms the nature of human action. An heir to the Enlightenment project of conquering nature by discovering the principles by which the material world is structured and by intervening with them, modern technology interferes in a similar way also with the human world where the person is both the subject and the object of technological intervention (Jonas, 1981). This transformation also affects the understanding of ethics: while traditionally ethics concerned itself with the world of human affairs and nature remained ethically neutral, a new ethics is necessary for situations in which human intervention in nature extends in scale and consequences and includes also intervention in humans. Many of the potential consequences of using new technologies to manipulate human nature are unforeseeable, and this should be a reason for responsible restraint to balance the enthusiasm for expanding the realm of medical possibilities. The dream of modern medicine is then to direct human evolution—to modify, enhance, and improve our own design.

Jonas, however, challenges this imperative of progress, asking whether we have the right to do so, and whether we are qualified for such a role. Who will be the image-makers, by what standards, and on what basis of knowledge? "If the new nature of our acting then calls for a new ethics of long-range responsibility, coextensive with the range of our power," writes Jonas (1981, p. 18), "it calls in the name of that responsibility also for a new kind of humility—a humility not like former humility, i.e., owing to the littleness, but owing to the excessive magnitude of our power, which is the excess of our power to act over our power to evaluate and to judge."

One of Jonas's important insights is that our power over nature also increases our power over one another and subjects us to a dependence on technology itself and the imperative of progress. This is evident most clearly in the area of biological engineering, genetics, and reproductive medicine (including prenatal or preimplantation screening), where also the question of whether we have the moral right to experiment on future human beings is raised. However, this power is enacted in more subtle ways in other areas, such as psychopharmacology. In an era that tends to consider a variety of natural but also behavioral, psychological, and social phenomena as a medical condition, this shift sanctions medically justified manipulation on the biological level. There is nevertheless an inherent danger in the technological transformation of human nature that threatens the very possibility of the ethical life. "Regardless of the question of compulsion or consent, and regardless also of the question of undesirable side-effects, each time we bypass the human way of dealing with human problems, short-circuiting it by an impersonal mechanism," Jonas (1981, p. 17) claims, "we have taken away something from the dignity of personal selfhood and advanced a further step on the road from responsible subjects to programmed behavior systems."

The dangers of reducing human life to its biological substrate and then exercising normative judgments on its value have also been exemplified by the various trajectories of eugenics movement (Kevles, 2004). The judgment that health is more desirable than disease—otherwise considered an unproblematic assumption of medicine—has the potential to become a judgment that healthy people are more worthy, desirable, or valuable than those affected by illness or disability, or those who are considered products of "defective genes." Although the excesses of eugenics in the first half of the twentieth century have been widely condemned, this argument continues to be exercised in the language of individualistic self-determination in the area of reproductive medicine and genetics (Sandel, 2009). Medicine that is unprotected by the commitment to universal human dignity can easily slide into being an instrument of social and political control—often underwritten by economic concerns (Foucault, 2006; Rose, 2006).

These thoughts bring me back to the opening paragraph of this section discussing anatomical dissection and its role in depersonalizing the patient. There is yet another aspect of this anatomical dissection that is worth noting since it discloses something about the other side of medicine. The ambivalent practice of opening and dissecting human corpses—unthinkable in other contexts—is legitimized in medicine since the knowledge about the human body is transformed into the power to heal, and therefore justified on utilitarian grounds. The corpses that indeed are available for the purpose of medical learning and research have—until relatively recent legal changes—been bodies of people who during their life were marginalized or excluded from human community: those of criminals, mentally ill, foreigners, and "unclaimed bodies" (Carlino, 1999; Richardson, 2000; MacDonald, 2010). These are the bodies of people whose human bonds have dissolved while they were still alive. This is an important reminder of the persistent tendency of medicine to enter the space of social exclusion for its own purposes. Such is also the origin of medical research conducted in public hospitals where disadvantaged patients with no means to pay for the care they received were used as subjects of medical research. Also, until 1960, a significant proportion of clinical research was conducted in prisons. Today this tendency continues in clinical trials often conducted on patients who cannot afford better care, especially in countries lacking resources and medical infrastructure (LaFleur et al., 2008; Petryna, 2009). However, this phenomenon is not limited to medical research, but it is also evident in clinical areas such as assisted reproduction and organ transplantation (Cohen, 1999; Sheper-Hughes and Wacquant, 2003). The tendency to use some individuals—with their autonomous consent—for the greater benefit of others is justified on utilitarian grounds. However, these practices seem to follow the dividing line of social inequalities, thus compromising the humanistic commitment to equality and justice.

The Institutional Context of Medicine

In his book *Mending Bodies, Saving Souls*, Günther Risse (1999) describes the history of hospitals in Europe. Examining the genealogy of these institutions, he notes that for most of European history hospitals were places of mercy, refuge, and also death. Hospitals were originally monastic shelters and infirmaries, where also the last sacraments were administered to believers expecting salvation, who—surrounded by prayerful caregivers—waited for their redemption: the church mediated between life and death. Recent centuries have witnessed a slow transformation of the ethical impulse to address the needs of others into various forms of secular institutions, including medicine. The limits of medicine have shifted significantly over the past century with the advent of new preventative and therapeutic approaches, which have increased life expectancy and enabled more people to live healthier lives (Porter, 1999).

The provision of medical care has long been the domain of those who had sufficient means, while those who could not afford were at the mercy of municipal hospitals and various charitable organizations. After World War II, many states in Europe introduced universal healthcare based on the assumption of social solidarity and the principle of the social contract. Although recently often argued for in terms of individual human rights, universal healthcare is indeed rooted in the ethical notion of responsibility and indebted to the principle of justice (Daniels, 2008). However, healthcare also became part of what has been called the medico-industrial complex, which has significant implications for the practice of medicine (Relman, 1980). Medicalization — as evident in expanding criteria of various conditions—also contributes to the widening sphere of healthcare, which in most contexts became part of the for-profit ethos of the market economy. This tendency nevertheless runs counter to the fundamental ethical principle of not benefiting from someone else's suffering.

Over the past century, the ways in which medical care is provided has changed significantly (Cooter and Pickstone, 2002). Medicine has long ceased to be a matter solely of doctors and their patients: nurses, medical researchers, and many other professions now contribute to the provision of healthcare. As a complex of social institutions, medicine simplifies the interactions among patients, physicians, and caregivers to role performances. Although in recent decades the move from medical paternalism to patient autonomy has influenced clinical practice, medicine is still practiced within the cultural context of social hierarchies and the asymmetrical relationship and distinct social status of patients and physicians—which remains a source of discontent (Tauber, 2005). The call for responsibility thus goes much further than fulfilling socially prescribed roles.

The etymology of the word "hospital" is closely linked with hospitality, offering refuge and providing care to those in need. This ethical impulse of compassion—which represents an essential component of various religious traditions—was in medieval times considered an exercise in virtue. In the *Summa Theologiae*, Thomas Aquinas describes "Mercy" as "the compassion in our hearts for another person's misery, a compassion which drives us to do what we can to help him." Although mercy is related to the virtue of charity as a spontaneous act of sympathy toward others, mercy is also an act of justice. The impulse to relieve others of their misery is exemplified in the corporal works of mercy: to feed the hungry, to give drink to the thirsty, to clothe the naked, to harbor the harborless, to visit the sick, to ransom the captive, and to bury the dead. These acts address the physical and material needs of the other persons, and they are complemented by seven spiritual acts of mercy that attend to their soul.

The distinction between the corporeal—the realm of the body—and the spiritual—the realm of the soul—exerted significant influence in European culture. The religious and the secular have thus intertwined in the spaces of illness and healing. In an interesting formulation from the Fourth Lateran Council of 1215, these realms are regulated respectively:

[W]hen physicians of the body are called to the bedside of the sick, before all else they admonish them to call for the physician of souls, so that after spiritual health has been restored to them, the application of bodily medicine may be of greater benefit. (Canon 22)

189

With the rise of natural sciences—science itself originally considered a form of virtue and spiritual exercise, as well as a way to repair and heal a fallen and fractured world (Harrison, 2007)—medicine was one of the institutions to provide care and possibly a cure for the ailments of the body, while religion was left to take care of the soul. The noble ambition of medical science to understand the origins and physical causes of maladies, to intervene in the pathological processes and to invent cures for diseases, and to add the virtue of "cure" to the list of the works of mercy has significantly transformed the landscape of human suffering.

However, the realms of religion and medicine have intertwined both in the domain of ideas about the origins and nature of illness and in patient care and treatment. The concept of the soul has since changed significantly and, with increasing secularization, medicine claimed more of the territory of what was traditionally understood as a soul. With the rise of psychiatry, psychology, and neuroscience—which now offer explanations for the inner life in terms of neurobiological processes in the brain—the concept of the soul has been emptied or rather annihilated (Zimmer, 2004; Porter, 2004). It is therefore not surprising that contemporary medicine is often criticized for the lack of attention to the personal aspects of illness and suffering and their meaning in human life. The fragmentation of person and subsequent establishment of specialized institutions devoted to care of the respective dimension of human life—physical, psychological, social, and spiritual—often obscure the uniqueness and singularity of the individual human being. The limitations of this approach, however, became clear—especially in the area of chronic illness, psychiatric conditions, and incurable diseases, as well as the frailty of aging and the process of dying.

Currently, sophisticated methods are used for the diagnosis and treatment of diseases that threaten the integrity of the person. However, with increased intensity we observe that disease and suffering are two distinct phenomena that in some cases merge and in others do not. There are many conditions (such as diabetes, hypertension, etc.) that are diagnosed merely on the laboratory values and treated to prevent the occurrence of clinical symptoms (Greene, 2009). On the other hand, there are conditions (chronic pain, depression, etc.) that still lack clear understanding of their pathophysiology and yet significantly affect the patient's life (Good et al., 1994). The attention directed toward other aspects of disease, other than the medical, and developed mainly in the areas of primary and palliative care, is slowly making its way into mainstream medicine. The concept of "bio-psycho-social" model of illness, as well as "patient-centered" approach has been influential in attempts to transform medicine and the provision of healthcare (Engel, 1977).[1] The focus on the subjective experience of illness that transforms the lifeworlds of the patients has inspired both clinicians and social scientists to turn to the narrative as an essential instrument for medical practice (Kleinman, 1989; Good, 1993; Frank, 1997; Greenhalg and Hurwitz, 1998; Mattingly and Garro, 2001; Charon, 2008). This literature makes it clear that in the perception of patients, illness represents a disruption of life's trajectory and a crisis of personal identity, and that it raises questions of meaning of illness and suffering. The factual inevitability of death that evades the taken-for-granted certainties of life is a situation that many patients have to face. These evoke a wide range of feelings and despite the new situation being incomprehensible the death becomes the new horizon for them. According to one patient,

> I have been trying to write down my feelings. But I simply don't have the energy or the concentration. I forget what I've gone through. All the hours in clinics and waiting rooms, the hospitalizations, one test result more depressing than the next. The inexorable course of things. The feeling there is something not me in me, an "it," eating its way through the body. I am the creator of my own destruction. The cancer cells are me and yet to me. I am invaded by a killer. I am become death. I really don't want to die. I know I must. I will. I am. But I don't want to. (Kleinman 1989, p. 148)

The experience of strangeness or estrangement and the problem of embodied identity and nonidentity in the experience of illness that transforms one's experience of selfhood have been insightfully described by many authors, such as Jean-Luc Nancy (2008) in his philosophical essay "The Intruder"—an account of heart transplantation; Robert Murphy (2001) in *Body Silent*—a narrative of progressive spinal condition; or Sarah Kane (2000) in her theatre piece *4.48 Psychosis*—the last play she wrote before committing suicide. These are situations, insights, and feelings that technological medicine is unable to address just because they are outside the narrow scope of its concerns.

According to some scholars, as a result of the medicalization of life and the hospitalization of those suffering, the subjective experience of pain and illness has also been transformed. In the words of Ivan Illich (2000, p. 140):

> When cosmopolitan medical civilization colonizes any traditional culture, it transforms the experience of pain. The same nervous stimulation that I shall call pain sensation will result in a distinct experience, depending not only on personality but also on culture. This experience, as distinct from the painful sensation, implies a uniquely human performance called suffering. Medical civilization, however, tends to turn pain into a technical matter and thereby deprives suffering of its inherent personal meaning. People unlearn the acceptance of suffering as an inevitable part of their conscious coping with reality and learn to interpret every ache as an indicator of their need for padding or pampering. Traditional cultures confront pain, impairment,

and death by interpreting them as challenges soliciting a response from the individual under stress; medical civilization turns them into demands made by individuals on the economy, into problems that can be managed or produced out of existence. Cultures are systems of meanings, cosmopolitan civilization a system of techniques. Culture makes pain tolerable by integrating it into a meaningful setting; cosmopolitan civilization detaches pain from any subjective or inter- subjective context in order to annihilate it. Culture makes pain tolerable by interpreting its necessity; only pain perceived as curable is intolerable.

Illich goes further in his critique of medicine as a denial of pain, suffering, and death that are inherent realities of human condition: only by responding to the challenges they present do we learn to live authentically, overcoming and transcending the limitations of our embodied, temporal lives. Although this radical critique needs a more nuanced assessment, Illich might be right that in its popular representations of medicine, contemporary culture ignores or even denies suffering and death and therefore people are unsure of how to face them when they become inevitable.

In his book *The Loneliness of the Dying*, Norbert Elias (1986) diagnoses the loneliness of death as a predictable and possibly inevitable consequence of the individualism characteristic of contemporary society, where the desire for autonomy affects the fabric of social relationships and may result in isolation. Illness is often experienced as estrangement, and the impersonal and bureaucratic regime of the hospitals contributes to it. As a result of an individualistic culture, psychological, spiritual, and social needs of patients are considered private by many in medicine, and, if discussed, often relegated to other professionals. Elias notes that illness and the closeness of death tends to isolate people from others as patients. Also, aging persons—who after the loss of their independence are relegated to the care of various institutions—gradually lose contact with others and therefore feel excluded from the community of the living. As Elias notes, the fulfillment of meaning for an individual is closely related to the meaning of one's life vis-à-vis other people. The emotional isolation in the hospital then makes the prospect of death even more difficult to face. Despite all the medical advances to treat and prevent diseases and to slow down the process of aging, the outer limit, death, nevertheless remains unavoidable, painful, and often cruel. For many, the moment of disclosure that there is nothing more that medicine can offer is often unpleasant and sometimes embarrassing. Death however comes only sometime after such pronouncement, and it is often this part of the journey that patients traverse alone. Moreover, physicians generally feel ill-equipped to deal with issues beyond their technical expertise, and some of them do not consider this aspect of life—dying—to be in the remit of their profession (Gawande, 2014).

The awareness of the unsatisfactory care for and treatment of dying patients inspired the hospice movement and the development of palliative care, beginning in the 1960s (Clark, 2005; Saunders, 2006). Acknowledging that in situations where there is no prospect of cure, especially in the terminal stages, the emphasis of hospice and palliative care is on pain relief, physical comfort, and a more personal approach to patients. The aim is also to allow patients to experience the last chapter of their life in an environment they prefer, often with their families present. However, living in the shadow or death is emblematic for many chronic conditions that tend to deteriorate over time. This emphasis on a comprehensive approach to patients' needs when facing death is something that other medical specialties should take seriously.

Phenomenological Philosophy of Existence

In this final section, I will introduce the perspective on human life in phenomenology and philosophy of existence as an alternative to the medical account of life, illness and death. Specifically, we shall consider texts by Martin Heidegger, Karl Jaspers, Viktor Frankl, Hannah Arendt, Emmanuel Lévinas, and Jan Patočka that allow us to understand the human condition from the perspective of temporality in terms of our presence in the world that inevitably entails suffering and death. Since we all share the human condition of vulnerability and finitude, the encounter between patients and their caregivers reveals the essentially ethical nature of medicine. I will argue that this approach is especially conducive for grounding medical humanism and an ethics of care within clinical practice.

The "phenomenology of existence" offers a perspective that aims to rescue the experiential mode from the objectifying tendency of science and technology. Phenomenologists draw on and respond to the work of Edmund Husserl, who distinguished the "theoretical attitude" and the "life-world." In a later work, *The Crisis of European Sciences*, Husserl (1970) advocates for the primacy of personal experience, namely, the intersubjective and pretheoretical over the objectifying approach of the sciences. This perspective represents a stark contrast to the scientific approach that operates in the "atemporal" perspective and is interested in aspects and traits that are generalizable to capture the uniqueness of individual human existence as it evolves. Simply, in contrast to the universals sought by science, Husserl highlighted the particularities of individual experience beyond the reach of the objective stance. This approach offers a perspective that emphasizes the temporal character of being human.

Heidegger articulated human temporality in a construction he called "Dasein" (being here, as well as being-in-the-world, and even dwelling), which seeks to capture human presence in the world as a temporal, embodied, situated, and intentional being (Jaspers, 1919; Heidegger, 2010). The emphasis on the temporality of the human presence in the world is crucial: "being" is understood as a verb rather than as substantive. The concept of Dasein also leaves aside the variations of anthropology based on dualism of body and soul/mind/spirit—a dichotomy that has plagued philosophy since Plato and, as already mentioned, served as the legacy of Descartes during the modern period. As Heidegger (2010, p. 47) writes:

> This question is about the being of the whole human being, whom one is accustomed to understand as a bodily-soul-like-spiritual unity. Body, soul, spirit might designate areas of phenomena which are thematically separable for the sake of determinate investigation; within certain limits their ontological indeterminacy might not be so important. But in the question of the being of human being, this cannot be summarily calculated in terms of the kinds of being of body, soul, and spirit which have yet first to be defined.

The concept of Dasein thus allows one to think of the physical, psychological, or spiritual aspects as distinct phenomena that characterize human existence—rather than as separate "substances." And of course, Dasein challenges the approach of medicine—entrenched in the tradition of the natural sciences derived from traditional ontology—that conceptualizes the human body as a physical substance. Consequently, aspects of human existence other than the physical seem to reach beyond medicine as typically conceived. However, since the individuality of being human is irreducible to the physical or material aspects of existence, a positivist approach is clearly insufficient when providing care for patients. In contrast, a philosophy of existence comes with the emphasis on human experience as primary, and it is this perspective that offers an alternative way to think of and to understand human life, illness, and death.

Dasein—Heidegger's attempt to characterize human presence in the world—has a beginning and an end. It develops, evolves, and engages with the world, and thus it relates to itself and to the world in various ways. Unlike natural sciences, which work in the mode of suspended time and where atemporal concepts endeavor to capture life processes in a specific moment, human life is experienced as it evolves in time. Temporality is of course impossible to conceive without reference to the physicality of experience. In other words, Dasein is embodied time. In this sense, the most general conditions of human existence are birth and death—two events that frame human life. Being born is the condition of possibility for experience. Although philosophers and particularly philosophers of medicine have devoted significant attention to the reality of finitude of human existence, to the facticity of death, the issues swirling around coming into existence have not gained the attention this central event deserves.

The acknowledgment of the unexpectedness of new life demands regard for human life, as well as for the finitude of human existence, in a new light, that is, with a positive rather than negative charge. Hannah Arendt (1998, pp. 177–78) took this challenge seriously and wrote:

> It is in the nature of beginning that something new has started which cannot be expected from whatever may have happened before. This character of startling unexpectedness is inherent in all beginnings and in all origins ... The new thus always happens against the overwhelming odds of statistical laws and their probability, which for all practical, everyday purposes amounts to certainty; the new thus always appears in the guise of a miracle.

It is rare for a philosopher to employ notions of miracle and mystery that are usually reserved for the realm of theology. However, it seems that few, if any, philosophical concepts are sufficient to capture the radical nature of such an event. Arendt goes even further in this direction when she claims:

> The miracle that saves the world, the realm of human affairs, from its normal, "natural" ruin is ultimately the fact of natality, in which the faculty of action is ontologically rooted. It is, in other words, the birth of new men and the new beginning, the action they are capable of by virtue of being born. Only the full experience of this capacity can bestow upon human affairs faith and hope. (p. 247)

She observes that faith and hope are ignored or disregarded by philosophy, although they do represent two essential characteristics of human existence: the openness to the future and the unpredictable and unconditioned.

Unlike Heidegger, for whom anxiety and death were the determining characteristics of Dasein, Lévinas insists that it is enjoyment, the happiness of life, that is determinative. "Life is activity and sentiment," insists Lévinas (1991, p. 115), "to live is to enjoy life. To despair of life makes sense only because originally life is happiness. Suffering is a failing of happiness; it is not correct to say that happiness is an absence of suffering." This is an important reversal. The primacy of the positive cannot be undone by the negative. It also allows the contemplation of suffering and death as a toll for life, for joy, rather than making life meaningless or absurd. Nevertheless, Lévinas (2003, pp. 69–70) also highlights another aspect of coming into existence:

> The banal observation that man is by birth engaged in an existence he neither willed nor chose must not be limited to the case of man as a finite being. He translates the structure of being itself. The fact of beginning to exist is not a matter of inevitability, for inevitability obviously already

presupposes existence. The entry into existence did not vex some will, since in that case the existence of that will would have come before itself . . . It is in the being that begins—not in its relations with its cause—that we find the paradox of a being that begins to be, or, in other words, the impossibility of distinguishing, in this being, what takes on the weight of being from that weight itself.

Lévinas is exposing the paradox associated with the core of human existence in which, in the very attempt to think of the beginning of our existence, the tension within the experience of oneself as a self—as an individual—rises to prominence. Not being the origin of ourselves, we have not chosen who we are or even that we are.

The situatedness of human life is captured by Heidegger's concept of "Geworfenheit" or being thrown. Being "thrown" into the world, Dasein finds itself in a specific situation—shaped by both biological and social historical forces. These forces, as well as the way in which Dasein understands and interprets them, determine the scope of projects that one is able to follow in life. This being-in-the-world is being-with-others. However, there is also the reality of solitude of Dasein, which becomes especially prominent against the horizon in which human life is framed: death. Death is the certain yet absent future that colors experience as temporary and transient. "Being-toward-death," as Heidegger (2010, p. 248) writes, "is grounded in care. As thrown being-in-the-world, Dasein is always already delivered over to its death. Being toward its death, it dies factically and constantly as long as it has not reached its demise." He defines the mode of "being-toward-death" as essentially an abiding anxiety. However, this reality of finitude tends to be obscured, forgotten, and disregarded by the everydayness of life. It is only in certain situations that the death enters conscious reflection, which for Heidegger is the source (as well as essential condition) of authenticity.

These encounters with death and its shadow over human life, experienced as suffering, were also the preoccupation of Jaspers when he introduced the notion of "limit situation." Specifically, there are experiences when suffering gains a new character as a situation becomes final, inevitable, and limiting (Jaspers, 1919, p. 222). He notes that there is always a tension in the situation Dasein finds itself in. This tension is created by antinomies of which the most fundamental are life and death, contingency and meaningfulness, fight and help, and guilt and forgiveness. These antinomies are constitutive of each other and while one of them has a positive and the other negative charge, it is impossible to have one without the other. Each is experienced as total in their character—there is no being outside of them with respect to personal experience. These situations in which we are faced with our essential limitations and finitude then represent a threshold, a demand for response. As Jaspers contends:

The shared characteristic of all limit experiences is that they cause suffering—but they also share the ability to awaken and cultivate strength that allows one to experience enjoyment, meaning and growth. Pleasure and pain, enjoyment and suffering are inextricably intertwined. Both of these are experienced as something final, overwhelming, unsurmountable, an essential part of our life situation. (pp. 218–19).[2]

This raises a characteristic theme of existentialism: the notion of human freedom. Although acknowledging the limitations imposed on us by external circumstances we still have a freedom as to how we respond to them, how we face the inevitable suffering. It was a motive elaborated by Frankl as the freedom to find meaning even in a hopeless situation. Based on his experience as a physician who survived the concentration camp, he observed that it was this attitude that made people "agree to life" despite the circumstances that inclined them to do otherwise. "When we are no longer able to change the situation—just think of incurable disease such as inoperable cancer—we are challenged," notes Frankl (2004, p. 116), "to change ourselves." Suffering, then, has the potential for transformation.

However, the tension of suffering is not necessarily the tension of the external situation; it might be experienced as internal tension, too. In an early essay entitled "On Escape," Lévinas (2003)—possibly in response to Heidegger—notes that while philosophy illuminated the tensions between the subject and the world, it still held as unproblematic our relationship to ourselves: we are and, at the same time, we understand ourselves and relate to ourselves in a certain way. This possibility of self-relation has been occasionally the focus of philosophy in the realm of ethics, as a mode of introspection of conscience. Lévinas nevertheless exposes this phenomenon of self-relation by examining the situations that awaken in us the acute feeling or desire to escape from ourselves.[3]

The desire for freedom upon which limits are imposed, not only by the world but also by our own embodied existence, is a motive around which Lévinas (2003) composed the essay "On Escape." To that end, he examines the phenomena of malaise, pleasure, and shame as situations of great intensity in which the "temporal existence takes on the inexpressible flavor of the absolute" (p. 52). The desire for escape is strongest while experiencing unbearable situations where one finds that it is impossible to "break the chains of the I to the self" for which it aspires. This then is the very definition of suffering: "It is not that the suffering with which life threatens us render it displeasing; rather, it is because the ground of suffering consists of the impossibility of interrupting it, and of an acute feeling of being held fast" (p. 52). This negativity is then surpassed in pleasure, which Lévinas describes as a "process of departing from being," of loosening of this malaise. Nevertheless, it is an escape that fails. "If like a process that is far from closing up on itself," asserts Lévinas, "pleasure appears in a constant surpassing of oneself, it breaks just at the moment where it seems to get out absolutely" (p. 62). This disappointment, the awareness of the failure, is then a source of shame as an incapacity for breaking with ourselves while being exposed and needing to excuse ourselves.

These phenomena crystalize in the experience of nausea. "Nausea," for Lévinas (2003, p. 68), "reveals to us the presence of being in all its impotence, which constitutes this presence as such. It is the impotence of pure being in all it nakedness." This very physical phenomenon then becomes emblematic of all experiences of suffering. The feeling of being exposed, the desire to revolt against oneself, and the impossibility of escape are intense in the experience of pain and physical illness. The unproblematic relation to oneself suddenly stands out as a heavy burden of suffering. The betrayal of the body is an assault on human freedom—an assault not from without but from within. Elsewhere, Lévinas (1987, pp. 68–69) formulates it accordingly:

> In pain, sorrow, and suffering, we once again find, in a state of purity, the finality that constitutes the tragedy of solitude. The ecstasis of enjoyment does not succeed in surmounting this finality …The content of suffering merges with the impossibility of detaching oneself from suffering. In suffering there is an absence of all refuge.

The experience of pain and suffering as an extreme and overwhelming passivity, enchainment, helplessness, abandonment, and solitude is then extended to the understanding of death.

In suffering there is the proximity of death. Lévinas (1987, p. 70) writes: "The way death has of announcing itself in suffering, outside all light, is an experience of the passivity of the subject." This "outside of light" means that death is something absolutely unknowable where we ourselves are seized. The relationship with death is a relationship with mystery.

> Death is a menace that approaches me as a mystery; its secrecy determines it—it approaches without being able to be assumed, such that the time that separates me from death dwindles and dwindles without end, involves a sort of interval which my consciousness can not traverse, and where a leap will somehow be produced from death to me. The last part of the route will be crossed without me. (Lévinas, 1991, p. 235)

Unlike Heidegger for whom death is the death of ourselves that we contemplate and that becomes the condition for the authenticity and freedom, Lévinas is concerned with the death of the Other as the source of the ethical.

In *Totality and Infinity*, Lévinas (1991) develops a phenomenology of the face, the primary organizing relation to the Other. The manifestation of the Other in the face constitutes the ethical relationship of responsibility. Face-to-face is the primordial situation where the Other presents as a demand, a call for response.

> The face in the nakedness as a face presents to me the destitution of the poor one and the stranger; but this poverty and exile which appeal to my powers, address me, do not deliver themselves over to the powers as given, remain the expression of the face. The poor one, the stranger, presents himself as an equal. (p. 213)

The face of the Other also signifies: "thou shall not kill" (Lévinas, 1987, p. 108). Lévinas thus grounds the most fundamental ethical command in the face-to-face encounter. Murder is the attempt of absolute negation, but there is always something that resists this negation and that is the Otherness that cannot be destroyed by any such means. Even if I do kill the Other, the Other remains, never fully subordinated or reduced to my will. The Other is irreducible to anything I can do to it, or what can I know about the Other. Because of this radical Otherness, the relationship with the Other also opens up the space of infinity, of transcendence, and of the ethical.

The Other for Lévinas is always someone in need, a stranger. The face is a demand not to remain indifferent to the suffering of the Other, to its possible death. This is for Lévinas (2006, pp. 80, 86) also the ethical grounding of medicine.

> Original opening toward merciful care, the point at which—though a demand for analgesia, more pressing, more urgent, in the groan, than a demand for consolation or the postponement of death—the anthropological category of the medical, a category that is primordial, irreducible and ethical, imposes itself. For pure suffering, which is intrinsically senseless and condemned to itself with no way out, a beyond appears in the form of the interhuman. The interhuman lies in a non-difference to one another, in a responsibility for one another.

The concern for the death of the Other thus comes before the care for the self or concern for one's own death. Lévinas does not present any form of theodicy, and for him suffering—the evil of suffering—remains intrinsically useless, "for nothing." The only way suffering can gain meaning is when it becomes suffering for the suffering of someone else. According to Lévinas,

> It is this attention to the suffering of the Other that can be affirmed as the very nexus of human subjectivity, to the point of being raised to the level of supreme ethical principle—the only one it is impossible to question— shaping the hopes and commanding the practical discipline of vast human groups. (p. 81)

The death that presents itself in suffering becomes the ethical moment. Being exposed to death the face of the Other also signifies "do not leave me alone in my death" (Lévinas, 2002, p. 145).

For medicine, which often perceives death as a failure of therapy, death is the ultimate limit. In a situation where technologies fail and medicine is left with only "instrumental" value, human presence reveals medicine's original ethical grounding. When there is nothing more to offer a patient from the medical perspective, the relationship, that is, the face-to-face encounter, remains as the primary ethical moment. It is a demand not to leave patients alone in their death. In acknowledging the moral imperative of the face, suffering is transformed and the space of transcendence opens. This opening is not a transcendence in a metaphysical sense but in terms of "beyond"—being more concerned with the suffering and death of the Other that takes priority over the concern with one's own demise. This is also the meaning of "humanity" that he calls goodness. "Goodness," for Lévinas (2002, p. 247), "consists in taking up a position in being such that the Other counts more than myself. Goodness thus involves the possibility for the I that is exposed to the alienation of its powers by death not to be for death."

The finitude of human existence is fundamental for grounding ethics. It is in the encounter with the Other as essentially exposed to death that ethics has its source. This again represents a shift from Heidegger for whom one of the characteristics of being-in-the-world is being-with-others. For Lévinas (2006, p. 188) this becomes "being-for-the other."

> The priority of the Other over the I, by which the human being-there is chosen and unique, is precisely the latter's response to the nakedness of the face and its mortality. It is there that the concern for the Other's death is realized, and that "dying for him," "dying his death" takes priority over "authentic" death. Not a post-mortem life, but the excessiveness of sacrifice, holiness in charity and mercy. This future of death in the present of love is probably one of the original secrets of temporality itself and beyond all metaphor.

Conclusion

In the previous sections, I described the tendency of medicine to objectify patients—by knowing, technological intervention, and impersonal care—which obscures the essentially ethical relationship of responsibility grounded in awareness of shared human condition as the origin of ethics. There is always a tension between the humanistic ideals and the complex cultural and socio-economic realities shaping the practice of medicine. However, in the situations that expose human vulnerability and finitude, awareness of this also provides a unique opportunity for humanity to flourish. Responding to the suffering of others does not only relieve their suffering, it also allows for the virtue of compassion of the caregiver and physician to be exercised and enables them to grow in their humanity.

Jan Patočka (1996) argues that the conception of ethics is grounded in the experience of "shaken-ness," the confrontation with the inherent fragility of human existence and the ethical responsibility that arises from this experience — solidarity of the shaken. In the final chapter of *Heretical Essays in the Philosophy of History*, Patočka portrays the twentieth century as a war, a state in which there is no outside but only a force that destroys life and leaves people shaken in their faith in the day, in life, and in peace (p. 134). He suggests that this state of absolute war can be overcome by the solidarity of those who are aware and acknowledge the inherent contingency of life, the vulnerability and finitude, the possibility of "shipwrecking." The awareness of the shared human condition is what grounds solidarity toward the Other, and the experience of being shaken has an ethical implication: having once experienced the war we become responsible for sustaining life and peace — the responsibility for the Other. This is what constitutes "living in truth": acknowledging our own limitations, taking seriously the finitude of our existence, and accepting the responsibility for the Other. For many, this is also what renders life meaningful.

Notes

1. Engel as well as other authors (Kleinman, 1989; Boyd, 2000) introduced the conceptual distinction between disease, as an objective entity, and illness, as a subjective experience. This distinction nevertheless does not necessarily have an equivalent in other languages.
2. The assistance of Asja-Ilka Tank with the translation is greatly appreciated.
3. These have been brilliantly portrayed in the accounts of Nancy (2008), Kane (2000), and Murphy (1990) as referred to previously.

References

Aquinas, T. *Summa Theologiae* II–II.30.1

Arendt, H. (1998). *The Human Condition*. The University of Chicago Press.

Boyd, K. M. (2000). Disease, illness, sickness, health, healing and wholeness: Exploring some elusive concepts. *Medical Humanities* 26: 9–17.

Canguilhem, G. (1991). *The Normal and the Pathological*. Zone Books.

Canon 22. (1215). Fourth Lateran Council.

Carlino, A. (1999). *The Books of the Body: Anatomical Ritual and Renaissance Learning*. The University of Chicago Press.

Cassell, E. J. (2003). *The Nature of Suffering and the Goals of Medicine*. Oxford University Press.

Charon, R. (2008). *Narrative Medicine: Honoring the Stories of Illness.* Oxford University Press.

Clark, D. (2005). *Cicely Saunders—Founder of the Hospice Movement: Selected Letters 1959–1999.* Oxford.

Cohen, L. (1999). Where it hurts: Indian material for an ethics of organ transplantation. *Daedelus* 128(4): 135–65.

Cooter, R., and Pickstone, J. (2002). *Companion Encyclopedia of Medicine in the Twentieth Century.* Routledge.

Daniels, N. (2008). *Just Health. Meeting Health Needs Fairly.* Cambridge.

Elias, N. (1986). *The Loneliness of the Dying.* Blackwell.

Engel, G. L. (1977). The need for a new medical model: A challenge for biomedicine. *Science* 196/4286: 129–36.

Foucault, M. (2006). *History of Madness.* Routledge.

Frank, A. (1997). *The Wounded Storyteller: Body, Illness and Ethics.* Chicago University Press.

Frankl, V. E. (2004). *Man's Search for Meaning.* Rider Books. [German original: *Trotzdem Ja zum Leben sagen: Ein Psychologe erlebt das Konzentrationslager.*]

Gawande, A. (2014). *Being Mortal: Medicine and What Matters in the End.* Metropolitan Books.

Goldstein, K. (2000). *The Organism.* Zone Books.

Good, B. (1993). *Medicine, Rationality and Experience: An Anthropological Perspective.* Cambridge University Press.

Good, M. J. V., Brodwin, P. E., Good, B. J., and Kleinman, A. (eds.) (1994). *Pain as Human Experience: An Anthropological Perspective.* University of California Press.

Greene, J. H. (2009). *Prescribing by Numbers: Drugs and the Definition of Disease.* John Hopkins.

Greenhalg, T., and Hurwitz, B. (eds.) (1998). *Narrative Based Medicine: Dialogue and Discourse in Clinical Practice.* Wiley.

Harrison, P. (2007). *The Fall of Man and the Foundation of Science.* Cambridge University Press.

Heidegger, M. (2010 [1927]). *Being and Time.* State University of New York Press.

Husserl, E. (1970 [1936]). *The Crisis of European Sciences and Transcendental Phenomenology: An Introduction to Phenomenological Philosophy.* Northwestern University Press.

Illich, I. (2000). *Limits to Medicine: Medical Nemesis, the Expropriation of Health.* Marion Boyars Publishers.

Jaspers, K. (1919). *Psychologie der Weltanschaungen.* Verlag von Julius Springer.

Jaspers, K. (1989 [1959]). Physicians in the technological age. *Theoretical Medicine* 10: 251–67.

Jonas, H. (1981). *Philosophical Essays.* University of Chicago Press.

Kane, S. (2000). *4.48 Psychosis.* Methuen Drama/Bloomsbury.

Kevles, D. J. (2004). *In the Name of Eugenics: Genetics and the Uses of Human Heredity.* Cambridge, MA: Harvard University Press.

Kleinman, A. (1989). *Illness Narratives: Suffering, Healing and the Human Condition.* Basic Books

LaFleur, W. R., Gernot Böhme, G., and Shimazono, S. (2008). *Dark Medicine: Rationalizing Unethical Medical Research.* Indiana University Press.

Landecker, H. (2010). *Culturing Life: How Cells Became Technologies.* Harvard University Press.

Lévinas, E. (1987 [1947]). *Time and the Other.* Duquesne University Press.

Lévinas, E. (1987 [1985]). Diachrony and representation. In *Time and the Other.* Duquesne University Press.

Lévinas, E. (1991 [1961]). *Totality and Infinity.* Kluwer Academic Publishing.

Lévinas, E. (2002). Intention, event, and the other. In *Is It Righteous to Be?* Stanford University Press.

Lévinas, E. (2003 [1935]). *On Escape: de l'evasion.* Stanford University Press.

Lévinas, E. (2006). Useless suffering. In *Entre Nous*. Continuum.

Lévinas, E. (2006). Dying for . . . In *Entre Nous*. Continuum.

MacDonald, H. (2010). *Possessing the Dead: The Artful Science of Anatomy*. Melbourne University Press.

Mattingly, Ch., and Garro, L. C. (eds.) (2001). *Narrative and the Cultural Construction of Illness and Healing*. University of California Press.

Murphy, R. F. (1990). *The Body Silent*. Norton.

Nancy, J. L. (2008). The intruder. In *Corpus*. Fordham University Press.

Patočka, J. (1996). *Heretical Essays in the Philosophy of History*. Open Court.

Pellegrino, E. D. (1979). *Humanism and the Physician*. University of Tennessee Press.

Pellegrino, E. D., and Thomasma, D. C. (1981). *A Philosophical Basis of Medical Practice: Toward a Philosophy and Ethic of the Healing Professions*. Oxford University Press.

Petryna, A. (2009). *When Experiments Travel: Clinical Trials and the Global Search for Human Subjects*. Princeton University Press.

Porter, R. (1999). *The Greatest Benefit to Mankind: A Medical History of Humanity. The Norton History of Science*. W. W. Norton & Company.

Porter, R. (2004). *Flesh in the Age of Reason: The Modern Foundation of Body and Soul*. W. W. Norton.

Relman, A. S. (1980). The new medical–industrial complex. *New England Journal of Medicine* 303: 963–70.

Richardson, R. (2000). *Death, Dissection and the Destitute*. Chicago University Press.

Risse, G. B. (1999). *Mending Bodies, Saving Souls: A History of Hospitals*. Oxford University Press.

Rose, N. (2006). *The Politics of Life Itself: Biomedicine, Power, and Subjectivity in the Twenty-First Century*. Princeton University Press.

Sandel, M. (2009). *The Case against Perfection: Ethics in the Age of Genetic Engineering*. Belknap Press.

Saunders, C. (2006). *Selected Writings 1958–2004*. Oxford.

Sheper-Hughes, N., and Wacquant, L. (2003). *Commodifying Bodies*. SAGE.

Tauber, A. I. (1999). *Confessions of a Medicine Man: An Essay in Popular Philosophy*. MIT.

Tauber, A. I. (2005). *Patient Autonomy and the Ethics of Responsibility*. MIT.

Zimmer, C. (2004). *Soul Made Flesh*. Free Press.

8 Phenomenology and Medicine

Fredrik Svenaeus

Introduction

The related traditions of phenomenology and hermeneutics provide theoretical tools to develop descriptions and concepts in which to grasp the nature and essence of illness as the suffering experienced by a person. Doctors and other healthcare professionals need to establish an understanding of the body- and world-embedded experiences of their patients if they are to help them in the best possible way. Medical practice, accordingly, is not only to be understood as applied medical science, but also as a kind of hermeneutics based on empathic, cultural, and communicative skills. Medical–scientific theories and technologies that change our view on and make us able to manipulate features of human biology are situated in a lifeworld of personal concerns that infuse theories and technologies with meaning. Phenomenology, I will argue, provides a way to understand and to evaluate critically new scientific–technological possibilities to heal our bodies, or even to enhance human nature, by taking such lifeworld meaning patterns into account.

In the chapter, I give references to and discuss contributions of phenomenologists who are central to the tasks and dilemmas of modern medicine: works by Maurice Merleau-Ponty, Martin Heidegger, Jean-Paul Sartre, and Hans-Georg Gadamer, but also contributions made by contemporary phenomenologists of medicine, such as Richard Zaner, Kay Toombs, Drew Leder, and Havi Carel.

Phenomenology of Medicine

Medicine is not only a scientific way of understanding and altering features of the human body; it is also a human practice with certain inherent goals, notably to heal and help suffering persons (Marcum, 2008; Pellegrino and Thomasma, 1981). As everyone who has pursued the field of philosophy of medicine knows, the exact nature and limits of medical activities has been a constant topic of debate in the field ever since the 1970s. Some philosophers defend a definition of medicine that stresses the *meeting* of healthcare professional and patient in an interpretative attempt to help and cure the ill and suffering party, whereas other philosophers would rather look for the essence of medicine in the *application* of medical knowledge in attempts to understand and alter the biological organism (Nordenfelt and Tengland, 1996). These two answers to the question of what medicine is need not exclude each other; they could be brought into dialogue, and the first answer could be made to include the second, just as the second answer could be complemented by the first (Svenaeus, 2000). The interpretative practice of understanding and helping the patient could, and, indeed, should, include biological knowledge, whereas the applied-biology paradigm would need to address, in some way, that the doctor sees a person and not only this person's body.

Despite the possibility of combining the two alternatives, where one puts the emphasis will be important, not only in answering the question of whether or not a particular activity is to be counted as a medical activity, but also in addressing ethical and political questions concerning the mission of medicine. If medicine is essentially a meeting between a medical professional and a patient aiming to restore or protect health and alleviate the suffering of illness, the practice itself has normative roots that need to be philosophically excavated in pursuing biomedical ethics. Whereas if medicine is basically the application of scientific knowledge in the clinical context, the ethical principles to be adhered to are not to be found by way of analyzing the structure of medical practice. As we will see the phenomenology–hermeneutics approach favors the first alternative and therefore assigns the ontology and epistemology of medical practice an important founding function in biomedical ethics. Further on, we will return to the issue of how to understand the nature of medicine, but first we need to say more about phenomenology.

Phenomenology is a tradition more than one hundred years old exploring and answering philosophical questions by proceeding from an analysis of everyday experiences; important classics are philosophers such as Edmund Husserl, Martin Heidegger, Maurice Merleau-Ponty, Jean-Paul Sartre, Hans-Georg Gadamer, Hannah Arendt, and Paul Ricoeur (Moran, 2000). Phenomenology relates and connects to the even older philosophical tradition of hermeneutics, in which some of the aforementioned figures are often assigned their major residence. The starting point for the phenomenologist (as well as the hermeneutist) is not the world of science, but the meaning structures of the everyday world, that which the phenomenologist calls the "lifeworld" (including communicative endeavors and textual artefacts).

Contemporary phenomenology has branched out into many different disciplines from the philosophical trunk provided by Husserl and his disciples in the beginning of the twentieth century. Scholars and researchers of art, literature, psychology, sociology, anthropology, pedagogy, history, and recently, also, nursing, and medicine have tried to make use of phenomenology in investigating phenomena of concern in their field. Phenomenology in these explorative endeavors may remain essentially philosophical or become more empirically applied in nature. In characterizing the ways of phenomenological analysis the idea of a certain *method* has been important from the Husserlian start, but more recently this philosophical methodology has by some scholars also been reformulated as a set of rules and tools for analyzing data gathered by way of, for example, interviews or field studies (van Manen, 2014). In both cases the phenomenologist aims to start her analysis in an unprejudiced manner, meaning a manner that is open to the meaning-structures of the lifeworld and not predetermined by scientific models of the phenomena she intends to study. In the phenomenological analysis—philosophical as well as empirically applied—the phenomenologist aims to focus by way of reflection on the meaning structures that make the experience of objects, other persons, and oneself in the world possible in the first place. What makes, for instance, a table appear as a table to us in everyday experience and how is the "tableness" in question dependent on the way we act in the world together with other persons (Ahmed, 2006)? Such questions will take us back to social and cultural traditions involving tables, but, even more fundamentally, they will address the way our embodiment is central to perceiving and making use of objects in the world.

The main topic of phenomenology of medicine and healthcare so far has been bodily experiences—experiences of phenomena such as illness, pain, suffering, disability, giving birth, and dying (Aho and Aho, 2008; Carel, 2006, 2008; Leder, 1990; Mol, 2002; Schott, 2010; Scullly, 2008; Slatman, 2014; Svenaeus, 2000; Toombs, 1992, 2001; Zaner, 1981; Zeiler and Käll, 2014). One finds elements of such analyses in the works of the major phenomenologists mentioned earlier, and, even more so, in some less-well-known figures of the tradition, such as F. J. J. Buytendijk, Hans Jonas, and Herbert Plügge. However, the idea of a phenomenology of medicine as a distinct field of academic studies was not formed until the 1980s when the discipline of philosophy of medicine gained increased attention in connection with the booming field of biomedical ethics. In this context the development of medical humanities in educational programs in medical schools during the same time should also be mentioned, since phenomenology and hermeneutics are firm members of the so-called continental tradition of philosophy in which the humanities are much more of neighbors than in the tradition of analytical philosophy that have long dominated the academic milieus of the United States and United Kingdom (Downie and Macnaughton, 2007). Long before the appearance of phenomenological studies of medicine in the 1980s and 1990s, however, phenomenology had executed a certain influence in one specific medical specialty—psychiatry—with major scholars such as Karl Jaspers, Erwin Strauss, and Henri Eye (Spiegelberg, 1972).

This influence, however, was, as in the case of Buytendijk, Jonas, and Plügge, mainly restricted to continental Europe.

The Lived Body

In phenomenological analysis, ever since the days of Husserl, the body is typically assigned a central place and function in all forms of human experiences. A basic distinction stressed in this context by the phenomenologist is between the body considered as an intentional structure in contrast to as a biological organism, often referred to as a distinction between the "lived," and the "living" body (Leder, 1990). The body already organizes my experiences and make them possible in a preconscious way that as a rule resides in the background of our attention. Proprioceptively it makes me present in the world, and kino-aesthetically it allows me to experience the things that are not me—the things of the world that show up to my moving, sensing body in different activities through which they attain their place and significance for me (Gallagher, 2005). The body is my zero *place* in the world, a point of access that makes spatial experience possible.

Normally the lived body remains in the background of our experience and our attention is instead focused on the things in the world that we are engaged with. In Merleau-Ponty (1962) and Sartre (1956), we find penetrating descriptions and conceptual analyses of such everyday experiences that are bodily in nature even though we are not focused on the body: seeing, listening, walking, talking, reading, and so on. In some situations, however, the body calls for our attention, forcing us to take notice of its existence in pleasant or unpleasant ways. This experienced body can be the source of joy, as when we enjoy a good meal, do sports, have sex, or are just relaxing after a hard day of work. However, the body can also be the source of suffering to its bearer, when a person falls ill or is injured and feels pain, nausea, or anxiety and experiences difficulties to perceive or to move (Aho and Aho, 2008; Carel, 2008; Leder, 1990; Svenaeus, 2009; Toombs, 1992). When I have a headache, the pain in question invades my entire world—my attempts to concentrate, perceive, communicate, move, and so on. If the doctors examine my body with the help of medical technologies, they may be able to detect processes going on in my brain and the rest of my body that are responsible for the pain in question, but they will never find my headache *experience*, the feel and meaning the pain has for me in my "being-in-the-world," to speak in a phenomenological idiom.

To suffer from a headache means to find oneself in a *first-person* perspective as regards the pain in question. To encounter another person having a headache means to perceive the headache from the *second-person* perspective: through the posture, gestures, facial expressions, ways of speaking and acting, and so on of the person in question. The *third-person* perspective on headache, on the other hand, in contrast to both the first- and the second-person perspective, is one from a neutral scientific party, who is interested in the biological, causal pathways that make the headache in question come into existence. We perceive other persons as directly connected to us through the lived expressions of their bodies, whereas our own body has an autonomous nature that is foreign to us in many ways and which can be studied by the doctor. Phenomenology starts out from the perspective of lived personal experience, but in this analysis it concerns the whole world of the embodied person, including the encounter with bodies of other persons and the possibility to adopt a scientific third-person perspective on any type of object appearing in view, including one's own body as a *living* thing—in this case studied by the very same *lived* body. In my overview of themes central to the phenomenology of medicine in this chapter, I will start out in the first-person perspective of the patient. I will then proceed to integrate also the second- and third-person perspective of the healthcare professional in the phenomenological–hermeneutical understanding of medical practice.

The difference between the first-person (and the second-person) and the third-person perspective on the body is an important one. It makes it possible to explain not only how human experience is meaningful and material simultaneously, but also how the body belongs to a person in a stronger and more primordial sense than a pair of trousers, a car, or a house. The body is not only ours, it is *us* and this insight will have important repercussions in facing ethical dilemmas associated with technologies that make it possible to transplant and cultivate parts of the body (Diprose, 2002; Leder, 1999). But even more important to medical practice than the contributions to bioethics in handling technological possibilities and dilemmas is the basic phenomenological analysis of the many situations in which the lived body plagues us in various ways: when we become ill.

As we have stressed earlier, the lived body performs its duties silently in the background of experience, not only proprioceptively and kino-aesthetically, but also as regards all the autonomic functions of our visceral life. We breathe, our hearts beat, our stomachs and bowels work without and beyond our conscious control and will. Sometimes, however, the body shows up in resisting and disturbing our efforts. It plagues us and demands our attention. A paradigm example is pain. If I have a headache, it becomes hard to concentrate and think. Even before my attention is directed toward the headache itself, the whole world and all my projects become tinted by pain. When I read, the letters become fuzzy, the text itself hurts when I try to understand it. This is Sartre's example from *Being and Nothingness*, published originally in 1943 (1956), so the phenomenology of illness, as the phenomenology of embodiment, actually goes back further than the contemporary studies mentioned earlier; another main source is Merleau-Ponty's *The Phenomenology of Perception* from 1945 (1962).

Illness and pain are never Sartre's or Merleau-Ponty's main objects of study; however, they are used mainly as examples to address questions about human nature in general (Svenaeus, 2009).

Illness as Unhomelike Being-in-the-World

Illness, as the headache example of Sartre shows, displays a "mooded" aspect tied to activities one is performing (Sartre, 1956, pp. 401 ff.). Other examples of illness moods are nausea, being too hot or cold, unmotivated tiredness, or the way the body resists the attempts to do different things—like when I try to climb the stairs and my chest hurts. Of course, there are distinctions to be made here. For most people, the chest starts to hurt after ten stairs of fast climbing, but when it does so more or less immediately or unexpectedly, it is a paradigm example of illness. According to another very influential phenomenologist, Martin Heidegger (1996, pp. 134 ff.), every experience we have is, as a matter of fact, attuned—"mooded"—but this attunement of our being-in-the-world normally, just like the embodied character of experience, stays in the subconscious background, not making itself known to us. In illness, however, the mood we are in makes itself known in permeating our entire experience, finally, when it becomes unbearable, bringing us back to our plagued embodiment, which now resists our attempts to act and carry out things, instead of supporting them in the unapparent manner of healthy being-in-the-world (Svenaeus, 2011).

Heidegger's (1996, pp. 184 ff.) analysis in *Being and Time*, his first major work, published in 1927, makes lucid how some feelings (moods) are world *constitutive* phenomena. Moods open up a world to human beings in which things *matter* to them in different ways. It is common in the contemporary philosophy of feelings to make a distinction between sensations, emotions, and moods (Goldie, 2000). Sensations have a distinct place in the body (pain), emotions have an object and are based upon beliefs (love or hate), whereas moods are not bodily and also lack a distinct object; they rather color the way everything appears to a person (joy or sadness). This schematization goes back all the way to the philosopher Aristotle and has been further developed in slightly different ways in the tradition of analytical philosophy. What is central to the distinctions is that certain feelings—emotions—have a cognitive content: feelings are not merely passions, which lead the rational agent astray in his search for knowledge; feelings are indeed forms of knowledge in themselves (Nussbaum, 2001).

Note, however, that this merely holds for emotions in this type of philosophy—in which an object of the feeling is involved—whereas in the case of sensations and moods the cognitive content is much harder to pin point and therefore tends to fall out of the analysis. This might appear rather adequate in the case of some sensations, in which the possible cognitive content is very meager in contrast to the content of typical emotions; for example, that I feel an itch on my back in contrast to my feeling envy in face of certain circumstances, an emotion that includes quite elaborate beliefs about the state of the world and the way I would like it to be. When it comes to moods, however, the lack of a distinct object of the mood in question seems to have forced the classic analysis in the wrong direction. Moods are, for sure, not something that contains thoughts in the same way that emotions do, but they are nevertheless determining which kinds of thoughts I will be able to develop by providing the general access to the way *all* things will appear to me in the world (Ratcliffe, 2008).

The experience of illness can be characterized as an "unhomelike" mood and way of being placed in the world (Svenaeus, 2009, 2011). The lifeworld is usually the home territory of the person, but in illness this homelikeness gives in and takes on a distinctly unfamiliar and uncanny character, rooted in thwarted ways of being embodied. The ways we inhabit the world, in homelike as well as unhomelike manners, are not only related to biological functions making us able to have experiences of and do things in the world, they are also related to social and cultural meaning patterns that doctors and other healthcare professionals need to study and understand if they are to help their patients. Especially in cases of chronic illness—when the biological functionality of the body cannot be fully restored—the difference between homelike and unhomelike being-in-the-world for the sick person will largely depend on changing the ways in which she leads her life on an everyday level and the ways in which she defines her life goals as the subject of a life story (Kleinman, 1988; Morris, 1998). We will return to these issues in addressing the meaning and nature of human suffering in what follows.

The concept of "being-in-the-world" was introduced by Heidegger in *Being and Time* (1996), and it was quickly picked up by other phenomenologists, such as Merleau-Ponty (1962) and Sartre (1956). In analogy to the way I *am* my body, in the phenomenological understanding I *am* my world, rather than just being placed in the world as a thing among other things. I am immersed in the lifeworld in a meaningful way, which connects its meaning patterns—and particularly the ones I am relying on in my most vital life projects—to my identity. The world is not merely a physically extended geography in which I happen to have a place among other things; being-in-the-world in phenomenology refers to the way human beings *inhabit* the world as a pattern of significance. As discussed earlier, this way of being-in-the-world always has a mooded aspect, even though this attunement might rest in the background of our activities, not being noticed by us until we turn to the mood explicitly. In illness, however, the mood in question has a tendency to *call* for our attention since it is unhomelike in character and makes us suffer. The homelikeness of health, in contrast to this, dwells in the background and is rarely paid attention to—we most often take the transparent, homelike being-in of health for granted until illness strikes us (Gadamer, 1996).

Unhomelike being-in-the-world is a wider characterization than illness, since external circumstances may render our being-in-the-world unhomelike in ways that are not cases of illness in themselves, even though they could, of course, lead to illness in the long run. To be locked up in prison for years and be exposed to harsh conditions is such an example. To experience the suffering of a war is another. Existential crisis suffered, for instance, after the loss of a loved one, a third. Remember, however, that it is the being-*in*-the-world of the person that counts as homelike or unhomelike in the phenomenological understanding. To live in an environment means to experience it and assign it meaning through feelings, thoughts, and actions. Thus the lifeworld of phenomenology is not identical to physical surroundings, but is a meaning pattern of human understanding. Whether being locked up in prison results in unhomelike being-in-the-world or not depends partly on the world that the person is situated in—its material as well as cultural characteristics—and partly on the way she projects this given world of necessities and possibilities in her life. The prisoner might in some cases be able to adjust to a homelike existence behind bars, although the conditions of imprisonment in most cases would offer too much resistance to allow this homelike reinterpretation of the person's life project (especially if the imprisonment is for life or for a very long time). The same goes for persons exposed to war or those experiencing the loss of loved ones.

It is important to stress the fundamental difference between a phenomenological *illness* concept and the concept of *disease* (Carel and Cooper, 2013). A disease is a disturbance of the biological functions of the body, or something that causes such a disturbance, which can only be detected and understood from the third-person perspective of the doctor investigating the body with the aid of her hands or medical technologies. The patient can also, by way of the doctor, or by way of medical theory, or, as often happens nowadays, by way of a webpage on the internet, adopt such a third-person perspective toward her own body and speculate about diseases responsible for her suffering. But the suffering itself is an illness experience of the person who is in a world, embodied and connected to other people around her. Illness has meaning, or, perhaps we should say instead, *disturbs* the meaning processes of being-in-the-world in which one is leading one's life on an everyday level.

Typically, when I suffer illness, my biological organism will be diseased, but there are possibilities of being ill without any detectable diseases, or of leading a homelike life, when suddenly the doctor finds a disease, for example, by way of a cancer screening. The phenomenologist would stress that the full importance and content of illness can be attained only if the doctor, in addition to being skilled in diagnosing diseases, also affords attention to the experienced suffering, the being-in-the-world, of the patient. The full life of the person and not only her biology is, as a matter of fact, the reason why diseases matter to us as human beings—because they can make our lives miserable and even make us perish. If this were not the case, we would not *care* so much about diseases. It is because we want to be at home in the world that we study disease-causing agents and try to find remedies for them, even though we will never succeed completely in this project, since illness and suffering are certainly necessary parts of a human life, too.

Human Suffering and the Goals of Medicine

Provided that the suffering of illness is to be understood as a mood, penetrating the being-in-the-world of a person, what is characteristic of such suffering-moods beyond the dimension of bodily ailments and difficulties to perceive and move in the world? Important examples of suffering-moods at play in illness are anxiety, fear, sadness, boredom, helplessness, despair, and shame. These moods would not be deprived of bodily aspects, but the pain that is involved in them would be of another type than physical distress only. As a matter of fact, the moods I just mentioned are all essential ingredients in the condition we call "depression," which can be regarded as exemplary for psychic suffering in gathering so many forms of suffering-moods. Many other psychiatric conditions are certainly also examples of suffering, but depression is exemplary because the moods to be found in depression are to such large extent part of everyday human sufferings that are not always debilitating to the point of being psychiatric disorders (cases of illness) (Ratcliffe, 2015).

By employing terms such as "mental suffering" or "mental pain" in contrast to "bodily suffering" or "bodily pain," we obviously do not want to introduce some kind of dualist philosophy. A dualist, just as a reductionist–materialist, view on the human mind are positions that the phenomenologist aims to overcome from the very beginning in approaching experience as embodied but yet lifeworld dependent in nature (Merleau-Ponty, 1962, pp. vii ff.). The point of proceeding from a phenomenology of moods in addressing illness suffering is exactly to show how bodily and mental suffering connect to each other and are part of one distinct phenomenon, namely, the being-in-the-world of a person.

Wishes and strivings for certain goals in life appear in the form of feelings, but as emotions they, in contrast to bodily sensations, include more or less specific *thoughts*, as explored earlier. Emotions are ways of presenting not only the whole world—as in moods—but also specific states of the world as those to be desired by the person who has the emotions. If I love a person, for example, I probably want to be with her and I also want her to be happy; this is what I desire by way of the emotion in question. To complicate matters, the way we live and embody life goals and life values is not always very well reflected or articulated. I may love a person without fully realizing this, because I resist this thought or because I have other competing feelings that block or become mixed up with the love in question, for example. The goals we have in life are not always fully clear to ourselves and they are rarely spelled out in any detail. Having said this, how are we to think about a "life plan" or a "life narrative" and the way they can be frustrated for a person in illness (Charon, 2006; Frank, 2013)? How explicit are the goals we set for ourselves in our lives and how cohesive is a life story?

Before attempting to spell out the phenomenology of suffering by way of moods and related emotions in more detail let us take into consideration a work that has been very influential in underlining the importance of a broader concept of suffering in medicine: Eric Cassell's book *The Nature of Suffering and the Goals of Medicine*, published originally in 1991 and then in a second, extended edition in 2004. Cassell's main message in the book is that medicine has been too preoccupied with the *causes* of pain and other bodily symptoms and is too ignorant of the way the symptoms attain *meaning* for the person suffering from them. Cassell defines "suffering" as a "state of severe distress associated with events that threaten the intactness of the person" (p. 32). The key concept here is, indeed, "person," which for Cassell involves a plethora of issues that he does not tie together neatly by means of any philosophical theory of personhood but nevertheless gives many examples and excellent discussions of in his book.

As regards definition, even more pressing than the concept of personhood, perhaps, are the terms Cassell uses to help us understand suffering as such; that is, the threatened "intactness" or, as he sometimes also puts it, "integrity" of the person. These concepts are put in place by Cassell to separate cases of suffering from other unpleasant, but not equally significant, processes that a person can go through in life, but they seem to imply that we know how to think about the person as a kind of *whole*, since it is the very holding together of the person that is threatened or broken down in suffering. The same issue comes up in the talk about life plans and life narratives in contemporary bioethics (DeGrazia, 2005). If life is a narrative, it is a whole in the sense of being stretched out in time with a beginning and an end and held together by some kind of plot. Another way of thinking about the cohesiveness of the person is to stress the experiential dimension, the holding together of a series of states of consciousness making up the self. Many issues in the philosophy of person- and selfhood come up here, but for reasons of space I will not deal with them directly in this chapter (Gallagher, 2011; Zahavi, 2006). Instead, I will now continue the phenomenological proposal for how we should conceptualize the suffering of persons by way of mood started out in the previous section on illness as unhomelike being-in-the-world.

Suffering due to a painful bodily condition involves a kind of potential *alienation* at the bodily level, making the person no longer able to be at home in and with her own body. This tends to lead to alienation at the levels involving the way a person acts in the world, relates to others, and realizes her core life values as well, because the mood invades the entire existence of the ill person. Self-understanding in these cases is linked to a temporal understanding of one's life, since the illness mood changes the way one approaches one's past and future. The past often becomes a paradise lost, whereas the future is more suffering to come or even an imminent, inevitable death (Charon, 2006; Frank, 2013; Kleinman, 1988; Svenaeus, 2011). However, there is certainly room for positive transformation in situations of very painful and life-threatening illness, too, particularly concerning core life values, since the seriousness of one's condition can make room for a more honest and true reflection upon what matters in life and who one wants to be (or to have been).

The typical illustration of that kind of rewarding suffering process is found in Leo Tolstoy's classic novel *The Death of Ivan Ilyich* (2013). However, in bringing up the transformative powers of severe illness, let us not forget the horrors suffered by the main character of this book, not only his bodily pains but also the disappointments brought upon him by his stupid family members and unfaithful friends in the story. Despite Ivan reaching a state of relative peace toward the end in facing his destiny, this is not the way many of us would like to end up, no matter how deeply deceived we may be about our life priorities and personal identity. If the transformation of one's core life values through suffering is to form an attractive alternative, we most often need more of a future to realize them in and somewhat less of bodily pains on the way to developing them.

Mental pains are not always easier to handle than bodily pains, but in most cases they are not as intense as the pains suffered by Ivan, who is dying from cancer of the intestinal tract. Whereas bodily alienation is often hard to make sense of and benefit from, the alienation that is caused by unwanted life events robbing the person of life meaning, rather than by pathological processes in her body, is more open to work on and change for the better. Transformative processes are in many cases an option here; one may find a new job, or a new partner, and go on to live a richer and more rewarding life. This may also happen in cases of somatic illnesses and injuries that are not life threatening, such as losing one's hearing or the ability to move one's legs as the result of an accident. In the latter cases the transformative change in question may be more of a coping than an empowerment process, but it could nevertheless include novel evaluations of one's life goals that make life more homelike again.

The moods we live in embody life priorities and evaluations by the way they make things in our life appear as more or less *significant* to us. Charles Taylor, in his book *Sources of the Self* (1989), argues that ourselves, our personal beings, are built up by means of such evaluations. Most important are the priorities he names "strong evaluations": evaluations *of* the things we more or less spontaneously desire and appreciate in life, such as food, sex, sleep, love, security, entertainment, and so on. These strong evaluations concern moral matters, the respect and responsibility we have for the life, integrity, well-being, and flourishing of other persons. They also concern questions about what a life worth living looks like and how I attain self-respect in this life together with others. These three zones of primal values are interconnected and they demand, at least to some extent, self-reflection. But the values of strong interpretation do not come about only through philosophical reflection; they become embodied by being-in-the-world with others from the very beginning of our lives. Evaluations, that is, the strong ones, are always dependent upon a life form, a horizon of attuned understanding that one has grown into by way of the support and influence of others.

Suffering can be brought about because of events that prevent one from realizing the values that are vital for one's life and sense of self-respect. The suffering-mood in question could be related, for instance, to no longer being able to do something that has been of utmost importance for one's sense of meaning in life—like listening to music, going for hikes, having sex, or drinking good wine. The suffering could also be related to events depriving the person of other persons that she loves and lives with. In all these cases the suffering would appear as a *mood* that the person lives in, and the mood in question would be related to a particular way of being-in-the-world and being-in-time, as well as being-in-the-body, that would be *alienated* in the sense of fundamentally *unhomelike* to the person in question. This is also the point at which we could talk about "broken" life narratives (Zaner, 2004). Such a suffering is not only or even fundamentally a case of having one or two particular wants in life frustrated; it is more like losing one's footing in the world and beginning to doubt that *anything* really matters anymore because the values in question are so central to one's life and identity.

Let us now conclude the phenomenological analysis of medicine developed in this chapter so far. The suffering of illness is an alienating mood overcoming the person and engaging her in a struggle to remain at home in the world in the face of loss of meaning and purpose in life. Illness involves painful experiences at different levels that are connected through the suffering-mood but are nevertheless distinguishable by being primarily about the person's embodiment, her engagements in the world together with others, and her core life values, respectively. The lifeworld is usually the person's home territory, but in illness this homelikeness gives in and takes on a rather *unhomelike* character, rooted in thwarted ways of being embodied. It is the mission of healthcare professionals to try to understand such unhomelike being-in-the-world and bring it back to homelikeness again, or at least closer to a home-being. This involves, but cannot be reduced to, ways of understanding and altering the biological functionality of the person who is ill. Healthcare professionals must also address the everyday world and core life values of patients with a phenomenological eye, addressing and trying to understand the being-in-the-world and story of the person's life, which has turned unhomelike in illness.

Hermeneutics of Medicine

As we have seen, human beings, according to a phenomenological analysis, understand and interpret themselves by manner of being placed in a context of meaning-relations referred to as their "being-in-the-world." At first sight Hans-Georg Gadamer's famous and extensive work in philosophical hermeneutics, *Truth and Method*, published originally in 1960 (1994), might seem rather remote from the phenomenology that Heidegger presents in his main work, *Being and Time*. Gadamer's book is divided into three parts; the first and second parts, which are by far the most extensive ones, deal with the work of art and with interpretation in the humanities, respectively. The third part of the book deals with the ontology of language and can be read as an articulation of the special pattern of understanding, which Gadamer has found to be present in the mentioned disciplines. As Gadamer (1994, pp. 254 ff.) acknowledges himself, however, and as I will attempt to elucidate further, *Truth and Method* is most accurately read as an extension of the phenomenological hermeneutics found in *Being and Time*.

As many readers have remarked, the title of Gadamer's book should properly read, "Truth or Method" and not "Truth and Method," since it is precisely the methodological conceptualization of hermeneutics, formulated by Friedrich Schleiermacher and Wilhelm Dilthey in the nineteenth century, that Gadamer is attempting to go beyond (Ricoeur, 1991). Truth in *Truth and Method* is meant as a basic experience of being together with others in and through language and not as a criterion for the correct interpretation of texts. This conception of truth is completely in line with Heidegger's interpretation of the concept in *Being and Time* as the openness or "disclosedness" of the self to the world of meaning in which things can be found and articulated *as* such and such things (as hammers, for instance) (Heidegger, 1996, pp. 213 ff.). Thus, for a sentence to describe, to correspond to, a state of the world—as, for example, in "the hammer is heavy"—this prior dismantling of the world as meaningful—a place where hammers can be too heavy—is necessary. Truth in Gadamer's philosophy, however, is to be understood primarily as openness to *the other* and *his* world and not only to *my own* world.

Language is emphasized by Gadamer as the key mode of human existence in being together with others. The form of language he concentrates his analysis on in *Truth and Method* is not, however, the spoken dialogue, but rather the reading of literature and other texts of the past. Historical texts are separated from us by a temporal distance, which makes the meaning incarnated in them more difficult to dismantle. Indeed, what does it mean to uncover the meaning of such texts? When we try to understand a historical document, our lifeworld and horizon of meaning is not identical with the world of the author of the document. Nevertheless, our horizons are not totally separated, but distantly united through the "history of effects"—of the document (Gadamer, 1994, pp. 300 ff.). It is consequently possible to bring the horizons closer together and reach an understanding of the document through that which Gadamer here calls a "merging of horizons."

The medical encounter can be viewed as such a coming together of the two different lifeworlds of healthcare professional and patient—in the language of Gadamer, of their different horizons of understanding—aimed at establishing a mutual understanding, which can benefit the health of the ill party. Doctors—as well as representatives of other healthcare professions—are thus not first and foremost scientists who apply biological knowledge, but rather interpreters—hermeneuts of health and illness. They address the suffering experienced by embodied and world-embedded persons and this necessitates a second-person perspective on health and illness guiding and substantiating the third-person perspective on diseases. Biological explanations and therapies can only be applied *within* the dialogical meeting, guided by the clinical understanding attained in service of the patient as a person and his health. The *lived* body is as important (or actually even more important) than the *living* body in medicine. Gadamer's philosophy of hermeneutical understanding, which has mainly been taken to be a general description of the pattern of knowledge found in the humanities, might thus be expanded to cover the activities of healthcare (Svenaeus, 2000).

Gadamer's (1996) late work *The Enigma of Health* supports this interpretation, addressing healthcare in a more direct way than the philosopher's earlier work. Medicine is characterized by Gadamer in this collection of papers as a dialogue and discussion by which the doctor and patient together try to reach an understanding of why the patient is ill. What is particularly obvious in the medical meeting is the *asymmetrical* relation between the parties. The patient is ill and seeks help, whereas the doctor is at home—in control by virtue of his knowledge and experience of disease and illness. This asymmetry necessitates *empathy* on the part of the doctor (Halpern, 2001). He must try to understand the patient, not exclusively from his own point of view, but through trying to put himself in the patient's situation. Consequently, that the doctor attempts to reach a new, scientifically informed understanding of the patient's illness in no way implies that he should avoid empathy. It is only through empathy that the doctor can reach an independent understanding that is truly productive, in the sense of shared *and* novel and in the sense of offering new perspectives on the patient's health problems.

At this point we may return to Gadamer's model of textual interpretation in *Truth and Method* to understand more in detail how the clinical understanding is developed. It is first and foremost the doctor who is the "reader" and the patient who is the "text." But since the meeting is dialogic, the reading is also a reciprocal process of questions and answers. The distance between the two parties is not a time-related distance as in the case of the reading of a historical text; it is rather a distance between two *lifeworld horizons*—the doctor's medical expertise of diseases and the patient's lived experience of illness—which can be narrowed down through the dialogue. This narrowing-down, this "merging of the horizons" of doctor and patient in the medical meeting, means that the horizons are brought into contact with each other, but nevertheless preserve their identities as the separate horizons of two different attitudes and lifeworlds (Svenaeus, 2000).

As several commentators have pointed out, Gadamer's project in *Truth and Method* is deeply indebted to the practical philosophy of Aristotle (Berti, 2003). Indeed, a discussion of "the hermeneutic relevance of Aristotle" is at the center of the chapter devoted to the problem of application in the second part of the book (Gadamer, 1994, pp. 312 ff.). When Gadamer chooses to continue his analysis of hermeneutic practice by turning to Aristotle and the *Nicomachean Ethics* (2002), he does so in order to underline the *normative* aspect of hermeneutics. The Greek concept rendered as "the virtue of moral knowledge" by Gadamer (1994, p. 324) is *"phronesis,"* often translated as "practical wisdom." It is thus clear that Gadamer intends his phenomenological hermeneutics to be a practical philosophy in the Aristotelian sense, and it is also clear that practical, phronetic wisdom is to be considered a hermeneutical virtue. Accordingly, *phronesis* is the mark of the good hermeneutist, and maybe, in particular, the good *medical* hermeneutist—the doctor. What does this mean in this context? And what conclusions can we draw, in the case of medicine, from such a strong link between Aristotle's concept of practical, moral wisdom and Gadamer's hermeneutics?

Phronesis for Aristotle is not a particular moral virtue, in the manner of fidelity, compassion, justice, courage, temperance, or integrity. It is rather an intellectual ability; however, as such, it informs the moral virtues in specific situations allowing the possessor of these virtues to make moral judgments. *Phronesis* is therefore in a sense a moral ability—despite being counted among the intellectual virtues by Aristotle—since it deals with practical decisions in situations in which not only abstract truths but also the concrete good are the matter at hand. The *phronimos*—the wise man—knows the right and good thing to do in *this* specific situation; in the case of medicine we would say that he knows the right and good thing to do for this specific patient at this specific time. This cannot be learned merely by applying universal, scientific truths, but only through long experience in concrete, practical matters of life (Svenaeus, 2014).

The hermeneutics of medicine is grounded in the *meeting* between healthcare professional and patient—a meeting in which the two different horizons of medical knowledge and lived illness are brought together in an interpretative dialogue for the purpose of determining why the patient is ill and how he can be treated. This has been one of the main points made from the very beginning of this chapter: medical practice is not merely applied science, but rather interpretation through dialogue in service of the patient's health. Within this interpretative pattern science and technology are made use of in various ways, but the pattern itself is not a set of scientific hypotheses or tools to be applied. Questions regarding the essence of the suffering that a particular person is going through demand a medical horizon that connects to and is able to incorporate life style and existential matters within its scope.

Phenomenology and Medical Technologies

The development of modern medical science during the past two hundred years or so has made it possible for humankind to intervene in our own biology in new and stunning ways (Reiser, 2009). Not only is it now possible to cure and prevent many diseases from which people previously died *en masse* or were crippled for life, it is also increasingly possible to enhance our biology beyond the borders of restoring normality (Agar, 2014; Buchanan, 2011). Medical technologies—gene technology and psychopharmacology, for instance—is now stepping onto the stage of self-transformation, making us become "better than well," to quote the title of a book by Carl Elliott (2003). This process is problematic and has given rise to high expectations as well as worries about the future of humankind. What contributions could phenomenology offer to this bioethical debate?

In its stress on encouraging doctors to focus on the ill person—the being-in-the-world of the patient—and not only on diseases, one can already sense a certain critique from the perspective of the phenomenologist toward a medicine in the hands of techno-science. The patient is, indeed, a *subject*, not only an object, and healthcare professionals must never forget this if they are to be successful in doing their job—helping sick people. This does not mean that a phenomenologist would recommend that doctors be less scientific in the sense of less knowledgeable in the field of diseases, only that the doctor must be able to establish contact between the medical, scientific gaze and the meeting with the patient as an ill person suffering an unhomelike being-in-the-world. Diagnostic and therapeutic technological devices and drugs that make doctors able to explore, control, and change features of our biology and embodiment must always ultimately be put in service of the patients and their everyday troubles.

However, new medical technologies have a tendency to bring with them not only new possibilities but also new norms that limit the scope of the healthy and good-enough life. New diagnoses are invented and the criteria for already existing diagnoses are expanded when, for instance, new pharmaceutical drugs are developed and enter the market (Angell, 2005; Horwitz, 2002). It is also very hard to resist the use of new medical technologies, since as soon as a technology has been introduced the situations in which we now make choices have already been altered. If we say no to a technology—for example, an early ultrascan test to detect a risk that a fetus might suffer from Down's syndrome—we must always do so from an analysis of what the technology in question *could* lead to. It could lead to a world with less tolerance for abnormalities and weaknesses when the number of persons being born with the chromosome deficiency declines. But, as the proponents of the technology will point out, the technology does not *have* to have these feared consequences; maybe many parents will choose not to have an abortion and they will now welcome the child with Down's syndrome out of a free and informed choice. The answer to this from the technology skeptic will be that, first, the parents are not really able to make any informed choices, lacking relevant experiences about the issue; and, second, in reality the risk assessment will lead not only to a world in which people with Down's syndrome will have less of a place, but also to a lot of fetuses being aborted without actually being afflicted by Down's syndrome, since any test of this type will produce a significant number of "false positives." Well, the proponent may admit, this is probably the price we will have to pay for putting the technology at use, but is it not far worse that people face unwanted situations, which they could have found a way out of if the technology had been made available? How could it be a fair move to restrict the freedom to have the kind of babies you want to have and avoid promoting biological abnormalities?

At this point, I think the phenomenologist could enter and make some valuable contributions. The evaluation of medical technologies must be supplemented by a different type of analysis than the moves found in the debate mentioned earlier, if we are to be able to understand what medical–technological developments mean and do to our society and culture. This analysis must focus on technologies as a part of our *mindset*; it must explore how the technologies and the driving forces putting them to work alter the lifeworld of people. One important force behind technology development is the market economy, but this is not all there is to the impact of new medical technologies in transforming our understanding of the world and ourselves. We are increasingly, doctors as well as patients, becoming objects of a medical–technological gaze, which we are making our own (Foucault, 1994). Heidegger (1977) already in the 1950s called this the "enframing" of our lifeworld by science through which everything consequently shows up as calculable and usable things. Heidegger, in his essays on technology, talked about hydroelectric plants and nuclear technology subjecting us to the "enframing" worldview (pp. 14 ff.), but the most acute extension of his analysis is the recent developments of gene technology, in which humankind itself is becoming the manipulated, not only the manipulator (Svenaeus, 2013).

A vital issue to contemporary phenomenological analyses in medicine is to not fall into the trap of fear and hostility toward all types of new technologies. It is so obvious that many medical technologies, if brought and kept within the bounds of sound judgment and application, are too valuable to our lives to be abstained from, although they do force people to take a stand on and possibly change their attitudes toward themselves and their own bodies. Organ transplantation is a good example. It harbors a tendency to resourcify and maybe even to commodify our bodies—or at least parts of them, the organs—but the possibilities it offers in saving and healing lives are too valuable to be abstained from (Svenaeus, 2010). The important thing in each case must be to make visible the mindset-transforming aspect of the technologies in question and relate this to the ethics and politics of technology use (Aho and Aho, 2008). "Control" appears to be a central concept in this phenomenological analysis. Who is in control of the technology? And how does the technology change our need to *be in control* of everything in our life? Can this urge for control also make our lives less worth living in the sense that we no longer have a place for the unexpected and unplanned? Or is it merely like making our roads safer by means of wider lanes, better fences, and speed limits, protecting ourselves from unwanted dangers, making our lives longer?

Two final obvious themes to point toward as essential for a phenomenology of medicine are birth and death. Or rather, since birth is never remembered and death itself can never be experienced, our "being-towards-death," human finitude, which is a key point for both Heidegger and Sartre in forming their philosophies (Heidegger, 1996; Sartre, 1956). We have once grown out of another body—the womb of the mother—and from birth we are marked by this togetherness of bodies, which makes us connected to other people in different ways throughout life (Diprose, 2002; Schott, 2010). The technological prospects of producing embryos in the laboratory by way of cloning and related methods, and the use of artificial wombs in which to grow babies outside the human body, would thus form fundamental turning points in the being-in-the-world we are presently all part of (Svenaeus, 2007). A person who has not been born but rather produced is still beyond the means of technological medicine, but a lot of philosophical interest has already been invested in understanding such a scenario (e.g., Buchanan, 2011), if rarely from a phenomenological point of view.

Things matter to us in the world because we are born and will die, and death is the ultimate thing we cannot control or postpone forever, even though medicine today, to some people at least, might harbor the promise of such post-human lives through biomedical enhancements and computerized extensions (Agar, 2014). The phenomenologist will point out in this context that death is an *existential*, and not only a biological, concept—just as life is, for that matter (Carel, 2006). Most of us will have no problems accepting that our bodies are vulnerable and ultimately will cease functioning, but, even so, we might have problems accepting that this will happen to *us*. I can learn everything there is to know about the biological processes of the cancer I have recently been struck by, but this will not stop me from asking "Why me?" and "Why now?" It may for some persons be possible to accept that death is soon to come, but in most cases this has very little to do with the dying person's being educated in and understanding more about biological processes (Tolstoy, 2013).

Persons, and not only their bodies, die—and they do so in relationships with other human beings. Nowadays, and for good reasons, this dying together and yet alone is a process that is taking place assisted by doctors and other healthcare professionals in or outside a hospital, and medicine therefore needs a phenomenological view on dying if it is not to fail in the difficult endeavor of helping those who are beyond hope in the medical sense (Bishop, 2011; Cassell, 2004). Being-toward-death is characterized by Heidegger (1996, pp. 246 ff.) as an experience, which is fundamentally unhomelike in character. This refers not to the final moments of life, but to the *acknowledging* that one is going to die. Being-toward-death is a death within life that we feel and discover at the very heart of our own being. Heidegger himself stresses existential anxiety as the ultimate unhomelike experience in his analysis, but our whole embodiment is a kind of existential mark of our finitude, making itself known to us through obstructions that plague us and that will finally bring us to death. To our final homecoming, one is tempted to say.

Conclusion

In this chapter, I have aimed to provide an overview of how phenomenology may enhance our understanding of themes central to contemporary medicine. The phenomenological analysis has taken into account the experience of illness, the meaning of suffering, the role of empathy and dialogue in the clinical encounter, the relationship between medical science on the one hand and medical practice on the other, and, finally, the impact of technology development on medicine. The related traditions of phenomenology and hermeneutics provide theoretical tools to develop descriptions and concepts in which to grasp the nature and essence of illness as the suffering experienced by a person. And doctors and other healthcare professionals need to establish an understanding of these body- and world-embedded experiences of their patients if they should be able to help them in the best possible way. Medical practice, according to the phenomeno-logical analysis, is not only to be understood as applied medical science, but also as a kind of phenomenological hermeneutics based in empathic, cultural, and communicative skills. Medical–scientific theories and technologies that change our view on human biology and make us able to manipulate features of it are always anchored in a lifeworld of personal concerns that provide the theories and technologies with meaning. In this manner, phenomenology paves ways to understand and to evaluate critically new scientific–technological possibilities to heal our bodies, or even enhance human nature, by taking human embodiment and lifeworld meaning patterns into account.

References

Agar, N. (2014). *Truly Human Enhancement: A Philosophical Defense of Limits*. Cambridge, MA: MIT Press.

Aho, J., and Aho, K. (2008). *Body Matters: A Phenomenology of Sickness, Disease, and Illness*. Lanham, MD: Lexington Books.

Ahmed, S. (2006). *Queer Phenomenology: Orientations, Objects, Others*. Durham: Duke University Press.

Angell, M. D. (2005). *The Truth about the Drug Companies: How They Deceive Us and What to Do about It*. New York: Random House.

Aristotle. (2002). *Nicomachean Ethics*. C. Rowe, trans. Oxford: Oxford University Press.

Berti, E. (2003). The reception of Artistotle's intellectual virtues in Gadamer and the hermeneutic philosophy. In *The Impact of Aristotelianism on Modern Philosophy*, ed. R. Pozzo. Washington, DC: The Catholic University of America Press.

Bishop, J. P. (2011). *The Anticipatory Corpse: Medicine, Power, and the Care of the Dying*. Notre Dame: University of Notre Dame Press.

Buchanan, A. E. (2011). *Beyond Humanity? The Ethics of Biomedical Enhancement*. Oxford: Oxford University Press.

Carel, H. (2006). *Life and Death in Freud and Heidegger*. Amsterdam: Rodopi.

Carel, H. (2008). *Illness: The Cry of the Flesh*. Stocksfield: Acumen Publishing.

Carel, H., and Cooper, R. (eds.) (2013). *Health, Illness and Disease: Philosophical Essays*. Durham, NC: Acumen Publishing.

Cassell, E. J. (2004). *The Nature of Suffering and the Goals of Medicine*, 2nd edition. Oxford: Oxford University Press.

Charon, R. (2006). *Narrative Medicine: Honoring the Stories of Illness*. Oxford: Oxford University Press.

DeGrazia, D. (2005). *Human Identity and Bioethics*. Cambridge, MA: Cambridge University Press.

Diprose, R. (2002). *Corporeal Generosity: On Giving with Nietzsche, Merleau-Ponty, and Levinas*. Albany: State University of New York Press.

Downie, R. S., and Macnaughton, J. (2007). *Bioethics and the Humanities: Attitudes and Perceptions*. London: Routledge.

Elliott, C. (2003). *Better Than Well: American Medicine Meets the American Dream*. New York: Norton.

Foucault, M. (1994). *The Birth of the Clinic: An Archaeology of Medical Perception*, A. M. Sheridan Smith, trans. New York: Random House (original work published 1963).

Frank, A. (2013). *The Wounded Storyteller: Body, Illness, & Ethics*, 2nd edition. Chicago: University of Chicago Press.

Gadamer, H.-G. (1994). *Truth and Method*, 2nd revised edition, J. Weinsheimer and D. G. Marshall, trans. New York: Continuum Publishing (original work published 1960).

Gadamer, H.-G. (1996). *The Enigma of Health: The Art of Healing in a Scientific Age*, J. Gaiger and N. Walker, trans. Stanford, CA: Stanford University Press (original work published 1993).

Gallagher, S. (2005). *How the Body Shapes the Mind*. Oxford: Oxford University Press.

Gallagher, S. (ed.) (2011). *The Oxford Handbook of the Self*. Oxford: Oxford University Press.

Goldie, P. (2000). *The Emotions: A Philosophical Exploration*. Oxford: Oxford University Press.

Halpern, J. (2001). *From Detached Concern to Empathy: Humanizing Medical Practice*. New York: Oxford University Press.

Heidegger, M. (1977). *The Question Concerning Technology and Other Essays*, W. Lovitt, trans. New York: Harper & Row (original work published 1954).

Heidegger, M. (1996). *Being and Time*, J. Stambaugh, trans. New York: SUNY (original work published 1927).

Horwitz, A. V. (2002). *Creating Mental Illness*. Chicago: University of Chicago Press.

Kleinman, A. (1988). *The Illness Narratives: Suffering, Healing, and the Human Condition*. New York: Basic Books.

Leder, D. (1990). *The Absent Body*. Chicago: University of Chicago Press.

Leder, D. (1999). Whose Body? What Body? The Metaphysics of Organ Transplantation. In *Persons and Their Bodies: Rights, Responsibilities, Relationships*, ed. M. J. Cherry. Dordrecht: Kluwer Academic Publishers.

Marcum, J. (2008). *An Introductory Philosophy of Medicine: Humanizing Modern Medicine*. Dordrecht: Springer.

Merleau-Ponty, M. (1962). *Phenomenology of Perception*, C. Smith, trans. London: Routledge (original work published 1945).

Mol, A. (2002). *The Body Multiple: Ontology in Medical Practice*. Durham: Duke University Press.

Moran, D. (2000). *Introduction to Phenomenology*. London: Routledge.

Morris, D. B. (1998). *Illness and Culture in the Postmodern Age*. Berkeley: University of California Press.

Nordenfelt, L., and Tengland, P.-A. (1996). *The Goals and Limits of Medicine*. Stockholm: AWI.

Nussbaum, M. (2001). *Upheavals of Thought: The Intelligence of Emotion*. Cambridge: Cambridge University Press.

Pellegrino, E. D., and Thomasma, D. C. (1981). *A Philosophical Basis of Medical Practice: Toward a Philosophy and Ethic of the Healing Professions*. New York: Oxford University Press.

Ratcliffe, M. (2008). *Feelings of Being: Phenomenology, Psychiatry and the Sense of Reality*. Oxford: Oxford University Press.

Ratcliffe, M. (2015). *Experiences of Depression: A Study in Phenomenology*, Oxford: Oxford University Press.

Reiser, S. (2009). *Technological Medicine: The Changing World of Doctors and Patients*. New York: Cambridge University Press.

Ricoeur, P. (1991). *From Text to Action: Essays in Hermeneutics, II*, K. Blamey and J. Thompson, trans. Evanston, IL: Northwestern University Press.

Sartre, J.-P. (1956). *Being and Nothingness*, H. E. Barnes, trans. New York: Washington Square Press (original work published 1943).

Schott, R. M. (ed.) (2010). *Birth, Death, and Femininity: Philosophies of Embodiment*. Bloomington: Indiana University Press.

Scully, J. L. (2008). *Disability Bioethics: Moral Bodies, Moral Difference*. Plymouth: Rowman & Littlefield Publishers.

Slatman, J. (2014). *Our Strange Body: Philosophical Reflections on Identity and Medical Interventions*. Amsterdam: Amsterdam University Press.

Spiegelberg, H. (1972). *Phenomenology in Psychology and Psychiatry*. Evanston, IL: Northwestern University Press.

Svenaeus, F. (2000). *The Hermeneutics of Medicine and the Phenomenology of Health: Steps towards a Philosophy of Medical Practice*. Dordrecht: Kluwer.

Svenaeus, F. (2007). A Heideggerian defense of therapeutic cloning. *Theoretical Medicine and Bioethics* 28: 31–62.

Svenaeus, F. (2009). The phenomenology of falling ill: An explication, critique and improvement of Sartre's theory of embodiment and alienation. *Human Studies* 32: 53–66.

Svenaeus, F. (2010). The body as gift, resource, or commodity: Heidegger and the ethics of organ transplantation. *Journal of Bioethical Inquiry* 7: 163–72.

Svenaeus, F. (2011). Illness as unhomelike being-in-the-world: Heidegger and the phenomenology of medicine. *Medicine, Health Care and Philosophy* 14: 333–43.

Svenaeus, F. (2013). The relevance of Heidegger's philosophy of technology for biomedical ethics. *Theoretical Medicine and Bioethics* 34: 1–16.

Svenaeus, F. (2014). Empathy as a necessary condition of *phronesis*: A line of thought for medical ethics. *Medicine, Health Care and Philosophy* 17: 293–99.

Taylor, C. (1989). *The Sources of the Self: The Making of Modern Identity*. Cambridge, MA: Harvard University Press.

Tolstoy, L. (2013). *The Death of Ivan Ilyich*, R. Nesbit Bain, trans. London: SoHo Books.

Toombs, S. K. (1992). *The Meaning of Illness: A Phenomenological Account of the Different Perspectives of Physician and Patient*. Dordrecht: Kluwer.

Toombs, S. K. (ed.) (2001). *Handbook of Phenomenology and Medicine*. Dordrecht: Kluwer.

van Manen, M. (2014). *Phenomenology of Practice: Meaning-Giving Methods in Phenomenological Research and Writing*. Walnut Creek: Left Coast Press.

Zahavi, D. (2006). *Subjectivity and Selfhood: Investigating the First-Person Perspective*. Cambridge, MA: MIT Press.

Zaner, R. M. (1981). *The Context of Self: A Phenomenological Inquiry Using Medicine as a Clue*. Athens, OH: Ohio University Press.

Zaner, R. M. (2004). *Conversations on the Edge: Narratives of Ethics and Illness*. Washington DC: Georgetown University Press.

Zeiler, K., and Käll, L. (eds.) (2014). *Feminist Phenomenology and Medicine*. New York: SUNY Press.

9 Gender Medicine and Phenomenological Embodiment

Tania Gergel

Introduction

Background to Philosophy of Gender, Medicine, and Embodiment

Gender has been the focus of considerable philosophical and general academic interest since the World War II. During the 1970s, in the wake of the intellectual and political revolutions of the 1960s, both gender studies and feminist philosophy emerged as academic disciplines that received increasing attention over the subsequent decades (Gould and Wartofsky, 1976; Zosuls et al., 2011). At the same time, postwar medicine itself became the focus of increased philosophical interest and scrutiny. On one side, philosophers of science, such as Boorse (1977, 1975) and Schaffner (1993), attempted to understand medicine and its processes within a value-free scientific framework. Meanwhile, others such as Engelhardt (1996) and Munson (1981) sought to draw attention to and to explain the evaluative and socially determined aspects of medicine. A philosophical examination of gender and medicine, then, considers the nature of the conceptual relationship between them, asking questions such as: What do we mean by "gender?"; What is the relationship between gender and the theory and practice of medicine?; Are there ways in which we might rethink our understanding of gender, which could help to overcome some of the difficulties surrounding gender with contemporary medicine?

Finally, there is the philosophical notion of embodiment, developed most extensively in the work of Merleau-Ponty. Phenomenology challenged conventional notions of objectivity, by making the first-person experience of phenomena primary within epistemology. Merleau-Ponty's (2002) particular challenge to objectivity stems largely from rejecting the assumption of the body as object, which he sees as central to Cartesian dualism. He proposes, instead, a unity of mind/soul and body, so that perception and therefore cognition and knowledge

227

of the world is truly embodied, rather than being absorbed through bodily perceptions that must then be discounted if we are to reach understanding:

> [T]he psycho-physical event can no longer be conceived after the model of Cartesian physiology and as the juxtaposition of a process in itself and a *cogitatio*. The union of soul and body is not an amalgamation between two mutually exclusive terms, subject and object, brought about by arbitrary decree. It is enacted at every instant in the movement of existence. (p. 102)

Simone de Beauvoir, most notably in *The Second* Sex—published in 1949 and heavily influenced by Merleau-Ponty's 1945 *Phenomenology of Perception*—took embodiment into the sphere of sex and gender. Like Merleau-Ponty, she argued that we engage with the world as embodied beings, but focused on the role of sex and gender within this process of engagement.

De Beauvoir's (2011) work has been seen as the origin of modern feminism, with her observations concerning the social construction of gender, which were central to the emergence of the sex/gender distinction within feminism and gender studies. Most famous, perhaps, is her pronouncement that "one is not born, but rather becomes, woman" (p. 330). De Beauvoir's main concern is with the disadvantages brought upon women through the ideas of otherness associated with the female gender. However, even if her primary focus is on the social context of embodiment, the overall principle of phenomenological embodiment means that there is no fundamental separation of biology and a social understanding of gender within her work. Aspects of female biology, along with how these are regarded and treated within the world of which a woman is a part, are all essential to the individual's understanding of the world and how they themselves are understood by others.

Some Central Distinctions in Gender and Medicine

In the late 1960s, psychologists started to differentiate between sex and gender in order to explain the difficulties faced by transsexuals, whose body and gender characteristics were felt to be in opposition. This distinction was then adopted within feminism to delineate the two ways of differentiating between male and female. "Sex" was understood as referring to the natural biological differences between the sexes, such as chromosomes, hormonal profiles, internal and external sex organs. "Gender" by contrast was understood as the characteristics attributed to "masculine" and "feminine" within society, and relates to social role, behavioral tendencies, and identity. This distinction became important in trying both to explain and challenge the roles and identities attributed to women and men within society. With its suggestion that many of the characteristics and roles attributed to women within society depend far more upon socially constructed notions of the "feminine" than on biology, it was used to challenge the biological determinism underlying much of the existing gender bias at the time (Mikkola, 2012; Zosuls et al., 2011).

While the sex/gender distinction has been both useful and influential, the notion that there are essential differences between the sexes has been criticized from various directions. Critics of gender realism argue that there is no essential feature or condition that is shared by all women as opposed to men and which can be seen as a fundamental gender difference. Spelman (1988), for example, argues that gender varies according to its social and cultural context, while Butler (2006) argues that feminist notions of what constitutes the female gender are, like other views of the feminine, normative rather than natural. Conversely, thinkers, such as Mikkola (2006), contend that such problems might not be reasons for rejecting gender realism tout court.

There have also been challenges to the notion that there are absolute and objective natural biological distinctions between the sexes. Jaggar (1983) and Fausto-Sterling (2005), for example, have both written extensively about how the social roles and expectations allocated to women influence their physiological development and contribute to the biological differences that emerge between the sexes.

Even though such debates continue to rage, there is general agreement that broad notions of the sex/gender distinction and what these terms conventionally entail are deeply entrenched and influential within contemporary society. The next stage, then, is to consider how these relate to medical theory and practice. In many ways, we can see the sex/gender distinction as correlating with the naturalist/normativist divide within philosophy of medicine (Carel, 2008, pp. 10–11), with sex as a "naturalist" and gender a "normativist" concept. Naturalist accounts of health and disease, usually associated with biomedical reductionism, present disease as some type of deficiency in the normal biological function of the body, an account fitting closely with the dominant medical model within contemporary Western medicine.

Challenges to the biomedical naturalist model have come from those who suggest that biomedical reductionism is not sufficient to account for our contemporary notions of health and disease. Normativist approaches suggest that our understanding of health, disease, and medicine are suffused with values and, to a large extent, socially and culturally determined. At the most extreme end, perhaps, were the bastions of postwar antipsychiatry, such as Szasz (1991, 2010), who saw "mental illness" as a myth created by society to control socially unacceptable patterns of behavior, rather than arising from any biochemical brain dysfunction.

Yet, normativist principles can also be seen as important within contemporary debate surrounding what seem, at first glance, to be purely biomedical

criteria. Recent controversies surrounding treatment and prophylactic maintenance strategies for high cholesterol, for example, point to the way in which a
diagnosis of high cholesterol and prescription of statins has become something
of a social phenomenon. They are often prescribed by doctors as an easier alternative to lifestyle change, even though emerging evidence suggests that this
strategy would have greater efficacy and less adverse effects in the fight against
heart disease. Critics suggest that the science of cholesterol management and
pharmacology has resulted from a change in approach to patient care among
clinicians, rather than stemming primarily from biomedical data and evidence
(Ornish, 2002; Sinatra et al., 2014). Similarly, criticisms of the widely used body
mass index (BMI) as the measure for obesity protest that such a measure is arbitrary, takes no account of body composition, and that, when other measures
are used, there may be, for example, significant changes in statistics relating to
ethnicity and obesity (Ahima and Lazar, 2013; Cawley and Burkhauser, 2006).
As we can see, there are arguments for questioning the "natural" status of even
the most seemingly biomedical of criteria. Within philosophy of medicine, as
with gender, the dominance of underlying assumptions based on naturalist/
normativist distinctions is recognized, but also widely challenged (Hamilton,
2010; Kingma, 2007).

Phenomenological approaches to medicine have also questioned both the
normativist and naturalist positions by applying aspects of phenomenological
philosophy to medicine. Most influential aspects are taken to be the importance
of the first-person subjective experience of illness for medical understanding,
the need to rethink theoretical assumptions, and, of particular relevance here,
the concept of embodiment as central to understanding the human experience
of illness and breaking down the distinctions such as subjectivity/objectivity,
body/mind, and naturalism/normativism (Carel, 2008; Gergel, 2012).

Medical Diagnosis and Gender Stereotypes—Over-, Under-, or Misdiagnosis?

Dominant Stereotypes of the Female Gender

Historically, the female gender has been associated with physical and psychological weakness and deficiency. Aristotle portrayed women as morally and
intellectually weaker than men: "a man would be thought cowardly if his courage were only the same as a courageous woman" (*Politics* 1277b); "the slave is
wholly lacking the deliberative element; the female has it but it lacks authority"
(*Politics* 1260a). Tragic heroines such as Electra are left to waste away in excessive outpourings of emotion, impotent to act without a male champion. While
Plato's acceptance of women as fit to occupy all social roles within his ideal

republic may seem progressive, Plato's Socrates still chastises the lamentations of his male companions at his impending death, saying that concern over such "absurd behaviour" was the reason why he sent the women away (117d). Female characters who defy such stereotypes are portrayed as male, while physical and, in particular, emotional weakness in men are labeled as female qualities. Finally, Seneca writes that, should he become ill, he will choose to do "nothing immoderately, nothing effeminately" (*Letters* 64.1).

Works such as de Beauvoir's *The Second Sex* trace the ways in which women have been defined as man's weaker counterpart throughout history, until the twentieth century. Micale (2009, p. 178) summarizes the views of the Austrian philosopher Weininger, at the end of nineteenth century: "there are 'laws' of masculinity and femininity, just as there are laws of physics, and these establish unmistakably the inferiority and insignificance of women." The influence of such gender norms and realism are clearly seen in the development of notions of psychiatric disorder. Hysteria, for example, was considered an exclusively female disease until Charcot and Freud (Tasca et al., 2012). Even then, diseases such as "male hysteria" and "shell-shock" were gendered and seen as manifestations of weakness and effeminacy (Micale, 2009, p. 162ff.).

Gender Stereotyping and Psychiatric Diagnosis

Even today, the influence of such gender stereotypes may well be felt in the gender disparity of certain psychiatric diagnoses, in ways which may be detrimental to both male and female patients for different reasons. According to the World Health Organization (WHO), unipolar depression is twice as common in women as in men, while alcohol dependence is more than twice as common in men than in women and men are three times more likely than women to be diagnosed with antisocial personality disorder. A recent WHO (2015) report on "Gender disparities in mental health" discusses how research reveals that gender bias and stereotyping in the treatment of female patients has been recorded since the 1970s and that women with similar symptoms to men are more likely to be diagnosed with depression than men and, once diagnosed, to be treated with psychotropic medication.

Moreover, women are more likely to seek help and disclose mental health problems to a primary care physician, while men are the principal users of specialist services and inpatient treatment. It seems that disparities in diagnosis and treatment may well be related to gender-based expectations:

> This suggests that gender based expectations regarding proneness to emotional problems in women and proneness to alcohol problems in men, as well as a reluctance in men to disclose symptoms of depression, reinforce

> social stigma and constrain help seeking along stereotypical lines. (WHO, 2015, pp. 8–9)

It seems that men may still be pressurized by gender expectations not to seek help until a mood disorder has emerged, to self-medicate through substance abuse, or to give expression to their problems through antisocial behavior.

For women, however, a diagnosis of depression or anxiety appears to be given all too easily, at a threshold where such symptoms would not be given the same diagnosis in a male counterpart. This may then result in physical disorders being missed. A commonly discussed example is the misdiagnosis of hyperthyroidism and hypothyroidism in women as psychiatric disorders. Klonoff and Landrine (1996) have written a guide for clinicians, detailing particular physical health problems that are likely to be misdiagnosed as psychiatric conditions. They maintain throughout that such a guide is necessary, since clinicians are led by gender-stereotyping to diagnose mood disorders where another medical explanation is correct. On the dangers of misdiagnosing thyroid disorders, Klonoff and Landrine write:

> Once misdiagnosed, these patients are then often treated with all "the right" pharmacological and psychotherapeutic interventions for a psychiatric disorder that the patients do not have. The patients therefore show no improvement in treatment, and that often leads to increasing the treatment. This aggressive treatment, as well as the failure to treat the disorder the patient actually has, then elicits additional symptoms and leads to patient deterioration or death. This unfortunate sequence of events is the logical and frequent outcome of assuming that depressed and anxious women necessarily have psychiatric disorders … this sequence is prototypical of responses to a diversity of other physical disorders. (pp. 18–19)

The phenomenon known as diagnostic overshadowing, in which a diagnosis of mental disorder leads to physical disorders being wrongly diagnosed as psychogenic (Jones et al., 2008; Nash, 2013), may well also be more common among women than men (Wilcox, 1992).

It seems that physical disorders are being missed or diagnosed as psychiatric because undue attention is paid to stress, as compared to men. A stressed or emotional woman is simply viewed as fulfilling their gender norm; an exceptionally stressed or emotional woman is fulfilling the more extreme version of a gender norm, which manifests itself as some form of mental disorder. At such times, it appears that gender stereotyping or even gender realism, which makes a fundamental connection between woman and excessive emotion or inability to cope, may be operating within a medical context. Illnesses may, effectively, be misdiagnosed because socially constructed beliefs about gender are taken as essential elements of normal function of the female sex, rather than extraneous social stereotypes, and symptoms are then understood within this framework (Munch, 2004).

Gender-based Disparities in Physical Healthcare

It appears that such problems are not restricted to mental or endocrine disorders, but may infiltrate into other areas of physical medicine, where there might at first seem to be little room for such confusion. For example, it has been widely reported that heart disease is misdiagnosed or underdiagnosed in women, as compared to men. Women are diagnosed later in the course of the illness and, consequently, there is increased mortality (Rogers, 2004, p. 56). Bess (1995, p. 41) described the growing evidence of gender disparities in heart disease treatment in the United States, suggesting that it was evident at every stage of the illness, to the point where "gender bias may result in delayed or inaccurate diagnosis, unequal medical interventions, and higher mortality for women who undergo invasive cardiac and surgical procedures." This phenomenon appears widespread. A 2002 Spanish study concluded that women receive treatment at a more advanced stage of heart disease than men, which may be attributed to "gender differences occurring in any (or all) phases of the disease process" (Aguilar et al., 2002, p. 557). A 2009 Italian study concludes that, in the early twenty-first century, "Italian women remain less likely than men to undergo surgical procedures for coronary artery disease," and this is consistent with the situation in the "US, UK and elsewhere." The Italian study shows that the "disparity persists even after taking account of differences in severity of illness" (Nante et al., 2009, p. 204).

For heart disease, it appears that women are still less likely than men to receive treatment or receive treatment later, even when there symptoms are of equivalent severity (Nante et al., 2009, p. 204). Numerous studies reveal treatment disparity elsewhere (Brezinka, 1995; Chang et al., 2007; Hochleitner, 2000; Hsich et al., 2014; Jibran et al., 2010; Kobashigawa, 2014; Regitz-Zagrosek and Seeland, 2012, p. 10; Zhang et al., 2013). In a recent survey of "sex and gender differences in clinical medicine," it is even noted that "undertreatment of women is most pronounced by male physicians" in the cardiovascular field, diabetes, and gynecology (Regitz-Zagrosek and Seeland, 2012, p. 16).

A variety of reasons are suggested for treatment disparity, and there are widespread calls for further research (Aguilar et al., 2002; Chang et al., 2007; Chiaramonte and Friend, 2006; Nante et al., 2009). The possibility that some of these disparities can be explained by a male bias within research, which fails to account for biomedical particularities of pathology and treatment of illness within women, is considered later. However, there have also been suggestions that gender stereotyping may well be a significant factor in generating gaps within diagnosis and treatment. How, then, might gender stereotypes influence diagnosis and treatment? And, are the influential stereotypes within this context consistent with general stereotyping of women in medicine and elsewhere?

A 2006 US study reveals interesting results, showing that both medical students and residents underdiagnosed heart disease in women compared to men, even when they had the same illness profiles, but only when the illness presented in the context of stress. This challenges the commonly held belief that men are more likely to receive the diagnosis because of the perception of heart disease as a male condition. Moreover, this was true regardless of study participants' own gender or attitude toward women. The 2006 study further developed the results that emerged from a 1998 study, revealing that "high-stress women consistently received lower cardiac attributions" and argues that "the main issue in the misdiagnosis of women is not the perceived incidence or prevalence of CHD as in the heuristic or stereotype model but the centrality given to women's stress and psychological symptoms" (Chiaramonte and Friend, 2006, p. 256). For men, by contrast, "stress symptoms may in fact be viewed as additional information (e.g. risk factor) and may augment and affirm, rather than detract from, the cardiac evaluation" (p. 257). The authors warn against drawing oversimplified or overly significant conclusions from their study and point to an urgent need for further research. Nevertheless, the results are striking and suggest a clinical tendency to perceive stress in men as more unusual and more likely to have an underlying physical cause than in women.

Gender disparities occur not only with heart disease, but also, for example, in stroke diagnosis, where it seems that early stroke symptoms are more likely to be missed among women (Newman-Toker et al., 2014; Smith et al., 2005) or in Parkinson's Disease (Saunders-Pullman et al., 2011). By contrast, fibromyalgia, a chronic pain disorder, with no obvious biomedical cause, is far more often diagnosed in women. It has been suggested that the prevalence of fibromyalgia diagnosis among women stems more from gender bias than from genuine biomedical phenomena (Katz et al., 2008, p. 152). A first study examining physician perspective in relation to the condition suggests that physicians will diagnose fibromyalgia more readily in women than in men and will seek additional physical explanations for symptoms when presented by men (Katz et al., 2010).

Some Conclusions on Gender and Diagnosis

Research reveals that particular conditions are diagnosed and treated more or less readily in males and females, even when there may be similar symptoms. While there is widespread consensus as to the need for further research into these gender divisions and possible biases, some preliminary conclusions can perhaps be drawn. It seems that certain beliefs about male and female characteristics and behaviors are playing a part in medical diagnosis and treatment, with potentially severe effects. For example, a view of women as more prone to emotional distress and less able to deal with pain may lead to overdiagnosis of mood disorders and apparently psychogenic conditions such as fibromyalgia, along with late or underdiagnosis of thyroid disorders or cardiovascular diseases, when the role of mental disorder or stress in the production of symptoms is overestimated, as compared to among men. Conversely, men may feel the pressure not to seek help and, consequently, not receive timely or appropriate treatment for psychological problems. It has also been suggested that the lower value placed on women by either themselves or others, as well as the pressure to perform a "caring" role may also lead to women's health problems being overlooked.

In view of all this, there appears to be sufficient evidence to suggest that deeply entrenched gender stereotypes are being taken as indicative of substantive differences between the sexes, and that this is still affecting medical diagnosis and treatment within contemporary medicine. Further research into gender discrepancies within medicine should explore the significance of such attitudes.

The Male Sex as Norm—Overdiagnosis and Exclusion of Female Biology

When it comes to biological differences between the sexes, often classified as "sex" rather than "gender" differences, one might imagine that the situation is more objective and less open to normative biases. Here, however, a different pattern seems to emerge. While physiological differences between the sexes may largely be a matter of natural biology, the normative evaluation and treatment of such differences seems laden with gender-based values.

Laqueur's (1992) "one-sex theory" account of the history of biological sex suggests that, from the Greeks to the Enlightenment, it was widely believed that there was only one sex and that women's sexual organs were an inverted version of men's. During the eighteenth century the model changed. While it was then accepted that there were distinct biological differences between the sexes, socially constructed gender differences and health differences rooted in sociocultural differences were then frequently attributed to "female reproductive anomalies" (Hammarström et al., 2014, p. 185). As de Beauvoir wrote in 1949, the female has, throughout history, been viewed as the "other," in relation to the male norm, and the dominance of such ideas still appears to manifest itself within medicine. I explore two different consequences of such dominance: first, the way in which normal biological phenomena exclusive to women, such as reproductive stages, are interpreted in terms of pathology and abnormality; second, the way in which male health and biology appear to be taken as the norms within evidence-based medicine (EBM), leading to the exclusion or deprioritization of women within research.

The Medicalization of the Female Life-stages

As women's societal roles within the developed world have become progressively less restricted by gender expectations, and female reproduction has become less of an impediment to gender equality, it appears that female biological life-stages have become increasingly medicalized. While much of this can be attributed to the availability of medical procedures that have led to a striking decrease in risk to mother and child through pregnancy and childbirth, for example, there is also an increasing focus on how excessive medicalization of such life-stages can in itself lead to problems for women.

Pregnancy and childbirth have come to be seen as a departure from a healthy norm. Mullin (2005, p. 54), for example, says that medicalized pregnancy "involves interpreting pregnancy itself as a disruption to health that necessarily requires expert medical intervention, and thinking of pregnancy as primarily about health and illness." Ironically, at the same time, medical explanations are increasingly sought for infertility, regarded as abnormal dysfunction of female biology (Greil and McQuillan, 2010, p. 138), so that it appears that both pregnancy and its absence are viewed as, in some way, biomedically dysfunctional.

While the advancement of obstetrics and better awareness of what substances or behaviors may be harmful to an unborn child have been enormously beneficial for pregnant women and fetuses, overmedicalization can be seen to engender excessive medical interventions or overly restrictive health recommendations in the absence of proper evidence. Certain practices, such as an increase in surgical births and episiotomy, have generated significant controversy (Demontis et al., 2011; Hartmann et al., 2005; Pietras and Taiwo, 2012).

Interestingly, overmedicalization of childbirth, in the absence of good evidence, may lead to converse, but deleterious, consequences. Feminist opposition to the medicalization of pregnancy may lead women to false expectations of childbirth and to underestimate legitimate dangers (Crossley, 2007). At the same time, significant difficulties arise from women requesting Caesarean rather than "natural" births, when there is no legitimate medical indication for such an intervention (Demontis et al., 2011; Kalish et al., 2008). Women may be exposing themselves and their babies to unnecessary risks, either through embracing an unsuitable medical model of a normal birthing situation or through rejecting the potential medical difficulties of an abnormal or a dangerous birthing situation, in an attempt to refuse what they perceive as the over-medicalization of women.

The situation during pregnancy is also complicated once a medical model of pregnancy is embraced. The notion of pregnancy as a high-risk health condition and the consequences of such a notion has received a great deal of critical attention, and there is a vast literature, both academic and popular, on this topic. Some of the most interesting analyses can be found in the work of Anne Lyerly. In her powerful coauthored 2009 report on "risk and the pregnant body," she identifies a number of key distortions that inform our risk-based perceptions and management of pregnancy. She describes medical intervention during pregnancy and birth as "Janus-faced," insofar as there is disproportionate attention given to any possible fetal risk of intervention compared to maternal risk of nonintervention, while the management of birth tends toward medical intervention, regardless of the potential burdens to mother and fetus which such interventions might incur. Outside of the clinical context, she argues that there is a "better safe than sorry," rather than evidence-based, attitude to lifestyle choices, such as diet and exercise. She suggests that medicalization and medical advice in this context may well stem more from gender-based ideas about "purity in pregnancy and control in birth," as well as "moral standards of sacrifice applied to mothers" (p. 3ff.).

For both Lyerly and many others, it seems that gender stereotypes associated with "ideal motherhood" or "female sacrifice" play a role within medical proscription of ordinary practices during pregnancy and the pregnant or breastfeeding woman's avoidance of legitimately prescribed medical treatment due to fears for the baby (McDonald et al., 2011). The medicalization of pregnancy and pregnant women leads to further concerns about erosion of female autonomy and equality, once matters of legal responsibility for choices that might affect the fetus are brought into consideration (Gonen, 1994). Some examples include "fetal protection" policies, which bar women of childbearing age from certain types of occupation (Gonen, 1994; Kenney, 1993), or prosecution of women for practices that may represent risk to the fetus. As Capron (1998, p. 33) argues, it would be difficult to limit the type of actions that could be prosecuted as "child endangerment" if such prosecutions were accepted: "failure to follow such advice [i.e. re drinking], or medical advice either to take or to refrain from taking prescription drugs or following other medical regimes, could thus lay the basis for a child endangerment prosecution if shown to have led to serious harm to a child."

Similar concerns have been raised over the potentially deleterious consequences of blanket medicalization of other female life stages, such as menopause or menstruation (Kaufert and Lock, 1997; Mackey, 2007; Meyer, 2001). "Women's health becomes dominated by 'reproductive biology.' Not only does this lead to excessive medicalization of reproductive biology, but may also lead to other aspects of women's health being overlooked" (Rogers, 2004, p. 55).

While medical advances in fields such as obstetrics may have made significant improvements to the health of mothers, babies, and women in general, it seems clear that there are dangers when legitimate medical problems and treatments concerning female life-stages give rise to their blanket medicalization. Medicalization of female reproductive phenomena may be another way of imposing "otherness" on the female sex, so with the ordinary aspects of female sexual biology rendered "abnormal" or "alien" through the process of pathologization. There seems to be a growing need for medicine to differentiate between ordinary female biological changes, which are part of ordinary human function, even if distinct from male biology, and legitimate cases of medical dysfunction in relation to such changes, which warrant medical intervention.

The Male Norm within Evidence-based Medicine

With the development of EBM, an increasing level of attention has been given to the way in which women are excluded or deprioritized within research at all stages (Goldenberg, 2006; Kim et al., 2010; Zucker and Beery, 2010). Rogers (2004, p. 60) writes:

> The gender bias amongst participants in clinical trials is well known. Women have been excluded from research for many years, for a variety of reasons including the alleged need for homogenous populations, the fear of harms to pregnant women, the cost of including women, and the purported difficulty of recruiting women.

While the exclusion of women from randomized controlled trials (RCTs) is often explained, for example, in terms of the risks of research for women of childbearing age, such reasons are insufficient to account for or to justify the lack of focus on women within EBM and the potential disadvantages this brings to women. While many of the arguments focus on the dangers of a research participant being or becoming pregnant, it is increasingly argued that even this is problematic for a number of reasons, such as the need to find effective treatment of pregnant women (Lyerly et al., 2008). While international ethical guidelines stipulate that pregnant women are eligible for participation in biomedical research, they are excluded, even though information surrounding safe and effective treatments cannot simply be extrapolated from "data on men and non-pregnant women." "This is ethically and medically unacceptable," according to Baylis (2010, p. 689), "for two reasons: pregnant women get sick and sick women get pregnant. Patients who happen to be pregnant are as entitled as anyone else to safe and effective treatments, yet they are denied this and will be for as long as pregnant women are excluded from clinical studies."

As Rogers (2004) points out, EBM can confer certain advantages on women, such as providing evidence of the dangers of overuse of episiotomy or a lack of evidence for fetal monitoring benefits. Nevertheless, EBM is seen as the gold-standard of current medical practice, creating the most statistically significant, objective, and generalizable research, despite the underrepresentation of women. Even phenomena such as the exclusion of the elderly from clinical trials could be seen to "further gender bias," insofar as women "form a greater proportion of the elderly population" (p. 62). Moreover, gender data are not routinely included within research, making it difficult to gather information about gender bias (Holdcroft, 2007; Rogers, 2004).

If, as suggested earlier, the biological male is viewed as the norm within clinical medicine, we can see how such exclusion or deemphasis of women might occur. Within this framework, it is likely that disease will be seen as the dysfunction of male biology. While ordinary aspects of female biology may then be pathologized, the primary model of disease itself will be male-orientated. Female particularities may well then come to be seen either as confounders within research, which distort a male-based understanding of how a medical intervention works, or as irrelevant, since there is an assumption that the male norm is straightforwardly generalizable to the female population in the most important respects. Rogers and Ballantyne (2008, p. 43) comment on the justifications given for excluding females from research: "The combination of these arguments demonstrates the traditional and paradoxical assumption that female hormones and other biological processes interfere with research to a sufficient degree to justify the exclusion of women, and yet males and females are homogeneous enough that research results from male studies can be generalized to women."

Strangely enough, we might even see this as suggesting a return to a "one-sex" type-model, in which there is one sex, typified by men, and shared by women. Female-specific differences are then interpreted either as irrelevant or as distortions of the male model, which will confuse scientific accounts.

Support for the idea of a dominant biological male norm within medicine can be found by considering examples of gender bias within EBM. Most well documented, perhaps, is the bias toward selection of male research participants. Despite regulations in a number of countries mandating inclusion of female participants, women continue to be underrepresented (Raz and Miller, 2012; Regitz-Zagrosek and Seeland, 2012). At the same time, as Raz and Miller (2012, p. 131) point out: "Around the globe, failure to understand and study female biology in medicine has resulted in higher mortality and co-morbidities in women." Sociocultural factors may also contribute, such as the underrepresentation of women among those setting research agendas, greater poverty, and lower social standing of women (Goldenberg, 2006; Holdcroft, 2007; Rogers, 2004). The problems lie not simply with participant selection, but also within failure to include or analyze gender data within research (Kim et al., 2010).

As we have seen an apparent gender bias within research appears to stem from some of the following assumptions:

- Medical interventions that work for men will work equally well or in the same way for women.
- Gender-based differences in symptoms and treatment are not significant elements within understanding health conditions and, thus, gender-based studies and gender data in research results are not a necessary element of good research practice.
- The need to protect pregnant women or even women of childbearing age from the risk of medical intervention is of primary importance, even when outweighed by factors such as the greater risk presented by lack of research on this group or the role of and the actual degree of risk from the trial and female rights and responsibility in ensuring that pregnancy is avoided during a trial in which a woman chooses to take part.
- The scientific validity of research agenda is unaffected by disproportionate representation of one gender among determining such agenda.

The notion that gender biases may play a role in the diagnosis and treatment of heart disease has already been discussed earlier. The context of research into heart disease also provides a useful example of where an overreliance on male biology can lead to gender-based problems within EBM, which appear to reflect some of the problematic assumptions laid out earlier.

A number of researchers have questioned the notion that male-based research is sufficient for understanding how women are affected by heart disease and point out the significantly higher representation of male participants or all-male studies within heart-disease research (Leuzzi et al., 2010; Regitz-Zagrosek and Seeland, 2012; Rogers and Ballantyne, 2008). For example, one 2012 paper discusses how women are underrepresented in RCTs for heart failure and notes that "although the population estimate among patients with Heart Failure in the United States is about 50%, only 17% to 23% of HF randomized controlled trials enrolled women" (Shin et al., 2012, p. 172). It goes on to suggest that more women need to be included in order better to identify and understand "sex-specific differences." Moreover, male bias appears to pervade every stage of the research process and even in the first stage of trials, "most research is done in male animals," despite the fact that "significant differences exist in the outcomes of male and female mice in models of myocardial infarction, pressure overload and genetic cardiomyopathies that are often not even considered by the researchers" (Regitz-Zagrosek and Seeland, 2012, p. 15).

Despite the widely acknowledged differences between how men and women are affected by heart disease, there is a lack of gender-specific research and research that provides gender data or analysis by gender (Rogers, 2004, p. 57; Shin et al., 2012). A male "norm" still appears to dominate. A 2010 article in *Nature*, for example, charges that differences between female and male experience of cardiovascular disease are "particularly acute." Nevertheless, typical early symptoms for women are "considered to be atypical because diagnostic standards were mainly established from research on men," while some of the diagnostic tests are also effective at detection in women (Kim et al., 2010, p. 688). As is the case more generally in medicine, heart disease within pregnancy or, as relating to other aspects of women's reproductive health, is underresearched. A clear lack of research into treatment and mechanisms of "pregnancy-related cardiovascular and metabolic and other diseases" has been identified, and there is also a need for research that acknowledges menopause specific factors (Regitz-Zagrosek and Seeland, 2012; Shin et al., 2012).

Although it is accepted that further research is needed, it has been suggested that the proportionately greater representation of men among those who are influential in determining research agendas may be one factor that leads to a greater focus on male health than female within research (Rogers, 2004, p. 60). It is not simply greater male representation within the scientific community that might lead to such problems, but also the EBM model itself. As Rogers, for example, has pointed out, EBM is "by and large located within a biomedical model in which identifiable causes lead to disease outcomes" and "a research agenda in which the immediate and identifiable causes are investigated and treated" (p. 68). Women globally are more likely to suffer from poverty and discrimination, all of which may have a major causal role in producing health inequalities and leading to illnesses such as heart disease (Chow and Patel, 2012). However, there is little room within EBM for consideration of such socio-economic factors, which are prevalent and may have major effects on health, but remain extremely difficult to measure, especially with a current EBM-type framework (Rogers, 2004, p. 67ff.).

Questioning the Biological Sex Divide—The Intersection of Sex and Gender?

It appears that many of the current problems and imbalances surrounding gender within medical research and treatment may stem from assumptions of male biology as the norm. Both within medical research in general and more specific contexts, such as heart disease, there are widespread calls for research that specifically targets gender-based differences in symptoms, presentation, and for treatment, which includes consideration of sociocultural factors. In addition, when it comes to reproductive biology, there is a general tendency to see female reproductive biology as a deviation from a healthy norm, leading to excessive general medicalization of pregnancy for example. Ironically, this appears to have the consequence that actual medical dysfunction within reproduction is inadequately provided for within healthcare and, particularly, within research. Here, it appears that a medicalization of pregnancy has led to exclusion of pregnant or potentially pregnant women from research, insofar as they are viewed as either an "at-risk" population or a population whose biological abnormalities may skew research findings.

If we stick to the conventional sex/gender divide, such phenomenon may seem hard to explain. Female biological differences are simply biomedical facts and research protocols such as EBM should therefore be more than adequate for taking such differences into account. However, medical data and phenomena do not exist in some type of biomedical vacuum. Sociocultural factors are inextricably tied to factors such as concepts of health and disease, selection of data, and research agenda; and it is here that we can see the limitations of a sex/gender distinction. While certain aspects of male and female biology may be biomedical "facts" or objective phenomena, how we, as humans, approach such biological phenomena is rooted in sociocultural context, attitudes, and the construction of norms.

Phenomenological Embodiment—A Way Forward

The Problems of the Sex/gender Distinction, in Theory and in Practice

The sex/gender distinction suggests that, as well as gender differences based on social and cultural attitudes and construction, there are also objective physiological differences between men and women. It is these latter sex-based differences that are assumed to be of relevance to medicine, rooted as it is in the scientific and objective analysis of medical symptoms and data.

Nevertheless, the limitations of the sex/gender distinction, as identified within a more general context, seem more relevant to medicine that one might at first suppose. Even within our basic concepts of health and illness, it is undeniable that normative factors play an important role in terms of determining which symptoms and phenomena are to be deemed healthy or unhealthy. It appears that sex-based differences are no exception. On the one hand, certain characteristics associated with a particular gender are invested with a level of realism, which means that they influence medical diagnosis. Meanwhile, the dominance of the male model within society means that male biological phenomena are understood as the "real" biological norm.

We seem to have a situation where the dominant biomedical model rests on the supposition that it concerns itself with the natural and objective biological realities of medical data, including sex-based differences. However, there is a failure to recognize that clinicians, researcher, and patients are situated within a sociocultural context, which is bound up with its own gender-based assumptions even at the level of determining what constitutes biological realities.

Phenomenology, Gender, and Embodiment

It appears that the sex/gender distinction is subject to the same limitations within the medical context as elsewhere, and that there is need for a model that can transcend the problems engendered by this distinction. The difference between sex and gender rests on a distinction between objective biological "facts" and subjective socioculturally determined attitudes. Within philosophy of medicine, one influential way of challenging this subjective/objective, perceptual/biological distinction is to adopt a phenomenological approach.

Phenomenology gives epistemological primacy to first-hand experience of phenomena. Between us, and through a process of intersubjectivity, we arrive at collective accounts. However, these are always mediated through our own first-hand experience and the notion that some attainable and essential reality beyond such experience is rejected. In as much as one can generalize about phenomenology, the phenomenological project is one of trying to come as close as one can to the raw personal experience of phenomena and to free oneself from the theoretical standpoints, which have become entrenched within us and which we use to filter our experiences (Gergel, 2012). Nevertheless, as Heidegger wrote, we are inextricably situated within our own temporal and cultural contexts, and our experiences will be filtered through such contexts. This was then taken further by Merleau-Ponty, who saw experience as "embodied" and rejected the notion that we have some purely mental level of contemplation or experience. Not only is our experience of phenomena enmeshed in our sociocultural context, this experience is also enmeshed within our physical body.

Although the potential value of embodiment is a way of approaching gender issues within medicine, it has been argued that phenomenological approaches to embodiment are distinct from other approaches and lack the gender and social–structural dimensions found elsewhere (Hammarström et al., 2014). It may be true that Merlau-Ponty himself was not directly engaged with gender-specific issues and focused more heavily on breaking down the internal mind/body divide, rather than its social situatedness. However, Merleau-Ponty's individual is seen as firmly embedded within their sociocultural context and the space for gender considerations within the framework he suggests are clearly evidenced by the subsequent thinkers who concentrate more directly on such matters.

For de Beauvoir, embodiment and the integral connection between mind, body, and social context was a way of achieving a fuller explanation of the disadvantages women have experienced through the ages. For her successors, the phenomena of embodiment was not only a way of understanding such disadvantages, but also challenging the dominance of the male model in a way that incorporated all elements of female experience (Mikkola, 2012).

However, rather than seeing gendered embodiment as necessarily entailing positive or negative consequences in itself, we might productively view it here as a notion with a strong explanatory value when considering issues of sex and gender within medicine. Rather than trying to deal with the seemingly intractable problems of attempting to explain medical phenomena either in terms of detached sex-based biological data or purely gender-based phenomena, the notion of embodiment suggests that such distinctions are based on a flawed separation of mind and body and of person from environment.

The complexity of understanding the role that gender differences play, for example, in heart disease leads to a number of questions. Do women present with different symptoms from men, or is it just the case that the same symptoms are judged differently? Are women's judgments concerning the abnormality of their own physiological experiences more readily questioned than men's? If female symptomatology is different, is this because of internal biological phenomena, or is this due to the external influence of gender-based models of behavior? If heart disease is underresearched in women, is this due to women's attitude to research participation, men's attitude to the importance of female inclusion or male bias in setting a more male-orientated research agenda? Do male and female differences in pathology of heart disease and receptivity to treatment or diagnostic tests mean that more emphasis should be given to gender-specific or gender-sensitive research?

Phenomenological embodiment suggests that such questions are interrelated. If we are truly to understand male/female differences in relation to health problems, such as heart disease, embodiment would allow us not only to see the relevance of all these questions, but also to provide a basis for their interrelation, which might give a more comprehensive explanation of the phenomena. If we can develop some type of embodiment-based framework for exploring medical phenomena, might this help us reach a clearer understanding of the essential interrelationship of all elements, both internal and external, bodily and psychological, of the experience of health and illness? It is beyond the scope of this chapter to develop such a framework. Nevertheless, if it is the case that many gender-related difficulties within medicine may stem from positing too rigid a separation between such elements, it seems that such a framework may have important explanatory potential within medicine.

References

Aguilar, M. D., Lázaro, P., Fitch, K., and Luengo, S. (2002). Gender differences in clinical status at time of coronary revascularisation in Spain. *J. Epidemiol. Community Health* 56: 555–59.

Ahima, R. S. and Lazar, M. A. (2013). The health risk of obesity—better metrics imperative. *Science* 341: 856–58.

Baylis, F. (2010). Pregnant women deserve better. *Nature* 465: 689–90.

Beauvoir, S. de (2011). *The Second Sex*. New York: Vintage Books.

Bess, C. (1995). Gender bias in health: A life or death issue for woman with coronary heart disease. *Hastings Women's Law J.* 6: 41.

Boorse, C. (1975). On the distinction between disease and illness. *Philos. Public Aff.* 5: 49–68.

Boorse, C. (1977). Health as a theoretical concept. *Philos. Sci.* 44: 542–73.

Brezinka, V. (1995). Gender bias in diagnosis and treatment of women with coronary heart disease: A review. *Z. Für Kardiologie* 84: 99–104.

Butler, J. (2006). *Gender Trouble: Feminism and the Subversion of Identity*, new edition. New York: Routledge.

Capron, A. M. (1998). Punishing mothers. *Hastings Cent. Rep.* 28: 31–33.

Carel, H. (2008). *Illness*. Durham, UK: Routledge.

Cawley, J., and Burkhauser, R. V. (2006). Beyond BMI: The Value of More Accurate Measures of Fatness and Obesity in Social Science Research (Working Paper No. 12291). National Bureau of Economic Research.

Chang, A. M., Mumma, B., Sease, K. L., Robey, J. L., Shofer, F. S., and Hollander, J. E. (2007). Gender bias in cardiovascular testing persists after adjustment for presenting characteristics and cardiac risk. *Acad. Emerg. Med. Off. J. Soc. Acad. Emerg. Med.* 14: 599–605.

Chiaramonte, G. R., and Friend, R. (2006). Medical students' and residents' gender bias in the diagnosis, treatment, and interpretation of coronary heart disease symptoms. *Health Psychol. Off. J. Div. Health Psychol. Am. Psychol. Assoc.* 25: 255–66.

Chow, C. K., and Patel, A. A. (2012). Women's cardiovascular health in India. *Heart Br. Card. Soc.* 98: 456–59.

Crossley, M. L. (2007). Childbirth, complications and the illusion of "choice": A case study. *Fem. Psychol.* 17: 543–63.

Demontis, R., Pisu, S., Pintor, M., and D'aloja, E. (2011). Cesarean section without clinical indication versus vaginal delivery as a paradigmatic model in the discourse of medical setting decisions. *J. Matern.-Fetal Neonatal Med. Off. J. Eur. Assoc. Perinat. Med. Fed. Asia Ocean. Perinat. Soc. Int. Soc. Perinat. Obstet.* 24: 1470–75.

Engelhardt, H. T. (1996). *The Foundations of Bioethics*. Oxford University Press.

Fausto-Sterling, A. (2005). The problem with sex/gender and nature/nurture. In *Debating Biology*, eds. G. Bendelow, L. Birke, and S. Williams. Routledge.

Gergel, T. L. (2012). Medicine and the individual: Is phenomenology the answer?: Medicine and the individual. *J. Eval. Clin. Pract.* 18: 1102–109.

Goldenberg, M. J. (2006). On evidence and evidence-based medicine: Lessons from the philosophy of science. *Soc. Sci. Med.*, Part Special Issue: Gift Horse or Trojan Horse? Social Science Perspectives on Evidence-Based Health Care Part Special Issue: Gift

Horse or Trojan Horse? Social Science Perspectives on Evidence-Based Health Care 62: 2621–32.

Gonen, J. S. (1994). Women's rights vs. "fetal rights." *Women Polit.* 13: 175–90.

Gould, C. C., and Wartofsky, M. W. (1976). Women and philosophy: Toward a theory of liberation. Putnam.

Greil, A. L., and McQuillan, J. (2010). "Trying" times: Medicalization, intent, and ambiguity in the definition of infertility. *Med. Anthropol. Q.* 24: 137–56.

Hamilton, R. P. (2010). The concept of health: Beyond normativism and naturalism. *J. Eval. Clin. Pract.* 16: 323–29.

Hammarström, A., Johansson, K., Annandale, E., Ahlgren, C., Aléx, L., Christianson, M., Elwér, S., Eriksson, C., Fjellman-Wiklund, A., Gilenstam, K., Gustafsson, P. E., Harryson, L., Lehti, A., Stenberg, G., and Verdonk, P. (2014). Central gender theoretical concepts in health research: the state of the art. *J. Epidemiol. Community Health* 68: 185–90.

Hartmann, K., Viswanathan, M., Palmieri, R., Gartlehner, G., Thorp, J., and Lohr, K. N. (2005). Outcomes of routine episiotomy: A systematic review. *JAMA* 293: 2141–48.

Hochleitner, M. (2000). Coronary heart disease: Sexual bias in referral for coronary angiogram. How does it work in a state-run health system? *J. Womens Health Gend. Based Med.* 9: 29–34.

Holdcroft, A. (2007). Gender bias in research: How does it affect evidence based medicine? *J. R. Soc. Med.* 100: 2–3.

Hsich, E. M., Starling, R. C., Blackstone, E. H., Singh, T. P., Young, J. B., Gorodeski, E. Z., Taylor, D. O., and Schold, J. D. (2014). Does the UNOS heart transplant allocation system favor men over women? *JACC Heart Fail.* 2: 347–55.

Jaggar, A. (1983). Human biology in feminist theory: Sexual equality reconsidered. In *Beyond Domination: New Perspectives on Women and Philosophy*, ed. C. C. Gould. Lanham, MD: Rowman & Littlefield Publishers, Inc.

Jibran, R., Khan, J. A., and Hoye, A. (2010). Gender disparity in patients undergoing percutaneous coronary intervention for acute coronary syndromes—does it still exist in contemporary practice? *Ann. Acad. Med. Singapore* 39: 173–78.

Jones, S., Howard, L., and Thornicroft, G. (2008). "Diagnostic overshadowing": Worse physical health care for people with mental illness. *Acta Psychiatr. Scand.* 118: 169–71.

Kalish, R. B., McCullough, L. B., and Chervenak, F. A. (2008). Patient choice cesarean delivery: Ethical issues. *Curr. Opin. Obstet. Gynecol.* 20: 116–19.

Katz, J. D., Mamyrova, G., Guzhva, O., and Furmark, L. (2010). Gender bias in diagnosing fibromyalgia. *Gend. Med.* 7: 19–27.

Katz, J. D., Seaman, R., and Diamond, S. (2008). Exposing gender bias in medical taxonomy: Toward embracing a gender difference without disenfranchising women. *Women's Health Issues* 18: 151–54.

Kaufert, P. A., and Lock, M. (1997). Medicalization of women's third age. *J. Psychosom. Obstet. Gynaecol.* 18: 81–86.

Kenney, S. J. (1993). *For Whose Protection?: Reproductive Hazards and Exclusionary Policies in the United States and Britain.* Ann Arbor: University of Michigan Press.

Kim, A. M., Tingen, C. M., and Woodruff, T. K. (2010). Sex bias in trials and treatment must end. *Nature* 465: 688–89.

Kingma, E. (2007). What is it to be healthy? *Analysis* 67: 128–33.

Klonoff, E. A., and Landrine, H. (1996). *Preventing Misdiagnosis of Women: A Guide to Physical Disorders That Have Psychiatric Symptoms.* SAGE Publications.

Kobashigawa, J. A. (2014). U.S. donor heart allocation bias for men over women? A closer look. *JACC Heart Fail.* 2: 356–57.

Laqueur, T. (1992). *Making Sex: Body and Gender from the Greeks to Freud*, new edition. Cambridge, MA: Harvard University Press.

Leuzzi, C., Sangiorgi, G. M., and Modena, M. G. (2010). Gender-specific aspects in the clinical presentation of cardiovascular disease. *Fundam. Clin. Pharmacol.* 24: 711–17.

Lyerly, A. D., Little, M. O., and Faden, R. (2008). The second wave: Toward responsible inclusion of pregnant women in research. *Int. J. Fem. Approaches Bioeth.* 1: 5–22.

Lyerly, A. D., Mitchell, L. M., Armstrong, E. M., Harris, L. H., Kukla, R., Kuppermann, M., and Little, M. O. (2009). Risk and the pregnant body. *Hastings Cent. Rep.* 39: 34–42.

Mackey, S. (2007). Women's experience of being well during peri-menopause: A phenomenological study. *Contemp. Nurse* 25: 39–49.

McDonald, K., Amir, L. H., and Davey, M.-A. (2011). Maternal bodies and medicines: A commentary on risk and decision-making of pregnant and breastfeeding women and health professionals. *BMC Public Health* 11(Suppl 5): S5.

Merleau-Ponty, M. (2002). *Phenomenology of Perception: An Introduction*, 2nd edition. London: Routledge.

Meyer, V. F. (2001). The medicalization of menopause: Critique and consequences. *Int. J. Health Serv. Plan. Adm. Eval.* 31: 769–92.

Micale, M. S. (2009). *Hysterical Men: The Hidden History of Male Nervous Illness.* Harvard University Press.

Mikkola, M. (2006). Elizabeth Spelman, gender realism, and women. *Hypatia* 21: 77–96.

Mikkola, M. (2012). Feminist perspectives on sex and gender. *Stanf. Encycl. Philos.*

Mullin, A. (2005). *Reconceiving Pregnancy and Childcare: Ethics, Experience, and Reproductive Labor.* New York: Cambridge University Press.

Munch, S. (2004). Gender-biased diagnosing of women's medical complaints: Contributions of feminist thought, 1970–1995. *Women's Health* 40: 101–21.

Munson, R. (1981). Why medicine cannot be a science. *J. Med. Philos.* 6: 183–208.

Nante, N., Messina, G., Cecchini, M., Bertetto, O., Moirano, F., and McKee, M. (2009). Sex differences in use of interventional cardiology persist after risk adjustment. *J. Epidemiol. Community Health* 63: 203–208.

Nash, M. (2013). Diagnostic overshadowing: A potential barrier to physical health care for mental health service users. *Ment. Health Pract.* 17: 22–26.

Newman-Toker, D. E., Moy, E., Valente, E., Coffey, R., and Hines, A. L. (2014). Missed diagnosis of stroke in the emergency department: A cross-sectional analysis of a large population-based sample. *Diagnosis* 1: 155–66.

Ornish, D. (2002). Statins and the soul of medicine. *Am. J. Cardiol.* 89: 1286–90.

Pietras, J., and Taiwo, B. F. (2012). Episiotomy in modern obstetrics—necessity versus malpractice. *Adv. Clin. Exp. Med. Off. Organ Wroclaw Med. Univ.* 21: 545–50.

Raz, L., and Miller, V. M. (2012). Considerations of sex and gender differences in preclinical and clinical trials. *Handb. Exp. Pharmacol.* 127–47.

Regitz-Zagrosek, V., and Seeland, U. (2012). Sex and gender differences in clinical medicine. *Handb. Exp. Pharmacol.* 3–22.

Rogers, W. (2004). Evidence-based medicine and women: Do the principles and practice of EBM further women's health? *Bioethics* 18: 50–71.

Rogers, W., and Ballantyne, A. (2008). When is sex-specific research appropriate? *Int. J. Fem. Approaches Bioeth.* 1: 36–57.

Saunders-Pullman, R., Wang, C., Stanley, K., and Bressman, S. B. (2011). Diagnosis and referral delay in women with Parkinson's disease. *Gend. Med.* 8: 209–17.

Schaffner, K. F. (1993). *Discovery and Explanation in Biology and Medicine.* University of Chicago Press.

Shin, J. J., Hamad, E., Murthy, S., and Piña, I. L. (2012). Heart failure in women. *Clin. Cardiol.* 35: 172–77.

Sinatra, S. T., Teter, B. B., Bowden, J., Houston, M. C., and Martinez-Gonzalez, M. A. (2014). The saturated fat, cholesterol, and statin controversy: A commentary. *J. Am. Coll. Nutr.* 33: 79–88.

Smith, M. A., Lisabeth, L. D., Brown, D. L., and Morgenstern, L. B. (2005). Gender comparisons of diagnostic evaluation for ischemic stroke patients. *Neurology* 65: 855–58.

Spelman, E. V. (1988). *Inessential Woman: Problems of Exclusion in Feminist Thought.* Beacon Press.

Szasz, T. S. (1991). *Ideology and Insanity: Essays on the Psychiatric Dehumanization of Man.* , Syracuse, NY: Syracuse Univ Press.

Szasz, T. S. (2010). *The Myth of Mental Illness: Foundations of a Theory of Personal Conduct,* anniversary edition. New York: Harper Perennial.

Tasca, C., Rapetti, M., Carta, M. G., and Fadda, B. (2012). Women and hysteria in the history of mental health. *Clin. Pract. Epidemiol. Ment. Health CP EMH* 8: 110–19.

WHO, 2015. Gender Disparities in Mental Health. World Health Organization: Department of Mental Health and Substance Dependence.

Wilcox, V. L. (1992). Effects of patients' age, gender, and depression on medical students' beliefs, attitudes, intentions, and behavior. *J. Appl. Soc. Psychol.* 22: 1093–110.

Zhang, B., Zhang, W., Huang, R.-C., Zhang, Y., Liu, J., Zheng, Z.-G., Jiang, D.-M., Sun, Y.-J., Ren, L.-N., Zhou, X.-C., and Qi, G.-X. (2013). Gender disparity in early death after ST-elevation myocardial infarction. *Chin. Med. J. (Engl.)* 126: 3481–85.

Zosuls, K. M., Miller, C. F., Ruble, D. N., Martin, C. L., and Fabes, R. A. (2011). Gender development research in sex roles: historical trends and future directions. *Sex Roles* 64: 826–42.

Zucker, I., and Beery, A. K. (2010). Males still dominate animal studies. *Nature* 465: 690.

10 Patient- and Person-Centered Medicine: Does the Center Hold?

James A. Marcum

Patient-centered Medicine: Does the Center Hold?

In the late 1960s, Michael and Enid Balint introduced the term "patient-centered medicine" (PatCM) to signify the centrality or importance of the patient in the delivery of healthcare. The Balints contrasted PatCM to "illness-centered medicine" in which clinicians through "scientific examinations" of a patient's body localize the disease to a particular body part and then prescribe treatment. The diagnosis and treatment are restricted simply to the diseased body part, with little concern for the patient as a "whole person." PatCM, however, is not only interested in localizing the diseased body part but doing so in the context of the patient as an intact individual. Its goal is to obtain an "overall diagnosis" of the patient's illness and to do so "should include everything that the doctor knows and understands about his patient; the patient, in fact, has to be understood as a unique human-being" (E. Balint, 1969, p. 269). To that end, PatCM includes the psychological dimensions of patients' illnesses.[1] It became part of the medical landscape in terms of Balint groups, which developed into an international movement.[2]

Besides the Balints, others began to develop medicine centering on the patient (Bardes, 2012; Grol et al., 1990; Laine and Davidoff, 1996). For example, Ian McWhinney (1988) emphasized the importance of the clinician focusing on the patient's overall illness experience. "The physician," according to McWhinney, "is enjoined to discover the patient's expectations, his feeling about illness, and his fears. He does this by trying to enter the patient's world and to see the illness through the patient's eyes" (p. 225). To that end, McWhinney and colleagues from the Department of Family Medicine at the University of Western Ontario developed a form of PatCM—which they call patient-centered clinical method (PCCM)—that combines the Balints' PatCM with Carl Rogers' client-centered therapy and Betty Newman's total person approach (Stewart et al., 2003, p. 8).[3] Importantly, PatCM or PCCM is not centered on disease, clinician, hospital, or technology.

PCCM and its practice are composed of six components (Stewart et al., 2003, pp. 33–148). The first is the assessment of the patient's presenting complaint, especially in terms of the patient's illness experience. The next component pertains to the integration the illness experiences with an understanding of the patient as a whole person, both in terms of individual and social contexts. The third component encompasses the identification of a common ground between patient and physician in order for the physician to access the information necessary to provide the best possible healthcare. To that end, the fourth component involves promoting patient–physician consultations, especially as an opportunity to encourage wellness. The penultimate component is establishing a robust patient–physician relationship, particularly through caring, compassion, and empathy on the part of the clinician. The final component is a realistic attitude to the limitations of modern medicine, especially given the complexities of medicine and the uncertainties involved in its practice.

At the center then of the therapeutic encounters for PatCM is the patient. This centeredness stems from the bioethical principle of patient autonomy in which healthcare professionals are to respect a patient's right for self-determination (Beauchamp and Childress, 2001). Moreover, a patient's preferences and values are what drive clinical encounters and decisions. In *Crossing the Quality Chasm*, for example, PatCM is defined as "care that is respectful and responsive to individual patient preferences, needs, and values, and ensuring that patient values guide all clinical decisions" (Institute of Medicine, 2001, p. 6). Debra Roter's (2000, p. 7) conceptualization of PatCM also emphasizes the centrality of the patient in the therapeutic encounter.

> Patients set the goal and agenda of the visit and take solo responsibility for decision-making. Patient demands for information and technical services are accommodated by a cooperating physician. Patient values are defined and fixed by the patient and unexamined by the physician.

In other words, patients are in control. Moreover, for clinicians to learn PCCM, they must suspend or relinquish their autonomy and control over patients (Stewart et al., 2003, p. 164).

Although patient-centeredness does empower patients, the question arises as to whether patients as the center can hold clinical encounters together. The emphasis of the patient at the center unfortunately can marginalize others, especially healthcare professionals, which might result in unintentional abandonment of and harm to patients. Alfred Tauber (2003, 2005), in reaction to emphasis on patients and their autonomy, claims that patients are generally left to their own resources and that autonomy can often interfere with a physician's fiduciary responsibility to treat and care for patients. He labels this type of autonomy as "sick," since it narrowly focuses on patients as individuals to the exclusion of their relationship with healthcare professionals. The result is loss of trust within the patient–physician relationship. According to Tauber (2003, p. 493), the solution is "one that configures a philosophy of medicine based on recognizing that the key issue in clinical care is not the protection of some severe form of individualism, but rather the exercise of autonomous choice within a moral context of trust, understanding, and enabling." Thus, the relational context of PatCM should be the center for the moral charge to medicine to benefit and care for patients.

Person-centered Medicine: Does the Center Hold?

While person-centered medicine (PerCM) has a long history, especially in terms of person-centered care, it has recently been championed within the healthcare literature (Cassell, 2010; Leplege et al., 2007; Slater, 2006; Snaedal, 2012). Although defining PerCM has presented a challenge, Stephanie Morgan and Linda Yoder (2012, p. 8) have recently proposed the following as "the most complete" definition. PerCM is

> a holistic (bio-psychosocial-spiritual) approach to delivering care that is respectful and individualized, allowing negotiation of care, and offering choice through a therapeutic relationship where persons are empowered to be involved in health decisions at whatever level is desired by that individual who is receiving the care.

Although their definition is certainly "complete" in the sense that it incorporates the biological, psychological, social, and even spiritual dimensions of the patient, it fails to provide a comprehensive definition of the human person or personhood per se.

Andrew Miles and Juan Mezzich (2011) have propounded a definition for PerCM that provides a more comprehensive definition of personhood. To that end, they begin with the following five key principles:

1. a wide, biological, psychological, sociocultural and spiritual theoretical framework;
2. attending to both ill health and positive health;
3. person-centered research and education on the process and outcome of the patient–family–clinician communication, diagnosis as shared

understanding, and treatment, prevention and health promotion as shared commitments;

4. respect for the autonomy, responsibility and dignity of every person involved &

5. promotion of partnerships at all levels. (p. 216)

These principles can be analyzed philosophically in terms of their ontological, epistemological, and ethical dimensions.

Ontologically, the first two of the five key principles attest to the nature of human personhood in health and illness, especially with respect to George Engel's biopsychosocial (BPS) model. Importantly, Miles and Mezzich include the spiritual dimension of personhood, which is generally overlooked or poorly developed in terms of the BPS model. The inclusion of the spiritual dimension is critical to a holistic definition of personhood, as noted earlier by Morgan and Yoder (2012). Importantly, these components of a person interact with each other and cannot be separated from one another ontologically; rather, each is interrelated and integrated with the other. In other words, what has an impact on one component has an impact on the others. PerCM's holism is certainly reminiscent of Francis Peabody's (1927, p. 878) reference to the patient as an "impressionistic painting"—"surrounded by his home, his work, his relations, his friends, his joys, sorrows, hopes, and fears."

Eric Cassell, whom Miles and Mezzich quote, also provides an ample notion of human personhood in holistic terms. "A person," according to Cassell (2010, p. 50), "is an embodied, purposeful, thinking, feeling, emotional, reflective, relational, human individual always in action, responsive to meaning, and whose life in all spheres points both outward and inward." Although this definition helps in explicating the nature of personhood in terms of responding to meaning, it must also be recognized that persons create or produce it. Indeed, the creation of meaning is an essential and a necessary quality of the human condition and is critical for determining a person's experience and understanding of either health or illness.

Julian Hughes (2001) also stresses the importance of a holistic approach to understanding human personhood, especially with respect to an embodied person's situatedness in various contexts—whether personal or social. According to Hughes, "[T]he person is best thought of as a human agent, a being of this embodied kind, who acts and interacts in a cultural and historical context in which he or she is embedded" (p. 87). For him, persons are agents who interact purposefully within a specific context particularly in terms of the creation of life's meaning and who then encode and incorporate that meaning within a personal narrative. Hence, a person's narrative and personhood go hand-in-hand and are vital for understanding the ontological nature of the human person.

Miles and Mezzich's second key principle pertains to the ontological dimension of health and illness. Unfortunately, little if any consensus exists within the philosophy of medicine literature over this dimension (Marcum, 2008). Positive health represents a person's well-being, especially in terms of the following characteristics:

(a) leading a life of purpose, embodied by projects and pursuits that give dignity and meaning to daily existence, and allow for the realization of one's potential; (b) having quality connection to others, such as having warm, trusting, and loving interpersonal relations and a sense of belongingness; (c) possessing self-regard, characterized by such qualities as self-acceptance and self-respect; and (d) experiencing mastery, such as feelings of efficiency and control. (Ryff and Singer, 1998, p. 69)

Illness, however, represents a disruption in a person's well-being. For example, Kay Toombs (1993, p. 81) claims that "illness must be understood not simply as the physical dysfunction of the mechanistic, biological body but as the disorder of body, self and world." Whereas positive health in terms of well-being permits a person to pursue life's goals and projects, illness obstructs such pursuits.

The third key principle is epistemological in nature, especially with respect to the knowledge about positive and ill health and how best to proceed when informed by such knowledge. Traditionally, this principle is generally construed in terms of a clinician's technical training and competence. However, for Miles and Mezzich's version of PerCM, it also requires the participation of patients. Specifically, clinical encounters require epistemically unrestricted and effectual communication between the clinician and patient in terms of making an accurate diagnosis and fashioning a shared treatment plan. As Miles and Mezzich contend, PerCM is not so much "based" on the empirical evidence derived from clinical trials as it is "informed" by it. Moreover, the evidence is not restricted to the evidence obtained just from clinical trials; but it also includes a clinician's expertise and knowledge of pathophysiological mechanisms, as well as incorporating the patient's illness narrative. Miles and Mezzich's PerCM, then, is evidence-informed rather than evidence-based epistemologically.

The final two key principles engage the moral or ethical nature of contemporary medicine, especially in terms of the patient–physician relationship. The fourth key principle particularly focuses on the respect persons deserve in terms of their autonomy and on the responsibility of moral agents to act in the best interests of one another. The physician should benefit rather than harm a patient, especially by including the patient's values and preferences into clinical judgments, to guide clinical decisions and actions. On the part of the patient, the clinician's experience should be trusted. Moreover, the patient should participate as actively as possible in the diagnostic process and in the treatment plan. Through mutual respect between the clinician and patient, the dignity of each is supported and not violated, so that the best clinical outcome is possible. Rather than a power disparity between clinician and patient, especially as often exhibited through institutional role playing, a mutual empowerment occurs in terms of the respect two persons have for one another to do what is right or beneficial and to avoid what is wrong or detrimental (Leplege et al. 2007, Morgan and Yoder 2012).

Finally, the fifth key principle refers ethically to the moral or proper duty of patients, physicians, and other healthcare professionals as persons participating in and contributing to clinical encounters. According to this principle, people should work together as partners toward an optimal clinical outcome. Importantly, the equality is not an identity of duties or obligations and it does not confuse institutional roles, for example, patients acting as physicians, but rather it requires respect for each member of the healthcare team, whether patients, family members, physicians, allied healthcare professionals, or even healthcare administrators. The principle specifically includes the values and mores that govern the behavior of those who work as a community committed to the best possible clinical outcomes. Moreover, it cannot be instantiated in terms of rigid rules of a deontological ethic but rather it should reflect the actions of authentic persons who desire to achieve what is genuinely good and beneficial—not just for the patient but also for those involved in the patient's care and treatment.

Based on the five key principles, Miles and Mezzich (2011, p. 216) provide the following four-part working definition for PerCM,

1. *of* the person (of the totality of the person's health, including its ill and positive aspects),
2. *for* the person (promoting the fulfilment of the person's life project),
3. *by* the person (with clinicians extending themselves as full human beings, well grounded in science and with high ethical aspirations) and
4. *with* the person (working respectfully in collaboration and in an empowering manner through a partnership of patient, family and clinicians).

Their four-part working definition can be analyzed philosophically in terms of its ontology, epistemology, and ethics, particularly with respect to the five key principles.

The preposition "*of*" signifies the ontological nature of the human person, since it attests to personhood from a holistic or global perspective. In terms of Cassell's notion of human personhood, personhood reflects a "totality" that includes the "embodied" and the physical, chemical, and biological mechanisms involved in health or illness—as derived from Miles and Mezzich's first two key principles. It also includes the psychological, such as "always in action" or behavioral, "thinking" or cognitive, and "feeling" or emotional, as well as the "relational" or cultural and social. Finally, it includes the transcendent or spiritual in which people forge meaning in their lives. These attributes are "*of*" the person, since possessing them are essential for defining who a person is. Moreover, they are also applicable to the clinician and other healthcare professionals. In sum, the embodied, psychological, cultural, social, and spiritual attributes of the persons participating in the clinical encounter converge to provide the best possible professional healthcare.

The preposition "*for*" also signifies the ontological nature of the human person, since it attests to the individuality of human personhood. A person's individuality—as derived from the first two principles, as well as the fourth key principle—refers to his or her unique life purpose and story, as well as to their realization. A person inhabits a distinct life-world, in which personal identity is shaped through the creation of meaning. A necessary precondition for shaping a meaningful life-world and a person's unique identity is self-knowing. According to Tanya McCance and colleagues (2011, pp. 2–3), self-knowing is "*being with self*, which emphasizes the importance of persons 'knowing self' and the values they hold about their life and how they make sense of what is happening to them" (emphasis in the original). Self-knowing, particularly with respect to personal preferences and values, is important for both patient and clinician. For the patient as an individual, healthcare must be designed to meet personal needs and not institutional convenience or profit. "Care should be organized by patients' personal needs and preferences," insist Morgan and Yoder (2012, p. 9), "instead of institutional standards of routine . . . because one size does not fit all." Moreover, clinicians must be self-knowing so as to meet not only their patient's needs but also their own professional and personal needs. Thus, "person-centredness means that the individual's [patient's or clinician's] subjective experience, personal history and emotion should be taken into account" (Leplege et al., 2007, p. 157).

The preposition "*by*" signals the cognitive faculty or epistemic capacity of the human person, whether patient or clinician. It is epistemological, as derived from the third key principle, in terms of knowing about health and illness and about how best to act when illness occurs. For patients as persons, such knowledge represents first-hand experience, especially with respect to the suffering and loss of dignity associated with illness. Physicians as persons certainly have first-hand knowledge about their personal illness experience. But for the patient's illness experience, they can only have second-hand knowledge, and the degree of that knowledge depends on their ability to empathize with the patient (Halpern, 2001; Hojat, 2010). An important feature of empathy is the common experience that patients and physicians share with respect to personhood. Last, as Miles and Mezzich emphasize, the epistemic dimension of clinical medicine is generally, if not always, associated with its ethical dimension.

Although technical competence is critical for delivering quality healthcare, such healthcare must comply with moral standards, which they explore in the final part of their working definition of PerCM.

The preposition *"with"* refers to the moral or ethical nature of the human person. Miles and Mezzich's last two key principles are essential for grounding relationships and interactions among persons with respect to acting or behaving properly. Appropriate action or behavior is essential for respecting people's dignity and aiding them in realizing their full potential as persons of value and worth. Such behavior is necessary not only for physicians in front of whom stand vulnerable patients, but also for patients in front of whom stand vulnerable physicians with respect to whether patients empower them to practice their trade. Patients and physicians deserve respect because of their fundamental value and worth. They cannot be reduced to their respective institutional roles, for to reduce them to such roles is to risk failing to empower each with the possibility of acting for the good of each other. The good for patients is generally the best possible clinical outcome, which might entail a cure, but it may also entail effective management of the illness, or possibly re-creating the meaning of their life story vis-à-vis their illness. The good for physicians is the opportunity to help patients, who trust in their clinical skills, as competent and compassionate healthcare professionals.

Although Miles and Mezzich's working definition of PerCM—based on their five key principles—provides a rather comprehensive definition, the major shortcoming is that they have insufficiently defined who the human person is in order to operationalize and justify PerCM (Griggs et al., 2014). Their conception of person, based on the work of Cassell and others, provides a good starting point but an inadequate means to complete the journey toward a robust model of PerCM. Without a satisfactory conceptualization of human personhood, the center of PerCM is in jeopardy of unraveling and not holding clinical encounters together. In the next section, healthcare personalism (HP), which conceptualizes personhood from ontological, epistemological, and ethical perspectives, is introduced in order to hold clinical encounters together. Moreover, it replaces the centeredness metaphor with a network metaphor in which centeredness is relativized to the needs of persons.

Healthcare Personalism

HP is an approach to clinical practice in terms of providing quality healthcare that focuses on the dimensions of personhood with respect to the healthcare team and not any one team member—whether patients or healthcare professionals (Marcum, 2015, 2016). In this section, the philosophy of personalism is used to provide a conceptual perspective for developing a dynamic notion of HP. To that end, personalism is first examined as a philosophical movement, followed by conceptualization of personhood based on Christian Smith's (2010) "critical realist personalism" framework. With this framework in place, the notion of HP is articulated in terms of the ontology, epistemology, and ethics of the human person. The section concludes with a discussion of the power of metaphor in medicine and with the substitution of HP's network metaphor for the centeredness metaphor of PatCM and PerCM, as well as for the foundational metaphor of evidence-based medicine (EBM). In sum, HP provides the means by which to sustain clinical encounters so to deliver quality healthcare in order to diminish human suffering caused by illness and to restore human dignity lost because of it.

Personalism

Personalism is a philosophy that has a rich historical tradition in almost every culture (Bengtsson, 2006, 2013). Thomas Williams and Jan Bengtsson (2014, p. 1), however, provide a sober caution concerning personalism.

> Personalism is a more diffused and eclectic movement and has no such universal reference point. It is, in point of fact, more proper to speak of many *personalisms* than one personalism. (Emphasis in the original)

These personalisms may include philosophical positions, such as idealism, phenomenology, existentialism, or Thomism. Moreover, they often have close nationalistic ties, whether European, American, Indian, Chinese, or Japanese. However, Williams and Bengtsson do identify several general characteristics that represent a common configuration for the different personalisms. These include the distinction between persons and nonpersons,[4] the nonreducibility of persons to their isolated parts, the dignity of persons, the subjectivity and self-determination of persons, and the social or relational dimensions of persons.

Moreover, Patricia Sayre provides a philosophical perspective that captures the main thesis of personalism. "Personalism, in its broadest sense," claims Sayre (2010, p. 151), "is a philosophical stance that takes the concept of personhood to be indispensable and central to a proper understanding of reality." Erazim Kohák fleshes out Sayre's perspective in terms of the personal and the communal dimensions of human existence. According to Kohák (1997, p. 11),

> [P]ersonalism is a philosophy committed to the *primacy of person-al (subject-related) categories of value and meaning*, to the mutual respect of all beings in a *reality experienced as a community of persons* who are convinced that

> subject-related categories are subjectival, not subjective in the sense of being private and arbitrary. (Emphasis in the original)

In other words, personalism envisions the individual not as subjective or isolated from others and the community but as subjectival or in relationship to others and the community.

Personalism, then, does not advance subjective (individual) or arbitrarily relative meaning and value concerning reality but rather "subjectival" meaning and value in the sense that a community is composed of persons who find meaning and value in their existence and relationships with one another (Kohák, 1988, 1997). Importantly, the relationship is genuine and authentic in that the individual's experience and understanding of others and the community are authentic and thereby genuine, that is, objective, and not skewed through personal bias or prejudice. According to Bengtsson (2013, p. 1727), "[P]ersonalism is ultimately about the quality of the life concretely lived by persons and in particular by persons-in-relation." For personalism at its source is about concrete persons embedded within a specific context who—through their relationships with others—strive toward authentic or sincere and genuine or reliable existence.

An important component of personalism, especially for developing HP, is that personalism counters or opposes impersonalism, which is the prevalent philosophical perspective in our contemporary technological society. In the Harris lectures delivered at Northwestern University, Borden Parker Bowne (1908) portrayed the "failure" of impersonalism accordingly.

> A human form as an object in space, apart from our experience of it as the instrument of expression of personal life, would have little beauty or attraction; and when it is described in anatomical terms there is nothing in it that we should desire it. (p. 270)

Particularly, Bowne criticized modern analytic philosophy and its impact on the nature of personhood, which degrades the person to a mechanistic machine. The person qua machine is composed of anatomical parts, which are quantified and averaged. As Kohák (1997, p. 50) so aptly articulates impersonalism, it reduces "personal being to an epiphenomenal reflection of 'objective' reality and moral concerns to private idiosyncrasies."

In place of impersonalism, Bowne (1908) proposed a "personal world." "If we are in a personal world," he insisted, "the final cause of nature must be sought in the personal and moral realm" (p. 324). He grounded his philosophy of personalism and its associated concept of personal world on two important dimensions of personhood. The first is that persons have thoughts and feelings that are indisputably theirs and simply cannot be invalidated by debasing them as subjective. The second is that persons cannot regard themselves as self-contained and autonomous in an unlimited or unqualified manner. They are part of larger communal or social networks and depend upon those networks for composing personal worlds that benefit not only themselves but also others making up the community. It is this tension between the person qua individual and the person qua community member in which a personal world is fashioned and reality is explicated and validated.

Richard Prust (1997) identifies three important elements that constitute Bowne's ontology of human personhood. The first is personal unity, which Prust claims represents a person's normative coherent narrative or what he calls a "story line." And it is through this story line that the second element of personhood arises, personal persistence and preservation, which represents a sequentially organized narrative—or what Prust calls "the way we coordinate our lives with stories" (p. 75). Personal persistence is the manner in which persons organize past events of their lives in the present through the stories they tell themselves and others, in order to project themselves into the future. The final element of personhood concerns personal responsibility, which pertains to accountability of persons for their own narratives. In other words, persons are responsible ultimately for who they are in terms of their personal narratives. Deeply rooted in personalism then is a moral obligation, to both the self and others, to relate these narratives truthfully, honestly, and with integrity.

Finally, Paul Schotsmans (1999) introduced personalism into medical ethics, which provides a generally framework for presaging HP generally. According to Schotsmans, "[T]he personalist approach offers a relational foundation for medicine as a healing profession" (p. 10). To that end, he identified three features of personalism. The first is the person as uniquely original, especially in terms of a life story or project. For healthcare, each patient has a unique illness narrative that the healthcare professional must incorporate into both diagnosis and treatment. Moreover, each healthcare professional has a unique life project that can have a significant impact on healthcare delivery. The next feature is the person as relationally intersubjective. Both the patient and healthcare professional certainly form a relational dyad, but holistically the dyad is composed of more than two elements. Rather, it represents a network of team members, each with their own unique life story and project. The final feature is the person as communicatively solidaritous, in which the relationship among members of the healthcare team qua persons forms a harmonious unity. In addition, each member of the healthcare team connects openly and honestly with one another. Finally, the value animating and supporting the features of HP is respect for the dignity of each person within the healthcare team. Although Schotsmans's notion of the person as uniquely original, relationally intersubjective, and communicatively solidaritous provides a general framework for HP, that notion is insufficient for developing a robust HP that can deliver quality healthcare, which reduces suffering and restores dignity.

Personhood

The notion of human personhood remains a contentious topic within philosophy, especially in philosophy of medicine and bioethics (Beauchamp, 1999; Gordijn, 1999; Hacker, 2007; Harré, 1984; Merrill, 1998; Seifert, 2004; Tooley, 2009). Ruth Macklin (1983, p. 35) provides a stern warning about explicating conceptually the notion of personhood, given its voluminous literature.

> The first and most apparent reason for the continuing controversy over the concept of personhood and the slim likelihood of ever reaching an agreement is that the antecedent values writers embrace determine the definition or criteria they arrive at by way of conclusion.

With this warning in mind, Smith's explication of the nature of personhood from a framework he calls "critical realist personalism" is presented in this section in order to formulate a robust notion of HP in the next section.

Smith constructs the framework not only on traditional personalism, as developed by Bowne and others, but also on critical realism and phenomenology. For Smith (2010, p. 197), personhood is

> a conscious, reflexive, embodied, self-transcending center of subjective experience, durable identity, moral commitment, and social communication who—as the efficient cause of his or her own responsible actions and intentions—exercises complex capacities for agency and intersubjectivity in order to develop and sustain his or her own incommunicable self in loving relationships with other personal selves and with the nonpersonal world.

In brief, a person is a "center with purpose" that emerges from the interactions of five different categories of capacities—Smith lists a total of thirty individual capacities. The "existence capacities" are the first category in which the person is at core not only a subconscious being but also a conscious being, who is aware of itself and its surroundings. The "primary experience capacities"—composed of an ability to comprehend quality and quantity, along with space and time, and to forge mental representations—are the next category. It also includes volition and practical consciousness. The "secondary experience capacities" are the third category, which include causal reasoning, interest formation, emotions, memory, and intersubjective understanding. The "creating capacities" are the next category, which range from creativity, innovation, and imagination to self-transcendence, language, narrative construction, and valuation, along with identity formation and self-reflexivity.

The "highest order capacities" are the final category, which include abstract reasoning and truth seeking, moral judgment and virtues, and aesthetic judgment. Importantly, the two most defining capacities of a person, according to Smith, are interpersonal communion and love. Interpersonal communion refers to mutual giving of one another in terms of fellowship for the good of each person. The good vis-à-vis human personhood is to flourish and to realize fully one's potential not only individually but also collectively as a highly functional and vigorous community. For Smith, human flourishing is the foundation for a "teleological personalist morality," especially in terms of the dignity of each person within society. Finally, love is what makes possible this self-giving for the good of the community and its members. For Smith (2010), it is not just limited to feelings of attraction, especially in terms of self-gratification. Rather, love pertains importantly to

relating to other persons and things beyond the self in a way that involves the purposive action of extending and expending oneself for the genuine good of others—whether in friendships, families, communities, among strangers, or otherwise. (p. 73)

Humans are persons, then, because they care authentically not just acting for themselves but also for others and the world itself through gifting themselves for the benefit or good of every person and thing.

Finally, Smith addresses the contentious notion—especially in the bioethics literature[5]—of human dignity.[6] For him, human dignity represents the sine qua non of personhood. Smith (2010, p. 471) defines "human dignity" as "an irreducible attribute of persons, proactively emergent as an ontologically real property at the level of personhood, not at the lower level of individual capacities." First, human dignity represents an "irreducible property" in the sense that it is "analytically irreducible" to any particularly property of human personhood (p. 443). Moreover, it is irreducible since it is a "proactively emergent" property in that it is a property inherent to the developing processes within a human person.[7] Thus, human dignity cannot be reduced to any particular capacity or sets of capacities since it transcends them. Human dignity is also "ontologically real," because "it does not require that people recognize it in order to exist" (p. 440).

In sum, human dignity, for Smith, represents "an inherent worth of immeasurable value ... [in that human] persons are creatures worthy of being treated with respect, justice, and love" (p. 435). Last, human dignity is an emergent property not only of the individual but also of human societies. For human persons to realize their full potential as dignified beings, they must recognize and attribute dignity onto others.

Personhood and Healthcare Personalism

The question arises as to how the nature of human personhood, as Smith explicates it, informs HP in order to deliver quality healthcare. In this section, that question is answered in terms of the ontology, epistemology, and ethics of personhood. Specifically, Smith's various capacities are used to articulate a notion of human personhood in order to develop a robust and comprehensive notion of HP. An important part of the motivation for developing HP is to accomplish two important goals of medicine. Although the main goal of the biomedical sciences is to cure disease in order to prevent the patient from dying—and this is certainly an admirable goal but not always attainable—for HP the first goal is to relieve or reduce suffering associated with illness. As Cassell (1982, p. 639) comments,

> The relief of suffering and the cure of disease must be seen as twin obligations of a medical profession that is truly dedicated to the care of the sick. Physicians' failure to understand the nature of suffering can result in medical intervention that (though technically adequate) not only fails to relieve suffering but becomes a source of suffering itself.

The other goal of HP is the restoration of human dignity often lost during the course of an illness. To achieve these goals, then, a comprehensive notion of personhood is developed in ontological, epistemological, and ethical terms.

Ontologically the human person is an embodied agent who is embedded holistically within biological and social contexts. There are two key ontological features of personhood. The first is embodiment, which reflects Smith's "existence capacity" of "subconscious being" and provides the necessary physicality or substrate for Smith's other capacities of personhood. There are two dimensions to embodiment. The first is biological in that embodiment qua physical body depends on—although it is not identical or restricted to—the human genome or genotype, that is, the set of genes and their products that make up the embodied human person. It is important to note that there is no ideal or normal genome but that genes do vary in terms of their composition, arrangement, and to some extent presence. A human person's genotype is *Homo sapiens* and not that of another biological species, even though there may be significant homology with them. Although a person's genotype and its expression (phenotype) do vary, personhood qua embodiment (at some level) cannot be ignored or denied.

One of the main issues for disease-centered medicine is determining what is normal so as to detect what is not, that is, what disease is. But what is normal in an absolute or precise sense is difficult to determine. For HP, health is not represented simply as a normal distribution of physiological parameters and disease a deviation from the normal. Rather, the normal with respect to health and the abnormal in terms of disease function as guides for setting parameters on how to proceed, especially therapeutically, but not in a deterministic sense. What needs to be incorporated is what constitutes the functioning level for the patient qua individual person. In other words, the patient's values and preferences have a significant impact on what constitutes health and disease for that particular patient. This also pertains to the genome as well, in that each patient's genome is unique, which can stipulate potentially biological parameters for health and disease but cannot dictate them essentially or deterministically. In other words, health and disease are not fixed ontologically to a rigid standard but fluid or variable in terms of the person's own unique genotype and its expression. For even genotype does not strictly define phenotype since a person's psychological, environmental, and social contexts can have an impact on gene expression.

The second dimension of embodiment is social in that a person is embedded within a community, which represents the communal body. Social embodiment pertains to a person's "being-in-the-world"—as Heidegger articulates it—which emerges from the interaction of biological and social dimensions (Svenaeus, 2000). In other words, a person's biological embodiment opens up possibilities for participating within the social realm. For HP, social embodiment signifies the collected and shared existence of embodied individuals—and not just patients but also healthcare professionals—within a healthcare system or network, in terms of the institutionalization of medicine. This then has an impact on what constitutes health and disease. Ontologically, health is the proper functioning, while illness is an improper functioning or dysfunctioning, of the person qua socially embodied and not just the person qua biologically embodied. Finally, for healthcare professionals qua socially embodied, their goal is to assist the patient in returning to some semblance of health.

While the first key feature of personhood is in terms of being, the second is in terms of doing or agency. In other words, a person is an agent for bringing about change, particularly as an efficient cause for transformation. According to Smith (2010, p. 42), agency reflects a person's "causal capacities," that is, "the ability to bring about changes in material and mental phenomena, to produce or influence objects and events in the world." Personal agency includes the capacity to function as an "efficient cause" of its own actions and interactions. For HP, agency is particularly important not only for healthcare professionals in terms of assisting patients medically but also for patients with respect to participating with healthcare professionals to bring about change vis-à-vis illness. To that end, agency depends on the existence capacity of "conscious awareness." For an agent must be aware of itself and its surroundings in order to bring about changes within them. Thus, for HP each person in the clinical encounter must be mindfully attentive to the needs of one another (Epstein, 1999).

Finally, as an embodied agent, a person exhibits several of Smith's "creating capacities," especially in terms of imagination and innovation. Creative imagination is at the root of bringing into existence that which did not exist before. According to Smith (2010, p. 47), "[P]eople can mentally innovate in order to visualize, dream, invent, connect, conceive, and envision ideas, possibilities, and images that do not yet exist in reality." Thus, creativity permits the embodied agent to be inventive and to shape both the material and cultural worlds at hand to solve pressing problems, particularly through technology. In a real sense, a person and its society are technological (Ellul, 1967; Jerónimo et al., 2013). For HP, technology is an important driving force for clinical advancement and practice, but it is not their sine qua non. If healthcare technology is not used humanely, that is, if it intervenes and separates the patient and clinician, causes additional pain and suffering, and violates human dignity, then it does not promote two of the chief goals of medicine—to reduce or relieve suffering and to restore human dignity—even though it may assist in curing the patient.

Epistemologically the person is an intelligent or epistemic agent, who exhibits perceiving or sensing and cognitive or rational/logical faculties and who can discern fact from fiction and truth from falsity. Epistemic agents rely then on two main faculties or processes. The first is perception and the second cognition (Goldstone et al., 2015). Perception involves the ability to sense or experience the world directly in an accurate and a reliable manner. Fundamentally, it involves Smith's primary experience capacity of observing and grasping spatial and temporal dimensions of the world, as well as its qualitative and quantitative properties. For HP, clinicians must be able to observe the patient's signs directly rather than read off laboratory results from a medical record—especially if composed by another. Abraham Verghese (2008, p. 2751) calls the latter patient an "iPatient" and warns that quality healthcare must include the "bedside ... the place where fellow human beings allow us the privilege of looking at, touching, and listening to their bodies." Besides clinicians, patients must also be able to observe and relate accurately and meaningfully their chief complaints and symptoms. Although this is difficult because of their illness, it aids clinicians in terms of making a proper diagnosis and proposing efficacious therapeutic options.

In terms of the epistemic agent's cognition, a predominant model is the dual process theory (DPT). According to DPT advocates, two systems—I and II—compose human cognition (Evans and Stanovich, 2013). System I is evolutionary old and shared with other sentient organisms. Its processes are relatively fast and almost automatic in terms of decision-making. It exhibits several of Smith's primary experience capacities. The first is "mental representation" and shapes the foundation for this system, with respect to portraying reality. The other primary experience capacity includes Smith's practical consciousness, which involves intuition or tacit knowing. System II is evolutionary recent and thought to be exclusively human. Its processes are relatively slow and deliberate, with respect to decision-making. Importantly, system II can override system I processes if error is detected or even suspected. It depends on several of Smith's secondary experience capacities, including "interest formation"—especially in terms of the well-being of self and others—and short- and long-term memory. It also depends on several creating capacities such as utilization of language, as well as signs and symbols, to communicate meaning. Its processes reflect several of Smith's highest order capacities, involving an ability to reason abstractly and a desire to know the truth. For HP, clinical decision-making relies on the proper functioning of the two cognitional processes. For example, clinicians can operate on system I processes to diagnose common illnesses but must rely on system II processes when confronted with uncommon ones.

Finally, the epistemic agent also exhibits Smith's highest order capacity of "forming virtues," particularly intellectual or epistemic virtues. Virtue epistemologists divide intellectual virtues into two categories (Baehr, 2011). The first are reliabilist virtues, which include virtues associated with an epistemic agent's dependable perceptual or sensory faculties and sound conceptual or cognitive faculties. The second category are responsibilist virtues, which involve an epistemic agent's virtuous traits or characteristics with respect to delivering the epistemic goods. Examples of these virtues include traditional intellectual virtues of *phronesis*, *episteme*, and *sophia*, and contemporary epistemic virtues of honesty, curiosity, and open-mindedness. For HP, the virtues animating the epistemic clinician are *phronesis* or practical wisdom (Pellegrino and Thomasma, 1993), as well as *sophia* or theoretical wisdom and epistemic courage (Marcum, 2009a). For the patient, intellectual virtues such as patience and perseverance ensure that the healthcare professional hears and understands the patient's illness story.

Ethically the person is a moral agent, who can discern right from wrong and good from bad (Hinman, 2013). The foundation of this moral agency is the person qua relational agent. Relational agency involves not simply an ability to form relationships with others, but rather it emanates from a relationship with the self and from that relationship emerges relationships with others. Central to a functional self-relationship is Smith's creating capacities, including "identity formation" and "self-reflexivity." "Identities are self-understandings," according to Smith (2010, pp. 50–51), "derived from occupying particular, stable locations in social, behavioral, mental, and moral space that securely define who and what somebody is, for themselves and for others." Functional identities depend on an ability to reflect insightfully into what or who constitutes the self. From an ability to identify the self and to reflect upon it, a person creates a personal narrative and can communicate it faithfully to others. For HP, relational agency is paramount to a successful and caring clinical encounter. Both healthcare professionals and patients must have well-formed self-identities, and they must be able to communicate their self-story honestly and effectively. Obviously, such relational agency is especially critical for the patient, who needs to communicate accurately and effectively the illness narrative to the healthcare professional.

Moral agency proper depends on several of Smith's capacities. The primary experience capacity of "volition" is foundational for the moral agent. If an agent is not free to make choices, then moral agency itself may be compromised or even abolished. As for Smith's secondary experience capacities, a moral agent's emotional experience has an impact on behavior and especially on intersubjective understanding, which is "the ability to at least somewhat correctly understand the subjective beliefs, thoughts, emotions, desires, intentions, goals, interests, moods, and meanings of other people" (p. 47). Both of these experience capacities form the basis for the creating capacity of "self-transcendence" in which the moral agent can step outside itself and attend to the needs of others. Thus, a self-transcendent moral agent can act for the good of others, who might require assistance. For HP, a healthcare professional's moral agency, especially in terms of self-transcendence, motivates the professional to address two of the important goals of medicine in terms of alleviating a patient's suffering as best as possible and certainly not adding to it, and with respect to restoring human dignity and not violating it. The patient must also transcend the self in terms of trusting the healthcare professional to provide the best healthcare care possible.

Moral agency also depends on another of Smith's (2010, p. 50) creating capacities: valuation, which is the ability "to assess in fairly abstract terms the relative goodness, rightness, worth, merit, importance, or virtue of various objects, situations, beliefs, or behaviors." This capacity allows the person to evaluate perceptions, concepts, and actions in a normative manner. And, it provides the foundation for two of Smith's highest order capacities: "aesthetic judgment and enjoyment" and "moral awareness and judgment." The former pertains to a person's ability to make judgments as to what is beautiful and attractive, while the latter to judgments of what is good and just. For HP, clinicians must be able to evaluate what is good and appropriate for patients in terms of treating them. As noted repeatedly, two of the chief goals of medicine are not to harm the patient any more than the suffering associated with the illness and not to violate the patient's dignity lost because of illness. For patients as moral agents, they must make sober and realistic judgments about what is best for them, as well as for others and society.

Finally, moral agency rests on two of Smith's highest order capacities. The first is the formation of virtues, especially moral virtues such as benevolence, caring, competence, courage, compassion and empathy, honesty, humility, integrity, respect, sincerity, and trust—to name a few (Marcum, 2012). The second is related to the moral virtues of "interpersonal communion and love," with the latter representing probably the chief virtue of a moral agent. As discussed earlier, interpersonal communion and love go hand-in-hand to ensure both personal and social flourishing. For HP, the chief virtue of healthcare professionals as moral agents is care, along with two associated virtues—compassion and competence. Through caring for the patient qua person the clinician qua moral agent is able to take care of the patient's healthcare needs. The chief virtue of patients is gratitude for healthcare professionals who strive to reduce their suffering associated with illness and to restore their dignity. In addition, respect is an important virtue, particularly as it pertains to the bioethical principle of respect for the patient as an autonomous agent, as well as respect for the autonomy of each healthcare professional involved in the patient's treatment.

Conclusion: Does the Center Hold?

Metaphors are powerful figures of speech or literary devices by which to clarify and support one concept through comparison with another (Kövecses, 2010; Ortony, 1993). They can function in terms of illuminating the meaning of a concept or sustaining a particular representation or understanding of it. As evident from contemporary medical pluralism, a number of metaphors, such as military, machine, spatial, and foundational metaphors, have been enlisted to help elucidate and defend a specific approach to medicine and its practice (Diekema, 1989; Hodgkin, 1985; Periyakoil, 2008). Obviously, two of the more popular medical metaphors are the foundational or "base" metaphor of EBM and the spatial or "centeredness" metaphor of PatCM and PerCM. In this concluding section, HP is distinguished from the foundational and spatial metaphors in terms of a network metaphor.

In contrast to EBM's metaphor, HP is nonfoundational with respect to evidence, especially in terms of quantitative laboratory results and randomized controlled trials. Although evidence is important, it is not HP's base. What is important for it is the person with a unique life story, such as the patient with an illness narrative or the healthcare professional with a career life project. For HP stresses the interrelationship among members of a clinical encounter with respect to a network. The philosophical implications of this metaphor vis-à-vis EBM's foundational metaphor are as follows. Metaphysically, as nonfoundational, HP replaces EBM's presupposition of reductionism with holism, which in general states that the whole is greater than the sum of its parts (Henning and Scarfe, 2013; Marcum, 2009b). In other words, for HP the person dwells contextually and not in isolation or as the patient anatomized. Consequently, quality healthcare requires incorporation of a person's life story and project, whether patient or healthcare professional. Epistemologically, as nonfoundational, HP replaces EBM's naïve empiricism or foundationalism with coherentism in which beliefs are justified by their consistency and cohesiveness with other relevant beliefs, as well as by their comprehensiveness (Audi, 1993). Last, HP replaces EBM's vertical metaphor of hierarchical evidence with a horizontal metaphor of relationships among persons (or evidence). In sum, by emphasizing the person in terms of the clinical encounter HP's network replaces EBM's impersonalism with personalism.

In contrast to PatCM's spatial metaphor of centeredness, HP does not privy the patient to the personhood of other healthcare team members. The personhood of everyone involved in the clinical encounter is required for meeting the goal of quality healthcare—the relief of human suffering and the restoration of human dignity. To that end, the network metaphor relativizes the absolute emphasis of PatCM on patient centeredness. In other words, the patient might be the center at one time while at another it might be the clinician or an allied healthcare professional—or even clinical evidence itself. Thus, for the HP network metaphor patients and other members of the healthcare team function as nodes or centers that are interconnected with one another and the nodal connections can fluctuate with respect to importance and strength.

In terms of the spatial metaphor of PerCM, especially Miles and Mezzich's version of it, HP's network metaphor again relativizes the centeredness of the relationships among members of the healthcare team. The metaphor has important implications with respect to the four prepositions of Miles and Mezzich's definition of PerCM. For HP, the person is the center "of" the healthcare encounter, not in terms of being an absolute center but a relative one in terms of the larger network of interactions. Again, each person in the healthcare encounter represents a provisional node around which interactions can be structured and arranged. The "for" preposition represents the purpose of the clinical encounter, which for the clinician is to treat or to care for the patient. Importantly, with these two prepositions Smith's definition of a person as a "center with purpose" is realized in that each member of the healthcare team has a particular role and purpose to play in the clinical encounter. In addition, the "by" preposition represents the notion of agency for HP, especially in terms of the clinician and/or patient as an efficient cause in promoting health and in treating illness. Finally, the "with" preposition reflects the relational context of HP in that the clinical encounter is interpersonal and thereby moral in nature. In sum, the HP network metaphor advances PerCM conceptually by providing a more comprehensive and realistic notion of human personhood vis-à-vis clinical encounters.

The HP network metaphor also elucidates more fully the five key principles Miles and Mezzich utilize to define PerCM. Specifically, HP clarifies conceptually these principles of PerCM in terms of their ontological, epistemological, and ethical dimensions. Ontologically, the person within HP is embodied not only in terms of the physical but also the psychological, spiritual, and social (principle 1). In addition, certainly the proper functioning (i.e., health) of the embodied or physical patient is paramount for HP and hence for PerCM but so is the proper functioning of the psychological, spiritual, and social aspects of the patient (principle 2). And to function improperly in any of these aspects, generally represents illness. HP's ontological nature of personhood then serves to expound the epistemological dimension of PerCM with respect to the information and knowledge associated with investigating human health and illness, and with treating the patient's illness (principle 3). For example, the healthcare professional represents an epistemic source for guiding the patient in terms of treatment options. To that end, HP advances the moral dimension of PerCM in terms of the patient's autonomy and dignity (principle 4). Last, HP grounds PerCM's moral dimension with respect to the relational agency of the clinical encounter (principle 5).

Finally, HP enhances PerCM in terms of one of the chief values animating healthcare—the dignity of each person involved in the clinical encounter. Human dignity is central to PerCM, although its advocates have not thoroughly developed it with respect to motivating the delivery of quality healthcare. For HP, human dignity is the motivating factor for delivering such care by treating patients as persons of value or worth. Specifically, persons have value because they are worthy of love and should be treated accordingly. To treat patients otherwise is to devalue them and open up opportunities for abuse, harm, and humiliation. And, in turn, patients must respect the dignity of clinicians and other healthcare professionals.

In conclusion, HP's notion of personhood in terms of its ontological, epistemological, and ethical dimensions is crucial for providing a philosophical framework to advance and elucidate more fully PerCM—especially in its effort to assure the delivery of quality healthcare. Moreover, HP's network metaphor is nonfoundational and relativizes centeredness in the sense that no one person or approach to providing healthcare suffices to bound or to restrict the clinical encounter. Rather, the encounter must be open to a wide range of possibilities for providing quality healthcare. Finally, a person is a loving agent who not only has self-respect and dignity but who also has respect for others and their dignity. Each person, then, in the clinical encounter, whether healthcare professional or patient, should respect the dignity or worth of each other in order to reduce the suffering associated with illness.

Acknowledgments

I thank Andrew Miles for encouraging me to explore philosophy of personalism in terms of analyzing person-centered medicine, which was published as Marcum (2015, 2016).

Notes

1. Interestingly, an important question Enid Balint (1969, p. 269) addressed with the distinction between illness-oriented medicine and PatCM was: "How does a practicing doctor avoid a split in himself? How can he avoid being a general practitioner to some of his patients and a competent psychotherapist to others?"
2. The website for the International Balint Federation is: http://www.balintinternational.com/.
3. George Engel's biopsychosocial model was also another patient-centered approach to medicine and served as a "template" for it (Epstein et al. 1993). Indeed, Nicola Mead and Peter Bower (2000) in their framework for defining PatCM list the "biopsychosocial perspective" as its first characteristic, along with patient and doctor as person, and sharing power and responsibility in terms of a therapeutic alliance.
4. For discussion of nonhuman personhood, see DeGrazia (2006).
5. Macklin (2003) precipitated quite a stir in the bioethics literature, claiming that the notion of dignity is simply too vague to be of any use (Jacobson, 2012; Rosen, 2012).
6. For additional discussion of human dignity, see Kateb (2011).
7. Smith (2010, pp. 86–88) contrasts a proactive emergent property to a responsive emergent property, which emerges in response to outside agency and not to internal agency.

References

Audi, R. (1993). *The Structure of Justification*. New York: Cambridge University Press.

Baehr, J. (2011). *The Inquiring Mind: On Intellectual Virtues and Virtue Epistemology*. New York: Oxford University Press.

Balint, E. (1969). The possibilities of patient-centered medicine. *British Journal of General Practice* 17(82): 269–76.

Balint, M., Ball, D. H., and Hare, M. L. (1969). Training medical students in patient-centered medicine. *Comprehensive Psychiatry* 10(4): 249–58.

Bardes, C. L. (2012). Defining "patient-centered medicine." *New England Journal of Medicine* 366(9): 782–83.

Beauchamp, T. L. (1999). The failure of theories of personhood. *Kennedy Institute of Ethics Journal* 9(4): 309–24.

Beauchamp, T. L., and Childress, J. F. (2001). *Principles of Biomedical Ethics*. New York: Oxford University Press.

Bengtsson, J. O. (2006). *The Worldview of Personalism: Origins and Early Development*. New York: Oxford University Press.

Bengtsson, J. O. (2013). Personalism. In *Encyclopedia of Sciences and Religions*, eds. A. Runehov and L. Oviedo. New York: Springer, pp. 1626–34.

Bowne, B. P. (1908). *Personalism*. Boston, MA: Houghton Mifflin.

Cassell, E. J. (1982). The nature of suffering and the goals of medicine. *New England Journal of Medicine* 306(11): 639–45.

Cassell, E. J. (2010). The person in medicine. *International Journal of Integrated Care* 10(Suppl): e019.

DeGrazia, D. (2006). On the question of personhood beyond *Homo sapiens*. In *In Defense of Animals: The Second Wave*, ed. P. Singer. Oxford: Blackwell, pp. 40–53.

Diekema, D. S. (1989). Metaphors, medicine, and morals. *Soundings* 72(1): 17–24.

Ellul, J. (1967). *The Technological Society*. New York: Random House.

Epstein, R. M. (1999). Mindful practice. *Journal of American Medical Association* 282(9): 833–39.

Epstein, R. M., Campbell, T. L., Cohen-Cole, S. A., McWhinney, I. R., and Smilkstein, G. (1993). Perspectives on patient–doctor communication. *Journal of Family Practice* 37(4): 377–88.

Evans, J. S. B., and Stanovich, K. E. (2013). Dual-process theories of higher cognition advancing the debate. *Perspectives on Psychological Science* 8(3): 223–41.

Goldstone, R. L., de Leeuw, J. R., and Landy, D. H. (2015). Fitting perception in and to cognition. *Cognition* 135: 24–29.

Gordijn, B. (1999). The troublesome concept of the person. *Theoretical Medicine and Bioethics* 20(4): 347–59.

Griggs, J. O., Barron, L. A., and Marcum, J. A. (2014). Operationalizing Miles and Mezzich's person-centered medicine. *European Journal for Person Centered Healthcare* 2: 98–105.

Grol, R., de Maeseneer, J., Whitfield, M., and Mokkink, H. (1990). Disease-centred versus patient-centred attitudes: Comparison of general practitioners in Belgium, Britain and the Netherlands. *Family Practice* 7(2): 100–104.

Hacker, P. M. S. (2007). *Human Nature: The Categorical Framework*. Oxford: Blackwell.

Halpern, J. (2001). *From Detached Concern to Empathy: Humanizing Medical Practice*. New York: Oxford University Press.

Harré, R. (1984). *Personal Being: The Theory of Individual Psychology*. Cambridge, MA: Harvard University Press.

Henning, B. G., and Scarfe, A. C. (eds.) (2013). *Beyond Mechanism: Putting Life Back into Biology*. Lanham, MD: Rowman & Littlefield.

Hinman, L. (2013). *Ethics: A Pluralistic Approach to Moral Theory*, 5th edition. Boston: Wadsworth.

Hodgkin, P. (1985). Medicine is war: And other medical metaphors. *British Medical Journal* 291(6511): 1820–21.

Hojat, M. (2010). *Empathy in Patient Care: Antecedents, Development, Measurement, and Outcomes*. New York: Springer.

Hughes, J. C. (2001). Views of the person with dementia. *Journal of Medical Ethics* 27: 86–91.

Institute of Medicine. (2001). *Crossing the Quality Chasm: A New Health System for the 21st Century*. Washington, DC: National Academy Press.

Jacobson, N. (2012). *Dignity & Health*. Nashville, TN: Vanderbilt University Press.

Jerónimo, H. M., Garcia, J. L., and Mitcham, C. (eds.) (2013). *Jacques Ellul and the Technological Society in the 21 Century*. New York: Springer.

Kateb, G. (2011). *Human Dignity*. Cambridge, MA: Belknap Press.

Kohák, E. (1988). Personalism: The next hundred years. *Personalist Forum* 4(2): 43–52.

Kohák, E. (1997). Personalism: Towards a philosophical delineation. *Personalist Forum* 13(1): 3–11.

Kövecses, Z. (2010). *Metaphor: A Practical Introduction*, 2nd edition. New York: Oxford University Press.

Laine, C., and Davidoff, F. (1996). Patient-centered medicine: A professional evolution. *Journal of American Medical Association* 275(2): 152–56.

Leplege, A., Gzil, F., Cammelli, M., Lefeve, C., Pachoud, B., and Ville, I. (2007). Person-centredness: Conceptual and historical perspectives. *Disability and Rehabilitation* 29(20–21): 1555–65.

Macklin, R. (1983). Personhood in the bioethics literature. *The Milbank Memorial Fund Quarterly. Health and Society* 61(1): 35–57.

Macklin, R. (2003). Dignity is a useless concept: It means no more than respect for persons or their autonomy. *British Medical Journal* 327(7429): 1419–20.

Marcum, J. A. (2008). *An Introductory Philosophy of Medicine: Humanizing Modern Medicine*. New York: Springer

Marcum, J. A. (2009a). The epistemically virtuous clinician. *Theoretical Medicine and Bioethics* 30(3): 249–65.

Marcum, J. A. (2009b). *The Conceptual Foundations of Systems Biology: An Introduction*. New York: Nova.

Marcum, J. A. (2012). *The Virtuous Physician: The Role of Virtue in Medicine*. New York: Springer.

Marcum, J. A. (2015). Healthcare personalism: A prolegomenon. *European Journal for Person Centered Healthcare* 3: 228–32.

Marcum, J. A. (2016). Healthcare personalism and the nature of the person: How can personalist thought advance the conceptual basis of person-centered medicine? Forthcoming in *European Journal for Person Centered Healthcare* 4(2).

McCance, T., McCormack, B., and Dewing, J. (2011). An exploration of person-centredness in practice. *Online Journal of Issues in Nursing* 16: 1–9. doi: 10.3912/OJIN. Vol16No02Man01.

McWhinney, I. R. (1988). Through clinical medicine to a more humane medicine. In *The Task of Medicine: Dialogue at Wickenburg*, ed. K. R. White. Menlo Park, CA: Henry J. Kaiser Family Foundation, pp. 218–31.

Mead, N., and Bower, P. (2000). Patient-centredness: A conceptual framework and review of the empirical literature. *Social Science & Medicine* 51(7): 1087–110.

Merrill, S. B. (1998). *Defining Personhood: Toward the ethics of Quality in Clinical Care*. Amsterdam: Rodopi.

Miles, A., and Mezzich, J. E. (2011). The care of the patient and the soul of the clinic: Person-centered medicine as an emergent model of modern clinical practice. *International Journal of Person Centered Medicine* 1: 207–22.

Morgan, S., and Yoder, L. H. (2012). A conceptual analysis of person-centered care. *Journal of Holistic Nursing* 30: 6–15.

Ortony, A. (ed.) (1993). *Metaphor and Thought*, 2nd edition. New York: Cambridge University Press.

Peabody, F. W. (1927). The care of the patient. *Journal of the American Medical Association* 88: 877–82.

Pellegrino, E. D., and Thomasma, D. C (1993). *The Virtues in Medical Practice*. New York: Oxford University Press.

Periyakoil, V. S. (2008). Using metaphors in medicine. *Journal of Palliative Medicine* 11(6): 842–44.

Prust, R. C. (1997). Soul talk and Bowne's ontology of personhood. *Personalist Forum* 13(1): 69–76.

Rosen, M. (2012). *Dignity: Its History and Meaning*. Cambridge, MA: Harvard University Press.

Roter, D. (2000). The enduring and evolving nature of the patient–physician relationship. *Patient Education and Counseling* 39(1): 5–15.

Ryff, C. D., and Singer, B. (1998). Human health: New directions for the next millennium. *Psychological Inquiry* 9: 69–85.

Sayre, P. A. (2010). Personalism. In *A Companion to Philosophy of Religion*, 2nd edition, eds. C. Taliaferro, P. Draper, and P. L. Quinn. Oxford, UK: Wiley-Blackwell, pp. 151–58.

Schotsmans, P. (2005). Personalism in medical ethics. *Ethical Perspectives* 6(1): 10–20.

Seifert, J. (2004). *The Philosophical Diseases of Medicine and Their Cure. Philosophy and Ethics of Medicine, Vol. 1: Foundations*. New York: Springer.

Slater, L. (2006). Person-centredness: A concept analysis. *Contemporary Nurse* 23(1): 135–44.

Smith, C. (2010). *What Is a Person? Rethinking Humanity, Social Life, and the Moral Good from the Person Up*. Chicago: University of Chicago Press.

Snaedal, J. (2012). Person centered medicine. *World Medical & Health Policy* 4(2): 1–14.

Stewart, M., Brown, J. B., Weston, W. W., McWhinney, I. R., McWilliam, C. L., and Freeman, T. R. (2003). *Patient-Centered Medicine: Transforming the Clinical Method*, 2nd edition. Oxon, UK: Radcliffe Medical Press.

Svenaeus, F. (2000). *The Hermeneutics of Medicine and the Phenomenology of Health: Steps Towards a Philosophy of Medicine*. Dordrecht: Kluwer.

Tauber, A. I. (2003). Sick autonomy. *Perspectives in Biology and Medicine* 46(4): 484–95.

Tauber, A. I. (2005). *Patient Autonomy and the Ethics of Responsibility*. Cambridge, MA: MIT Press.

Tooley, M. (2009). Personhood. In *A Companion to Bioethics*, 2nd edition, eds. H. Kuhse and P. Singer. Oxford: Wiley-Blackwell, pp. 127–39.

Toombs, S. K. (1993). *The Meaning of Illness: A Phenomenological Account of the Different Perspectives of Physician and Patient*. New York: Springer.

Verghese, A. (2008). Culture shock—patient as icon, icon as patient. *New England Journal of Medicine* 359(26): 2748–51.

Williams, T. D., and Bengtsson, J. O. (2014). Personalism. In *The Stanford Encyclopedia of Philosophy*, ed. E. N. Zalta. URL: http://plato.stanford.edu/archives/spr2014/entries/personalism/.

11 Health and Disease

Rachel Cooper

Introduction

In this chapter, I consider a range of issues surrounding concepts of health and disease. The literature on these concepts is extensive but hard to survey. Philosophers of science, medical ethicists, sociologists, medics, and others write on concepts of health and disease, but much of the writing has been produced in apparent isolation and is not situated in a broader literature. Here I start with an overview of the traditional debate regarding concepts of health and disease as it appears in the philosophical literature. This debate takes "disease," "disorder," or, occasionally, "malady" as an umbrella term to refer to all sorts of medical disvalued state (diseases in the narrow sense, injuries, wounds, disabilities, and so on). This usage will be employed in this chapter, and the terms "disorder" and "disease" will be used as interchangeable umbrella terms. The key question is what distinguishes pathological from nonpathological states (vices, normal variations, nonmedical problems). Can disease be understood purely in terms of biological dysfunction, or are diseases also necessarily bad? Must a condition be unexpected or unusual to count as a disorder? Are diseases essentially the sorts of things that medics treat? I end this section by considering recent suggestions that the traditional debate has become bogged down, and that a new approach is required. Maybe, for example, "disease" is best understood as a family resemblance term and no account in terms of necessary and sufficient conditions can be given.

The second section of the chapter focuses on mental disorder. How does mental disorder differ from physical disorder? The third section addresses emerging challenges: How can the philosophy of medicine become adequately responsive to the lived-experience of illness? How can philosophers of medicine respond to work in the sociology and history of medicine, which shows that concepts of disorder shift over time? Have philosophers been right in lumping diseases, injuries, and disabilities together? Or, should disability, in particular, be thought of quite differently?

The Traditional Dispute

How can We Distinguish the Pathological from the Nonpathological?

Whether a condition is considered a disease matters because we tend to think that the disordered should be treated differently from the nondisordered. Disorder can act to justify treatment, to excuse wrongdoing, and to elicit sympathy. As such, debates as to whether this or that condition is fairly considered a disorder are commonplace: are children with attention deficit hyperactivity disorder (ADHD) disordered or are they maybe just naughty? Is long-standing and intense grief to be considered pathological, or taken to be a normal response to loss? Should shyness be considered the sort of thing that might be treated with a pill? Through such examples, we can see that distinguishing disorders from other types of condition can become problematic along several different dimensions. Types of problematic case include the following:

- *Disorder versus moral failing*—problem cases include personality disorders, ADHD, alcoholism—in these cases we are unsure whether a condition is a disorder or a moral failing.
- *Disorder versus normal good variation*—problem cases include Deafness, dwarfism, asexuality—in these cases some claim that the condition is a good thing—and thus just a normal variation rather than a disorder.
- *Disorder versus normal unpleasant states*—problem cases include middle-aged male impotence, mild depression—these cases seem problematic because they seem too common to be considered disorders.

These examples illustrate why it is that deciding whether a condition is a disorder can frequently be problematic and the cause of controversy. An extensive philosophical literature now attempts to spell out the criteria according to which we might judge whether a condition is normal or pathological. Here I review common suggestions from this literature.

Are Diseases Biological Dysfunctions?

One of the best developed, and most discussed, accounts of disorder has been proposed by Christopher Boorse (1975, 1976a, 1977, 1997, 2011), who claims that diseases are simply biological dysfunctions. Others, most notably Jerome Wakefield, reject Boorse's claim that biological dysfunction is sufficient for disorder but continue to consider dysfunction to be at least necessary; in Wakefield's (1992a, b) account diseases are to be identified as harmful dysfunctions. Here we consider what it means to say that something is a biological dysfunction, and consider whether biological dysfunction can be considered either sufficient or necessary for disease.

Boorse holds that diseases should be identified with biological dysfunctions. He takes "dysfunction" to be a descriptive, value-free notion, and on his account whether a condition counts as a disease is thus purely a matter of biological fact. Boorse thinks of humans as being made up of numerous subsystems. Subsystems include organs, such the heart or kidneys, and more diffuse systems, such as the nervous system. Potentially, "mental modules" might also be considered as Boorsean subsystems. (Boorse (1975, 1977) restricts his account to physical disorders but for reasons that are unclear, Schramme (2010) discusses in detail whether the account can be extended to mental disorders.) Each subsystem has one or more natural functions. For example, a function of the lungs is to enable oxygen to be taken into the body. When each subsystem functions as it should, the person is healthy; when there is a failure in functioning, he or she has a disease.

The basic idea is clear enough, but to understand the account fully, and the problems it might face, we need to consider what is meant by "function" in greater detail.

Normal Functions

In the literature on functions in the philosophy of biology there are two main accounts (Aristotelian accounts of disease also consider diseases to be dysfunctions but offer a very different account of normal function and will be considered later). Robert Cummins (1975) suggests that we ascribe functions to a part or mechanism on the basis of the causal contribution it makes to the current goals that can be ascribed to some larger complex system. On such an account we might see existing human beings as complex systems that are goal-directed at reproduction and survival. We would then say that the function of the heart is to pump blood as this is what a heart usually does that supports these goals.

The other main account of functions, proposed by Larry Wright (1973), ascribes functions on the basis of history. In the case of biological and psychological functions this means evolutionary history. On such an account, the function of X is Z means:

(a) X has been naturally selected because it does Z
(b) Z is a consequence (or result) of X's being there.

Still, the function of the heart is to pump blood as this is what it does, and the fact that it does this explains why it is there (via natural selection). Very often exactly the same functions will be attributed to a subsystem irrespective of whether a Cummins or Wright account of functions is adopted.

On occasion, though, the accounts come apart. In some cases, a subsystem that evolved for one purpose may now be used for something else—consider whatever mental subsystems turn out to underpin our ability to read. In such cases, a Cummins account can see dysfunction whenever a system that usually currently serves some function fails to do so. Thus, dyslexia can straightforwardly be considered indicative of dysfunction. On a Wright-style approach, seeing something like dyslexia as a dysfunction is more problematic; it would require dyslexia to be linked to a failure of some evolved function.

Although Boorse (1976b) adopts a Cummins-style approach to functions,[1] most of those who have followed him in holding that diseases are dysfunctions go for Wright-style functions (Wakefield, 1992a; Papineau, 1994). As I shall show, either way, an account that claims that diseases are dysfunctions faces challenges. Boorse employs Cummins-style functions in the following way. If we want to know whether some bodily or mental subsystem is fulfilling its function, we need to compare the functioning to that which can be expected given the organism's "reference class." "Reference classes" are made up of organisms of the same basic design—basically the same age and sex. For each reference class, we figure out a range for the statistically normal functioning of the various subsystems—for, say, toddler boys we can conduct measurements and find out the normal range for blood pressure, height, hearing accuracy, and so on. A child with functioning within these normal ranges is healthy; a child where some subsystem falls below the typical range is disordered.

As Elselijn Kingma (2007) argues, a key difficulty with this account emerges if we question why it is that toddler boys are to be taken to form a reference class, whereas, say, toddler boys with Down syndrome are not. If toddler boys with Down syndrome were taken as a legitimate reference class then we might consider the IQ of a particular individual with Down syndrome, find it within the normal range for "toddler boys with Down Syndrome" and announce the child healthy. How can Boorse avoid this? It looks as if Boorse has no adequate answer—it's only by presupposing that Down syndrome (or any other condition) is pathological that one can rule out employing it as the basis of a reference class. Boorse's account thus becomes circular.[2]

This problem emerges because Boorse adopts a Cummins-style account of functions, which necessitates the comparison with a reference class to identify dysfunction. Many of those who agree with Boorse that disorders are dysfunctions have instead opted for a Wright-style approach to determining normal functions. On such an account, normal function is determined by evolutionary history. The big difficulty faced by such accounts is that selective pressures have commonly varied over time (Kitcher, 1993). A decision is thus required: are functions to be determined by original selection pressures, current selection pressures, or selection pressures within some specified period, say the "recent past?"

All options face difficulties. Suppose we take original selection pressures. Then we'll have problems with cases where an organ or behavior evolved for one purpose but now serves another. Maybe some insect wings originally evolved as heat regulating organs and only came to be used for flying much later. If we attribute functions on the basis of original selection pressures we are forced to the counterintuitive claim that an insect wing that regulates heat but is no good for flying is healthy.

If we say that functions should be attributed on the basis of current selection pressures, we also run into difficulties. Think of contemporary humans living in the developed world. It's plausible that whatever selection pressures there are line up only poorly with the conditions we consider diseases. Cavemen with asthma may once have been more likely to get eaten by lions. But for those living in modern environments, with modern healthcare, it seems likely that many diseases produce no selective disadvantage; asthma is controlled with inhalers, poor eye sight corrected with contact lenses, and so it is implausible that those with such conditions die younger or have fewer children.

The idea that normal functions might be attributed on the basis of selection pressures during some specified period, say "recent" selection pressures, is also problematic—what counts as "recent" is either underdefined or arbitrary. We can conclude that finding an account of function that can serve as the basis of disorder-as-dysfunction account thus faces difficulties (see also Amundson, 2000; Gammelgaard, 2000).

Is Dysfunction Sufficient?

Even if some acceptable account of normal functioning can be found, there are problems with claiming that dysfunction is either sufficient or necessary for understanding disorder. Boorse claims biological dysfunction is sufficient. He accepts that on his account disorder may not be a bad thing and may not need treating. To many, this consequence sounds counterintuitive. Many hold that it is conceptually necessary for a disorder to be a bad thing—only harmful states get counted disorders.

This concern came to the fore in debates over homosexuality. As is well known, homosexuality was considered a mental disorder not so long ago. The American Psychiatric Association eventually bowed to protests and deleted homosexuality from its manual in 1973 (for an account, see Bayer, 1981). Why the change? Not because homosexuality was shown to involve no biological dysfunction; the evolutionary origins of homosexuality remain unknown, and it remains conceivable that some biological dysfunction might be involved. Rather, the fundamental reason why homosexuality was declassified was that protesters argued that being homosexual was compatible with living a flourishing life. It was because most thought that only a harmful condition could be a disorder, and that homosexuality is not a bad thing, that homosexuality came to be normalized. For those who agree that disorders are necessarily harmful, biological dysfunction cannot be sufficient for disorder, as not all biological dysfunctions need be harmful.

Is Dysfunction Necessary?
Following the debates about homosexuality, many became attracted to Jerome Wakefield's (1992a, b) account of disease according to which diseases are harmful dysfunction. On Wakefield's account, in so far as homosexuality is not harmful, it does not count as a disorder. We will consider the harm element of Wakefield's account later. For now, we will just consider the acceptability of the idea that biological dysfunction is necessary for disease.

The main challenge for the idea that all diseases involve biological dysfunctions is that in some cases the genetic bases of conditions that we would normally class as disorders may confer an evolutionary advantage and thus be selected (Murphy and Woolfolk, 2000). Conditions might be adaptive in the present environment, or in some past environment, or via kin selection, and so on. Evolutionary psychologists have been struck by the fact that many mental disorders appear to have a genetic basis and yet occur at prevalence rates that are too high to be solely the result of mutations; examples include manic depression, sociopathy, obsessive-compulsivity, anxiety, drug abuse, and some personality disorders. This means that the genetic bases of these mental disorders must be promoted by natural selection, which implies that the genes are adaptive in some way or other. Such possibilities do not only arise with mental disorders; the "thrifty phenotype" account of type 2 diabetes suggests that the condition arises as a side effect of adaptations designed to deal with food shortages (Hales and Barker, 1992). Although it may be possible to develop some account of biological dysfunction that can account for such disorders, any successful attempt will be complex and risks being post-hoc. Evolved disorders pose a major challenge to the idea that biological dysfunction is necessary for disorder.

At the end of this section, we can see that the idea that diseases are biological dysfunctions faces challenges. It's not clear whether a satisfactory account of biological dysfunction can be developed. Nor it is clear whether biological dysfunction can be claimed to be either sufficient or necessary for disease.

Must Diseases Be Bad?

Many have suggested that diseases must be harmful (Clouser et al., 1981; Cooper, 2002, 2005; Foot, 2001; Fulford, 1989; Megone, 1998, 2000; Nordenfelt, 1987, 2000, 2001; Reznek, 1987; Wakefield, 1992a, b). In the philosophy of medicine it has been commonplace for authors to state that diseases must be harmful without going into detail about what counts as harm. Those who hold that diseases are harmful are often lumped together as holding "normativist" accounts. However, this labeling hides much diversity (Simon, 2007). "Normativist" accounts, once fully developed, will be highly divergent, as depending on how one conceives of harm, very different accounts of disease will ultimately be produced. To give some idea of the range of options we will here concentrate on neo-Aristotelian accounts, which think of harm as an objective matter of fact; and on Wakefield's account of harm, which sees it as being defined by social norms.

Aristotelian Accounts

Aristotelian accounts consider diseases to be biological dysfunctions but simultaneously hold that dysfunction is a normative concept. In being dysfunctions, diseases are thus naturally bad states. Aristotelian accounts have been proposed by a number of authors, most notably by Philippa Foot, in *Natural Goodness* (2001), and by Chris Megone (1998, 2000) in several influential papers.[3] Though Foot's work is well known she is concerned mainly with other issues and discusses disorder only briefly, and as such the discussion here focuses on Chris Megone's work.

In Megone's view, healthy human beings have a biology and psychology that increases their chances of leading a flourishing life. What makes a flourishing human life is supposed to be a natural fact about humans. In the same sort of way that is a fact about polar bears that they are naturally the kinds of creature that live well by roaming long distances and eating seals, it is taken to be a fact about human beings that we are creatures that need to have friends, to be engaged in meaningful activities, and to have fun.

Megone (1998) explores the flourishing life from two directions. His first approach treats human beings on a par with other natural kinds (pp. 194–95). Good members of a natural kind are those that undergo a series of characteristic changes that contribute to the cycle of development characteristic of members of the species "as they should be." So good acorns grow into saplings and then into adult oaks that themselves produce acorns. Similarly, good humans are those that develop physically and mentally in the ways that facilitate the continuation of the species. One difficulty for such an approach is that on the Aristotelian account "function" is taken to be a value-laden term—it is supposed to be a good thing for systems to function correctly. Whether the continuation of a species is good in the way required is by no means clear, however (Wakefield, 2000, p. 30). Furthermore, this biological interpretation of "human flourishing" leads to difficulties similar to those that afflict Wakefield's account. As discussed previously, there may be some diseases that contribute to the inclusive fitness of an organism. It is not clear how a reproduction-based Aristotelian account might accommodate such diseases.

At other points, Megone emphasizes the idea that the good human is one that has the attributes required for a "good life," which is taken to be a life that is "fully rational" (note that his Aristotelian notion of "rationality" is very broad, involving the ability to play as well as solve logic problems). Exactly what will contribute toward living a fully rational life will of course be controversial, but clearly more will be needed that mere reproductive success (Megone, 1998, p. 198). Plausibly a good life will include things like: freedom from subjectively unpleasant sensations (pain, panic, etc.); having friends; engaging in meaningful activities; and so on. However although there may be broad consensus about many of the ingredients of the "good life," some aspects will be controversial. Take having friends—most people like having friends, but a few may claim to have no need of social contact. The difficulty for the Aristotelian who seeks to establish the nature of the "good life" in objective facts other the purely biological is to determine exactly what these facts should be.

The Aristotelian vision of the good life risks being either too strongly linked to biology, or too ill-defined. All types of neo-Aristotelian approach, which take diseases to be harmful, and take harm to be an objective matter, face this difficulty.[4]

Harm According to Jerome Wakefield

For a quite different account of harm, consider the work of Jerome Wakefield, who holds that disorders are harmful dysfunctions. Wakefield (1992a, p. 373) tells us that "harmful is a value-term based on social norms." Harm is "a value term referring to the consequences that occur to the person because of the dysfunction and are deemed negative by sociocultural standards" (p. 374). That is, someone is harmed if their society judges their condition harmful.

In contrast to Megone's account, figuring out what counts as harmful on Wakefield's account is relatively unproblematic—one has merely to survey the value-judgments of the person's culture. The chief problem is that there are cases where it is extremely plausible that a cultural group can be mistaken about what is valuable (Cooper, forthcoming). Take the case of "pro-ana" groups, which are groups that promote the idea that anorexia is a good thing. Pro-ana groups are generally web-based. On their sites you can access chat rooms in which people swap diet tips, compare body statistics, and support each other during fasts. There are also galleries of "thinspiration" images, which are photos of very thin people looking beautiful. The members of pro-ana groups celebrate aesthetics of extreme thinness, they admire the control that is required to limit food intake, and they delight in the euphoric experiences that can be produced by fasting. One might argue that pro-ana groups do not form a culture—their members are dispersed and tend to communicate online. But suppose that members of a pro-ana group start a commune, and go and live together, in whatever numbers might be required to count as a proper community. In such a case a whole community would hold that anorexia is not bad but desirable. On Wakefield's account it looks like one is forced to say that as a cultural group values anorexia, there is no harm in being anorexic. But this seems the wrong thing to say. Regardless of the opinions of their peers, anorexia looks to be bad; anorexic people tend to have a constricted range of interests, with lives revolving around food and its avoidance, and risk death. All accounts of harm which rely on the judgments of actual people lead to similar difficulties—actual people—whether individuals or whole societies can plausibly make mistakes in their judgments[5]

General Comments about Harm

The discussion of Megone and Wakefield should help bring out the divergences between different normative accounts. Different types of normativist disagree about what counts as "harm" and so end up with very different accounts of disorder. While Megone and Wakefield have problems in defining "harm," note that so too does everyone else. Figuring out what makes up the "good life" is, of course, one of the most long-standing and contentious of philosophical questions. Although various accounts of the good for an individual have been proposed, all are problematic (for an in depth overview, see Griffin, 1986).

Normativist accounts do not just differ in their accounts of harm. Further diversity among value-laden approaches emerges as most theorists will add extra criteria that a condition must satisfy in order to count as a disease. Value-laden accounts of disease agree that diseases are bad things, but of course there are many bad states that are not diseases (illiteracy, selfishness, homelessness) and so value-laden accounts have to say something about which sorts of bad state they consider to be diseases. While harm may be necessary for disorder, no one considers it sufficient. A normativist account must thus employ other criteria to distinguish those harmful states that are disorders from other types of harmful state. Some of the most popular of these—that the condition must be appropriately medically treatable, or statistically unusual—are considered shortly. Different normativists pick different additional criteria thus giving rise to a diversity of normativist accounts.

Even once an account of harm has been developed, and whatever other criteria might be required for a condition to count as a disorder determined, normativist accounts still face one further difficulty. There are cases where some find it plausible to say that there is a disorder but no harm. Among the most plausible cases are tic disorders (Cooper, 2015). Some people have tics that do not bother them. Still, in so far as such conditions plausibly result from a neurological dysfunction, and have a similar cause to severely disabling tics, many tic researchers would consider even harmless tics to be disorders. Such intuitions threaten the idea that harm is a necessary criterion for disorder.

Must Diseases Be Unusual or Unexpected?

Why do ringworm, panic disorder, and impacted wisdom teeth count as disorders, but wrinkles, menstruation, and teething do not? We have strong intuition that a condition can only be a disorder if it is somehow unusual or unexpected.

We only consider someone to be disordered if they could reasonably have hoped to have been otherwise. Thus, teething is unpleasant but not pathological, because it happens to all babies. Similarly menstruation happens to most women and so is not considered a disorder. However, cashing out this intuition is surprisingly problematic. The difficulties arise because it proves extremely hard to flesh out the idea that diseases are in some sense unusual or unexpected, but also to support the intuition that occasionally everyone can suffer from a disease, for example, in a pandemic, or in the case of near universal conditions such as dental caries.

The idea that a condition must be statistically infrequent in order to be a disease (as held by Taylor, 1976; and Kendell, 1975) is clearly inadequate, as it cannot accommodate the possibility of a pandemic. A variant might seek to say that a disease is statistically infrequent most of the time, or in most environments. But it is doubtful whether this will quite do either. Post-nuclear war it seems that disorder might come to be the norm for most humans for quite some time.

Boorse's approach employs a variant of the claim that disorders must be statistically infrequent and faces the same challenges. In Boorse's account, the idea that diseases must be unusual is built into his notion of dysfunction. For Boorse, a subsystem dysfunctions when it fails to fulfil whatever functioning is statistically normal for similar organisms. Thus, it is only because my blood pressure is high compared to that of other middle-aged women that I count as having a disorder. This approach faces difficulties dealing with pandemics; as it seems plausible that all the organisms in my reference class might suffer a dysfunction at the same time (Kraemer (2013) attempts to get round this problem).

If we give up on the idea that statistics can inform the distinction between what is normal and what is disorder, we might try adopting a modal approach. Modal approaches deal better than statistical approaches with the possibility of pandemic: suppose that I have bird flu in a bird flu pandemic. My condition is not statistically rare—everyone has bird flu. However, I am still justified in considering myself unlucky—I know that it is possible that none of us has bird flu. There are many nearby possible worlds that are full of healthy possible people.

Still, figuring out exactly how a modal approach to defining unluckiness might work requires work. Genetic disorders pose particular problems. Some philosophers would hold that one's genetic make-up is essential to one's identity. If so, in the case of a genetic condition, such as Down syndrome, there are no possible worlds in which that individual exists but does not have Down syndrome. One might argue that even so there are possible worlds that contain people relevantly like the afflicted people but who are healthy. This approach, though, risks falling into all the problems regarding reference classes that caused problems for Boorse's account.

Even once an account has been developed of what it means to say that a condition is unusual or unexpected, the question of how unusual a condition must be to count as a disorder remains. Such issues are discussed by Andrew Stark in *The Limits of Medicine* (2006). Stark adopts a statistical approach, but similar problems would emerge with a modal approach to unluckiness. Stark notes that many biological features are normally distributed (height and IQ, for example). A normal curve supplies no objective grounds on which a certain part of the curve might be cut off and considered abnormal. He concludes that we might equally well consider the extreme 1 percent, or 5 percent, or any other percent, of the population to be abnormal. As a consequence, Stark suggests, all those on any part of a normal curve, with the exception of the very best off, are free to choose whether to consider themselves normal or in need of treatment. Stark's position has some consequences that I consider counterintuitive. Suppose that I am very well off in some respect—I have a near perfect nose. Stark claims that, because there are still some humans who have nicer noses than I, I may consider myself abnormal and seek treatment. Now, while it seems there is reasonably room for debate on the question of whether we should consider the extreme 5 percent or 10 percent or 20 percent of the population to be abnormal, for there to be some leeway in cut-off point surely need not mean that all choices are equally justifiable. To hold that 95 percent of the population might fairly be considered abnormal seems counterintuitive. Yet, if we reject Stark's approach we are left with the problem of determining how we might decide which proportion of the population can fairly be considered disordered. If 95 percent of a population is too many to count as disordered, how many is fair?

Must Diseases Be Medically Treatable?

Disorders must be distinguished from other types of misfortune—economic problems, educational problems and so on, and also from vices. Those who believe that disorders are necessarily biological dysfunctions can use this notion to draw the line, but those who reject the claim that dysfunctions are necessary for disorder need some other means of distinguishing disorders from other type of problems. To this end, some have claimed that the idea that a disorder is a condition that might be appropriately medically treated plays an essential role.

Laurie Reznek (1987) and Rachel Cooper (2002, 2005) both hold that for a condition to be disorder it must be such that it could potentially be appropriately medically treated. A cure need not be presently available, but the condition must be such that there is reasonable hope that a medical treatment might become available in the future. Whether a condition might be appropriately medically treated also depends on social and moral constraints. As Reznek points out, even if violent impulses might technically be prevented by brain surgery, because we think such surgery morally inappropriate we would not think of violence as being a disorder.

If, having said that diseases must be potentially medically treatable, one went on to define "medicine" as the art of treating diseases, such accounts would be circular. However, there are other ways of giving content to "medicine" (although the major challenge for Reznek and Cooper is that many find neither of their suggestions palatable). Reznek suggests that "medical intervention" can be defined via enumeration; a list of medical treatments can be given. Cooper suggests that medicine is practiced by doctors and other medical personnel, and suggests adopting a sociological approach to deciding who counts as "doctors and other medical personnel."

Debates among those who advocate competing accounts of disorder continue, with no end in sight. Recently, a number of authors have suggested that the traditional debate has run out of steam and can only be resolved if the debate is reconceptualized.

Moving on from the Traditional Debate

Compatibility of Descriptive and Normative Approaches

Kingma (2013) argues that seeing naturalist and normativist accounts of disease as being opposed to each other, and construing debates about the concept of disorder as a choice between the two, is a mistake. She employs Ian Hacking's (1999) work on social constructivism to show how social constructivism can be used to provide a way of combining key insights from both the naturalist and normativist analyses of disease. Following Hacking, Kingma characterizes the social constructivist as insisting that the concepts we employ are historically contingent. Both normativism and naturalism about health and disease are consistent with this claim. The normativist can insist that values play a role in explaining why we have the concepts of health and disease that we do. At the same time the naturalist can insist that the categories that we employ reflect a natural structure and can be described in value-free terms. Thus, one might claim, for example, that the class of conditions that our historically produced values have led us to focus on can be defined in terms of biological dysfunction. Kingma concludes that a long-standing debate in the philosophy of medicine is something of a red herring—we should not see naturalism and normativism as being opposed.

Disease as a Wittgensteinian Family Resemblance Term or Roschian Concept

There may be no satisfactory account of disease that can be given in terms of necessary and sufficient conditions. Some hold that "disease" is a family resemblance term. Wittgenstein (1953, §66) pointed out that many concepts, such as "game," cannot be characterized by sets of necessary and sufficient conditions but are instead held together by networks of family resemblances. Those who claim that disorder is a family resemblance term similarly think that whether a condition should count as a disease depends on it being similar enough to accepted central examples. Prototypical diseases cause suffering, and possibly death, are caused by viruses or bacteria, are treated with drugs, are unusual, are treated by medics, and so on. Conditions that share enough of these features will be considered diseases. Suggestions that disorder is a Roschian concept are in a similar vein. The psychologist Eleanor Rosch (1975) argues that we classify particular cases on the basis of their similarity to prototypical examples of a kind. In a well-known article, Scott Lilienfeld and Lori Marino (1995) suggest that "mental disorder" is best understood as a Roschian concept, and although they focus on mental disorders their approach might be generalized to all disorders.

Multiple Accounts of Disorder

Jeremy Simon (2007) suggests that there may not be one unitary concept of disease but rather a family of related concepts. We can think of disease qua the object of medical research, qua states that legitimize treatment, qua states that imply that a sufferer can legitimately enter the "sick role," and so on. Simon thinks that distinct philosophical accounts of disease may be required to account for each of these various, though related, concepts.

Doing without Accounts of Disorder

Germond Hesslow (1993) argues that we do not need to clarify our concept of disease because the concept has no legitimate role to play in medical practice or policy. In Hesslow's view, if we want to know whether some condition can legitimately be treated, whether it can excuse wrongdoing, justify disability payments, or any other question that might be of interest, we should directly consider the relevant ethical, pragmatic, and political issues; asking whether the condition is a disease is a red herring. Along somewhat similar lines, Marc Ereshefsky (2009) suggests that rather than arguing over whether this or that condition is a "disease," we should switch to talk explicitly about what might actually be at issue, which might be the "state description," that is, the description of the condition under consideration, or some normative concern.

287

Mental versus Physical Disorder

There is a long tradition of theorists who take mental health to be problematic in a way that somatic disorder is not. The antipsychiatry movement of the 1970s was perhaps the most visible manifestation of such thinking. The antipsychiatrists were a loose collection of thinkers whose only point of agreement was that they all considered mental disorders to be only dubiously disorders. Thomas Szasz (1972) noted the political and social usefulness of psychiatric diagnoses; labeling as "mad" those who are difficult, disagreeable, or challenging facilitates their silencing and removal from everyday society. Michel Foucault (1971) traced the historical origins of concepts of "mental disorder." In his work, thinking of madness as a form of disorder is a rather recent conceptualization, and is historically contingent in the sense that if history had worked out somewhat differently we might today think of forms of mental distress quite differently, in say religious or moral ways. R. D. Laing (with coauthor A. Esterson) (1964) studied the speech of those diagnosed with schizophrenia and showed that when properly contextualized their words could sometimes be construed as rational. In other work, and drawing on existentialist philosophy and mystical thinking, Laing (1967) suggested that schizophrenia might facilitate access to a "higher form" of rationality. Rosenhan (1973) showed that psychiatrists could be tricked into diagnosing those who merely pretended to hear voices, and claimed that psychiatrists could not distinguish mental disorder from normality. For a time, antipsychiatry seemed to pose a threat to the social legitimacy of psychiatry.

Since the early 1970s, however, the dominant paradigms within psychiatry have become more biologically based. While the mechanisms underlying most mental disorders remain obscure, the idea that some sort of brain dysfunction is involved has become dominant within the mental health professions and has also won wide public acceptance. Still, while "antipsychiatric" thinking is less prominent than it once was, some important thinkers still argue for key claims made by the antipsychiatrists, for example, that at least certain forms of mental distress might be conceptualized in ways other than as disorder, and that "mental illness" can be used as a label by the powerful to discredit a point of view (see, e.g., Bentall (2004) and Bracken and Thomas (2005)).

These days, while many have doubts about the legitimacy of some of the conditions that psychiatrists treat (mild depression, say, or antisocial personality disorder), few would go so far as to hold that "mental illness is a myth" (as the title of Szsaz's 1972 book famously proclaimed). Those who hold that there are some legitimate mental disorders are faced with the challenge of determining whether and how such conditions differ from somatic disorders.

While talk that implies that somatic and mental disorders are importantly distinct is commonplace, finding a criterion for distinguishing mental and physical disorders has proved problematic. Splitting disorders on the basis of whether they have physical or psychological causes will not work, as many disorders are affected by both psychological and physical causal factors. For example, many somatic conditions are made worse by stress. Conversely, one's risk of developing schizophrenia is increased by social stressors, and also by drug abuse, birth complications, and genetic factors. Nor can mental and physical disorders be distinguished on the basis of their having either somatic or psychological symptoms, as again many conditions have both physical and psychological effects; depression makes people miserable, but also often causes sleep disturbances, multiple sclerosis causes physical problems but also often emotional changes.

Furthermore, when one considers lists of those disorders that are traditionally classed as "mental" and disorders that are classed as "physical," one can see that the distinction between the two is often somewhat arbitrary. As Dominic Murphy (2006, p. 70) points out, neurosyphilis is now considered a neurological disorder, while Huntington's chorea is still taken to be psychiatric, although both have known physical causes. Murphy also discusses the case of blindness (pp. 55–56). In so far as vision is a psychological process one might suppose that problems with vision would be considered mental disorders, which, of course, is not the case.

Reznek (1991, p. 174) suggests that mental disorders have to affect *higher* mental processes (thinking and feeling) and thus visual problems are not considered mental disorders. But psychiatrists do treat disorders linked to problems with some "lower" mental processes, for example, disorders related to sleep and sexual function. It looks as though whether a disorder is today considered mental or physical depends in large part on which medical specialty treats it, and this depends on contingent historical factors. No plausible way of cleanly distinguishing mental and physical disorders has been proposed, and there is considerable overlap between mental and physical disorders. This being said, in Cooper (2013) I argue that among those disorders that are considered mental are a disproportionate number that are only dubiously disorders, either because they shade into normality or because it is unclear whether they should be considered disorders or moral failings. I take this to explain, at least partially, why it is that "mental disorders" as a class have come to seem unusually problematic.

Emerging Challenges

The philosophical literature on concepts of health and disease has tended to assume a particular framework. The literature tends to tacitly adopt a third-person perspective—we assume the viewpoint of a clinician or scientist considering what has gone wrong with the mechanism of some organism. Diseases are thought of ahistorically—all people at all times, the philosopher assumes, have been afflicted by much the same sorts of diseases. The paradigmatic case of disease has generally been taken to be a condition that affects otherwise healthy people, that with luck and medical treatment, is then overcome. The adequacy of these traditional philosophical assumptions can be challenged.

Accommodating the Lived-experience of Illness

Thinking of disease from a third-person perspective risks missing out what is most important about disease. Diseases cause us problems; they may produce pain, fatigue, or nausea, or threaten our autonomy, agency, or rationality. Work on the phenomenology of illness considers what it is like to be ill from a first-person perspective.

In *Illness* (2008) Havi Carel writes from her own experiences as a person with a long-term and life-threatening lung condition. She considers how serious and long-term illness changes a person's experiences of the world; space and time contract, possibilities close down, the body can no longer be taken for granted. At the same time, the experience of illness need not be wholly negative. For example, illness can force people to appreciate current experiences and activities, and to relate with greater authenticity to others. Other key work on the phenomenology of illness includes that by Svenaeus (2000a, b) and Toombs (1988).

Work that analyses the experience of illness is clearly important. Thinking about how disorders affect people plays a key role in thinking through how we should respond to illness, at both a personal and societal level. The phenomenology of illness is a rapidly expanding and exciting area. One thing that is currently unclear is the extent of the challenge that phenomenological work poses to traditional third-person approaches to disease—can a first-person perspective simply be added to philosophical work that to date has adopted a third-person perspective? Or is a radical restructuring of thinking about health and disease required?

Understanding Medicalization and Demedicalization

In constructing accounts of disease, philosophers have standardly appealed to "our intuitions" regarding the disease status of this or that condition. However, work by sociologists and historians of medicine makes it clear that the boundaries of disorder have shifted over time. The idea that there are relatively stable concepts of health, disease, or illness is thus thrown into doubt.

"Medicalization" has led to the reconfiguring of various conditions that would previously have been considered "problems in living" as disorders. It occurs in part because people are treated differently depending on whether they are thought of as disordered. As such various groups have an interest in making sure that we apply the term in various ways. For example, in general, a drug treatment can only be sold if the condition that it treats is thought of as a disease. This motivates pharmaceutical companies to launch marketing campaigns to encourage us to think of more and more conditions as diseases. In recent years, for example, such marketing campaigns have been used to make sure that we come to think of "Social Anxiety Disorder" as a disorder rather than simply seeing it as extreme shyness (Lane, 2007). Similarly the manufacturers of Viagra have been keen to stress that male erectile dysfunction is a medical condition, and that Viagra is thus a necessary treatment, as opposed to a life-style drug (Conrad, 2008).

Others also have an interest in how we think of health and disease. For example, patient lobby groups seek to influence public opinion in various ways. In *The Harmony of Illusions* (1997), Allan Young documents how lobbying by organizations of Vietnam Veterans played a key role in post-traumatic stress disorder (PTSD) coming to be recognized as a disorder. This lobbying was in part motivated by the fact that as a combat-related condition, a diagnosis of PTSD would facilitate disability payments and provision for treatment.

At the same time that medicalization has increased the medical domain in some areas, the influence of medicine has decreased in other areas. Homosexuality is the best-known example of a condition that was once thought to be a medical disorder and is now considered normal. The disability rights movement has had also some success in demedicalizing certain forms of disability—the idea that disabled people are not ill and do not need medical care is becoming more widespread.

It is now well established that medicalization and demedicalization happen, and future philosophical work on disease needs to become more sensitive to the fact that intuitions as to whether this or that condition is a disorder or normal shift over time.

The Variety of Medical Conditions

When seeking to define disease, it has been normal for philosophers to take the term "disease," "disorder," or occasionally "malady" to be an umbrella term that includes illnesses, disabilities, injuries, and diseases in the narrow sense. Although plausibly justifiable for certain projects, in lumping all medical conditions together, work in the philosophy of medicine misses much detail. Much more philosophical work is needed that focuses on the differences between the various concepts related to health and disease. Among others, the following distinctions are plausibly significant.

Disabilities

Philosophers of medicine have tended to consider disabilities alongside acute conditions (for exceptions, see Amundson (1992), Kristiansen et al. (2009)). Much work in disability studies criticizes this move. Some argue that disability should not be considered as being primarily a medical problem at all. On the social model of disability, a woman born without legs is not disabled by her body, but by deficiencies in the material and social environment (classic formulations of "the social model" can be found in Finkelstein (1980) and Oliver (1990)). If ramps became more commonplace, as a wheelchair-user, she would no longer be disabled, but as mobile as anyone else.

The social model of disability raises many interesting philosophical questions. What does it mean to say that disability is "caused by" environmental deficiencies? Is this a descriptive or a political claim? (I begin to address these questions in Cooper (2007).) If a social model of disability is adopted, what are the implications for thinking about chronic illness or old age? Some claim that disability and chronic illness are quite distinct states (Amundson, 1992); others contest this (Wendell, 1996). On one view, acute illnesses (which are clearly appropriately medically treatable), shade into chronic conditions, which shade into disabilities (which the social model considers nonmedical problems). Where then should the line between disease and disability be drawn?

Diseases versus Risk Factors

More and more medical treatment aims at managing "risk factors." Those with elevated blood pressure or cholesterol are monitored and may take pills. How should we think of such risk states? Those who are at elevated risk of developing disease seem to fall into a grey zone between disease and health—they are not quite healthy, but they are not yet ill either (and if the preventive therapy works, or they are lucky, they may never become ill). Risk states are hard to conceptualize, and challenge the assumption made in much philosophical work that disease and health are mutually exclusive concepts. For further discussion on how risk factors might be conceptualized, see Pelters (2013).

Old Age

It is unclear whether old age should be considered pathological. The difficulty is that we want to acknowledge that increasing frailty among the elderly is to be expected, and so normal, and yet we also want to allow that certain conditions, such as mild dementia, might be both extremely frequent and yet still pathological. Getting an account that can respect both these intuitions is extremely problematic; for further discussion, see Caplan (1981) and Schramme (2013).

Problems Faced by Artificial Organisms

Current literature on the concepts of health and disease generally supposes that healthy organisms are "natural," in the sense that organisms are assumed to be purely biological and to have an evolutionary history. However, not all organisms can reasonably be judged by considering how well they fit some "natural" design (Holm, 2014). Genetically engineered or technologically enhanced organisms may be designed to be "unnatural." It is unclear what sort of account might be given for the problems faced by such organisms. What should we make of health problems that might be faced by a genetically engineered organism? As a related issue, how should we think of the failures of artificial body parts? Are faults in pace-makers and artificial hips medical or engineering problems?

Notes

1. Boorse (2002) presents his account of function and Cummins's account as distinct and opposed accounts. I consider his account Cummins-like in so far as it accounts for functions in terms of current typical causal relationships, as opposed to history.
2. Boorse's response to this and other objections can be found in Boorse (2002).
3. For a related approach, see Sade (1995).
4. For further criticisms of the Aristotelian approach, see Cooper (2007).
5. In a 2013 commentary, Wakefield shows sensitivity to this sort of case, and starts to move away from the view that initial social judgments alone determine harm. Examples like the foot binding case now prompts Wakefield to concede that "To this extent, my (Wakefield, 1992) claim that harm is judged by social values was overly simplistic."

References

Amundson, R. (1992). Disability, handicap, and the environment. *Journal of Social Philosophy* 23: 105–19.

Amundson, R. (2000). Against normal function. *Studies in History and Philosophy of Science Part C: Studies in History and Philosophy of Biological and Biomedical Sciences* 31: 33–53.

Bayer, R. (1981). *Homosexuality and American Psychiatry: The Politics of Diagnosis.* Princeton: Princeton University Press.

Bentall, R. P. (2004). *Madness Explained: Psychosis and Human Nature.* London: Penguin

Boorse, C. (1975). On the distinction between disease and illness. *Philosophy and Public Affairs* 5: 49–68.

Boorse, C. (1976a). What a theory of mental health should be. *Journal of Social Behaviour* 6: 61–84.

Boorse, C. (1976b). Wright on functions. *Philosophical Review* 85: 70–93.

Boorse, C. (1977). Health as a theoretical concept. *Philosophy of Science* 44: 542–73.

Boorse, C. (1997). A rebuttal on health. In *What Is Disease?*, eds. J. Hunter and R. Almeder. Totowa, NJ: Humana Press, pp. 1–134.

Boorse, C. (2002). A rebuttal on functions. In *Functions: New Essays in the Philosophy of Psychology and Biology*, eds. Andre Ariew, Robert C. Cummins, and Mark Perlman. Oxford: Oxford University Press, pp. 63–112.

Boorse, C. (2011). Concepts of health and disease. In *Philosophy of Medicine*, ed. F. Gifford. Oxford: Elsevier, pp. 13–64.

Bracken, P., and Thomas, P. (2005). *Postpsychiatry: Mental Health in a Postmodern World*. Oxford: Oxford University Press.

Caplan, A. (1981). The "unnaturalness" of aging—a sickness unto death? In *Concepts of Health and Disease*, eds. Arthur L. Caplan, H. Tristram Engelhardt, Jr., and James J. McCartney. Reading, MA: Addison-Wesley Publishing Company, pp. 725–37.

Carel, H. (2008). *Illness: The Cry of the Flesh*. Stocksfield: Acumen.

Clouser, K. D., Culver, C. M., and Gert, B. (1981). Malady: A new treatment of disease. *Hastings Center Report*, 11: 29–37.

Conrad, P. (2008). *The Medicalization of Society: On the Transformation of Human Conditions into Treatable Disorders*. Baltimore, MD: John Hopkins University Press.

Cooper, R. (2002). Disease. *Studies in History and Philosophy of Science Part C: Studies in History and Philosophy of Biological and Biomedical Sciences* 33: 263–82.

Cooper, R. (2005). *Classifying Madness: A Philosophical Examination of the Diagnostic and Statistical Manual of Mental Disorders*. Dordrecht: Springer.

Cooper, R. (2007). Can it be a good thing to be deaf? *Journal of Medicine and Philosophy* 32: 563–83.

Cooper, R. (2013). What's special about mental health and disorder? In *Arguing about Human Nature*, eds. E. Machery and S. Downes. New York: Routledge, pp. 487–500.

Cooper, R. (2015). Harm in the DSM: Must disorders cause "distress or impairment"? In *The D.S.M.-5 in Perspective*, eds. P. Singy and S. Demazeux. Dordrecht: Springer.

Cooper, R. (forthcoming). On harm. In *Defining Mental Disorders: Jerome Wakefield and His Critics*, eds. I. Faucher and D. Forest. Massachusetts: MIT Press.

Cummins, R. (1975). Functional analysis. *Journal of Philosophy* 72: 741–65.

Ereshefsky, M. (2009). Defining "health" and "disease." *Studies in History and Philosophy of Science Part C: Studies in History and Philosophy of Biological and Biomedical Sciences* 40: 221–27.

Finkelstein, V. (1980). *Attitudes and Disabled People*. New York: World Rehabilitation Fund, Inc.

Foot, P. (2001). *Natural Goodness*. Oxford: Oxford University Press.

Foucault, M. (1971). *Madness and Civilisation*. London: Tavistock. (First published in French as *Histoire de la Folie* in 1961. First published in English 1967.)

Fulford, K. W. M. (1989). *Moral Theory and Medical Practice*. Cambridge: Cambridge University Press.

Gammelgaard, A. (2000). Evolutionary biology and the concept of disease. *Medicine, Health Care and Philosophy* 3: 109–16.

Griffin, J. (1986). *Well-Being*. Oxford: Clarendon Press.

Hacking, I. (1999). *The Social Construction of What?* Cambridge, MA: Harvard University Press.

Hales, C. N. and Barker, D. J. (1992). Type 2 (non-insulin-dependent) diabetes mellitus: The thrifty phenotype hypothesis. *Diabetologia* 35: 595–601.

Hesslow, G. (1993). Do we need a concept of disease? *Theoretical Medicine* 14: 1–14.

Holm, S. H. (2014). Disease, dysfunction, and synthetic biology. *Journal of Medicine and Philosophy* 39: 329–45.

Kendell, R. (1975). The concept of disease and its implications for psychiatry. *British Journal of Psychiatry* 127: 305–15.

Kingma, E. (2007). What is it to be healthy? *Analysis*, 67: 128–33.

Kingma, E. (2013). Health and disease: Social constructivism as a combination of naturalism and normativism. In *Health, Illness and Disease: Philosophical Essays*, eds. H. Carel and R. Cooper. Durham, NC: Acumen, pp. 37–56.

Kitcher, P. (1993). Function and design. *Midwest Studies in Philosophy* 18: 379–97.

Kraemer, D. M. (2013). Statistical theories of functions and the problem of epidemic disease. *Biology & Philosophy* 28: 423–38.

Kristiansen, K., Vehmas, S., and Shakespeare, T. (eds.). (2008). *Arguing about Disability: Philosophical Perspectives*. Abingdon: Routledge.

Laing, R. D. (1967). *The Politics of Experience and the Bird of Paradise*. Harmondsworth: Penguin.

Laing, R. D., and Esterson, A. (1964). *Sanity, Madness and the Family, Volume 1: Families of Schizophrenics*. Tavistock.

Lane, C. (2008). *Shyness: How Normal Behavior became a Sickness*. New Haven: Yale University Press.

Lilienfeld, S. O., and Marino, L. (1995). Mental disorder as a Roschian concept: A critique of Wakefield's "harmful dysfunction" analysis. *Journal of Abnormal Psychology*. 104: 411–20.

Megone, C. (1998). Aristotle's function argument and the concept of mental illness. *Philosophy, Psychiatry and Psychology* 5: 187–201.

Megone, C. (2000). Mental illness, human function and values. *Philosophy, Psychiatry and Psychology* 7: 45–65.

Murphy, D. (2006). *Psychiatry in the Scientific Image*. Cambridge, MA: MIT Press.

Murphy, D., and Woolfolk, R. L. (2000). The harmful dysfunction analysis of mental disorder. *Philosophy, Psychiatry, & Psychology* 7: 241–52.

Nordenfelt, L. (1987). *On the Nature of Health*. Dordrecht: D. Reidel.

Nordenfelt, L. (2000). *Action, Ability, and Health*. Dordrecht: Springer.

Nordenfelt, L. (2001). *Health, Science and Ordinary Language*. Amsterdam and New York: Rodopi.

Oliver, M. (1990). *The Politics of Disablement*. Houndmills, Basingstoke: Macmillan.

Papineau, D. (1994). Mental disorder, illness and biological dysfunction. *Royal Institute of Philosophy Supplement* 37: 73–82.

Pelters, B. (2013). Doing health. In *Health, Illness and Disease: Philosophical Essays*, eds. R. Cooper and H. Carel. Durham: Acumen, pp. 197–210.

Reznek, L. (1987). *The Nature of Disease*. London: Routledge and Kegan Paul.

Reznek, L. (1991). *The Philosophical Defence of Psychiatry*. London: Routledge.

Rosch, E. (1975). Principles of categorization. In *Cognition and Categorization*, eds. E. Rosch and B. Lloyd. Hillsdale, NJ: Lawrence Erlbaum, pp. 27–48.

Rosenhan, D. L. (1973). On being sane in insane places. *Science* 179: 250–58.

Sade, R. M. (1995). A theory of health and disease: The objectivist–subjectivist dichotomy. *Journal of Medicine and Philosophy* 20: 513–25.

Schramme, T. (2010). Can we define mental disorder by using the criterion of mental dysfunction? *Theoretical Medicine and Bioethics* 31: 35–47.

Schramme, T. (2013). "I hope that I get old before I die": ageing and the concept of disease. *Theoretical Medicine and Bioethics* 34: 171–87.

Simon, J. (2007). Beyond naturalism and normativism: Reconceiving the "disease" debate. *Philosophical Papers* 36: 343–70.

Stark, A. (2006). *The Limits of Medicine*. Cambridge: Cambridge University Press.

Svenaeus, F. (2000a). Das Unheimliche — Towards a phenomenology of illness. *Medicine, Health Care and Philosophy* 3: 3–16.

Svenaeus, F. (2000b). The body uncanny — Further steps towards a phenomenology of illness. *Medicine, Health Care and Philosophy* 3: 125–37.

Szasz, T. (1972). *The Myth of Mental Illness*. London: Paladin

Taylor, F. K. (1976). The medical model of the disease concept. *British Journal of Psychiatry* 128: 588–94.

Toombs, S. K. (1988). Illness and the paradigm of lived body. *Theoretical Medicine* 9: 201–26.

Wakefield, J. (1992a). The concept of mental disorder—On the boundary between biological facts and social value. *American Psychologist* 47: 373–88.

Wakefield, J. (1992b). Disorder as harmful dysfunction: A conceptual critique of D.S.M-III-R's definition of mental disorder. *Psychological Review* 99: 232–47.

Wakefield, J. C. (2000). Aristotle as sociobiologist: The "function of a human being" argument, black box essentialism, and the concept of mental disorder. *Philosophy, Psychiatry, & Psychology* 7: 17–44.

Wakefield, J. (2013). Addiction, the concept of disorder, and pathways to harm: Comment on Levy. *Frontiers in Psychiatry* 4 (published online May 14, 2013): 34. doi: 10.3389/fpsyt.2013.00034.

Wendell, S. (1996). *The Rejected Body: Feminist Philosophical Reflections on Disability*. New York: Routledge.

Wittgenstein, L. (1953). *Philosophical Investigations*. Oxford: Blackwell.

Wright, L. (1973). Functions. *Philosophical Review* 82: 139–68.

Young, A. (1997). *The Harmony of Illusions: Inventing Post-traumatic Stress Disorder*. Princeton, NJ: Princeton University Press.

12 Causation in Medicine

Brendan Clarke and
Federica Russo

Understanding Medicine

Our aim in this chapter is to discuss causation in medicine. One key claim for us here is that there are different ways of understanding causes, and these different ways of understanding causes are more or less useful depending on the medical context. One difficulty at the outset is to try and describe the range of contexts that we are interested in. We locate our interest in medicine within the philosophy of science in practice tradition. This means that our foremost aim is to engage with the details of scientific practice. However, what kind(s) of scientific practice does this chapter therefore choose to engage with? We can think of no generally recognized piece of terminology that picks out our field(s) of interest. Rather than invent a new word, for the purposes of this chapter, we will instead define "medicine" in the broadest possible terms to include all clinical, scientific, and political forms of engagement with health and disease. We recognize, however, that our *medicine* is a disunion, with the consequence that our definition might well include forms of practice that not all would recognize as *medicine* in some more restrictive way. Specifically, here, we are thinking of fields such as:

- Clinical practice, including primary care and hospital medicine;
- Preventive medicine and public health (more policy-oriented);
- Epidemiology.

Just as these fields are many, so are their theories. Again, while our broad definition might include a few marginal accounts of how health and disease should be understood, we aim to capture the several more major theories found in contemporary medicine. In this chapter, we intend to involve and encompass several of these, including, for instance:

- Evidence-based practice and associated practice like guideline development and evidence reviews;
- Narrative medicine;

- Personalized medicine;
- Gender medicine;
- Alternative, or complementary medicine.

It is worth being inclusive here because, although some of the accounts mentioned earlier may be perceived as too heterodox to be included in "medicine," in their attempt to understanding causes and effects of health and disease, they may eventually feed more mainstream medical approaches.

For instance, according to well-accredited evidence-based medicine (EBM) approaches to evidence, narrative medicine fares rather poorly. However, we want to leave the door open in case we develop methods for evaluating evidence of mechanisms that makes patients' or doctors' narratives useful. Likewise, we want to leave the door open for alternative or complementary medicine, in case they manage to provide sound (scientific) evidence for the efficacy of treatments that are currently nonstandard. It is worth emphasizing that this does not allow an "anything goes" kind of argument. We agree that for some of the aforementioned accounts we currently lack explanations of health and disease that are also compatible with our best scientific theories. However, as history of science (and of medicine) teaches us, knowledge is not a simple, progressive accumulations of facts. We had to go through wrong theories and concepts to make progress in our understanding of the natural and social world, and of the functioning of the body. Conversely, many of the concepts and theories that today are considered well established were not received positively by the scientific communities of the time. Examples abound. So while we do want to be cautious about what counts as a *scientific* approach to studying causes and effects of health and disease, we do *not* want to adopt a narrow-minded attitude that a priori excludes an approach, just because *today* it does not fit with our best science. In this sense, history of science (and of medicine, for the matter) is an integral part of the philosophy of science—as well as of the scientific practices we engage with (Chang, 1999).

In sum, in this chapter we would like to include any scientific approach that engages with health, disease, and well-being of individuals and populations. These two groups—one of kinds of practice, the other of theories of practice— are each large and disparate. However, for our purposes, they have one goal in common: in whole, or in part, they involve reasoning about the *causes and effects* of health and disease. Here, we are trying not to presuppose that a particular way of understanding how this reasoning about cause and effect should be privileged. Commonly used umbrella terms, such as "biomedicine," emphasize one part of medicine in a way that is unhelpful to us. Biomedicine, as the name might suggest, emphasizes the biological aspects of medicine, while "medical practice" emphasizes the clinical aspects of medicine at the expense of policy or of fundamental research. We think that very different ways of reasoning about cause and effect are found in the many practices that each of these umbrella terms picks out.

For example, the rise of evidence-based approaches over the past 20 years has prioritized causal strategies capable of demonstrating the efficacy of a treatment (cause) with respect to an outcome measure (effect). If we treated evidence-based practice as if it were all of medicine (in our broad sense), our approach would be dominated by approaches that emphasize efficacy over other goals of causal analysis, such as the search for causes of effects. But this, as Miriam Solomon (2011) has argued, would be to mistake a mode of reasoning that is common with one that is universal. This worry is our motivation for our inclusive approach, and possibly explanatory of our earlier terminological quibbling.

On our part, this claim about the universality of causation remains controversial, in that causal language or concepts may not be explicit in many areas of medical practice. The best example that we know of is the move toward describing the *risk factors* of a disease, rather than their causes. This is a change that began in academic epidemiology during the 1970s, but has become very widely adopted in this medicine that we describe here. While some medical doctors and epidemiologists have been explicit in defending and discussing a causalist approach in medicine (see, e.g., Vineis, 2003; Vandenbroucke, 2009), there also have been much more skeptical attitudes. Russo and Williamson (2007) review some of these skeptical approaches and instead argue in favor of including causal notions explicitly in medical theory and practice.

Our aim in what follows is to try and understand causation in medicine by looking at some of its manifestations in practice. These, which we have dubbed "episodes of medical causation," aim to show what causation looks like all over the (deliberately) broad field of medicine as we understand it. We will then try to come to some more general understanding of causation. However, as we have already written, it would be misleading to claim that this process of moving from accounts of causes in medicine to an account of causation in medicine more generally will be simple. Medical practices differ from each other, and the causal problems of one field may be very unlike those found elsewhere. Anything like a simple accumulation of lessons learned about causes won't do here. Instead, we introduce a central metaphor—that of the *causal mosaic*—in order to try and assist us draw some general lessons from these particular cases. Our intention here is to use this central metaphor as a way of understanding the ways that causal thinking might work in different contexts.

Philosophical Theorizing about Medical Causation

As just mentioned, this chapter makes use of "episodes of medical causation" to come up, at the end of the chapter, with a general approach to causation in medicine, one that hinges upon the metaphor of building a mosaic. An important source of inspiration in this is the work of Jonsen and Toulmin (1988). In this book, they describe an ambitious project to resuscitate one of the dirtiest words in moral philosophy: "casuistry." This practice of basing moral decisions largely on the details and contingencies of individual cases has been viciously attacked as a philosophical stance that is itself "an invitation to excuse the inexcusable" (p. 11).

In their 1988 book, Jonsen and Toulmin instead argue that thinking about cases is a necessary component of effective moral reasoning. Inflexible rules cannot account for all moral decisions; some flexibility is needed; the bounds of this flexibility are formed by the details of the case in question. This is the role for casuistry outlined here: as shock-absorber between inflexible moral rules and flexible nature:

> [A]nyone who has occasion to consider moral issues in actual detail knows that morally significant differences between cases can be as vital as their likenesses. We need to respect not only the general principles that require us to treat similar cases alike but also those crucial distinctions that justify treating dissimilar cases differently. (p. 14)

Here, Jonsen and Toulmin are interested in the way that the details of individual cases interact with general moral principles. We aim to achieve a similar project for causation by thinking carefully about the roles, methods, and practices of causal reasoning in medicine. We select these from different contexts — research and clinical, preventive and curative, commonplace and oddball. They also come from different geographical locations and different times (although, admittedly, with a modest bias toward the contemporary) and have different implications for involved actors. What unites them, though, is that each of these episodes are defined by a central problem: reasoning about causes and effects of health and disease, of one kind or another.

Each of these episodes points to important and controversial issues that emerge in medical practice (but not exclusively there) and that are debated in the philosophy of causality.

We use different episodes, rather than one single "toy" example, because causal questions, while often formulated as "Does *C* cause *E*?" do not, in fact, reduce to this one. There are instead a plethora of issues involved, all causal, one way or another. Illari and Russo (2014) distinguish five scientific challenges that causal theory is confronted with: inference, explanation, prediction, control, and reasoning. Episodes of medical causation are also confronted with different challenges, but not all at *one* time. Explaining disease is not the same as formulating prognosis; reasoning about causes and effects of health and disease can take different forms, depending whether at stake is individual diagnoses, epidemiological studies, or other.

This is also reflected in the various methods used in medicine. In the previous section, we highlighted that medicine constitutes an umbrella term including areas as diverse as clinical medicine, epidemiology, EBM, and so on. It is therefore not surprising that, in the selection of the episodes discussed later, we have been inclusive also with respect to their methods. Some of them employ statistical methods, whether observational or experimental (e.g., randomized controlled trials (RCTs)), others rely on experiments done in labs, some others employ case reports, and so on. Each method has its own virtues and vices, but we will not enter this debate here. The form of causal pluralism that we defend toward the end of the chapter goes hand in hand with a form of *methodological* pluralism, that we also embrace, and for which arguments have been offered elsewhere (for a discussion, see, e.g., Illari and Russo, 2014; Russo, 2009, 2014). In a nutshell, such form of methodological pluralism holds that there is not a fixed and immutable ranking of methods from best to worst. Differently put, there is not a gold standard that any other method is supposed to reach, as any method has to be assessed taking into account the specific scientific challenge it is designed to address.

Thus, for instance, RCTs are not intrinsically better than observational studies. A well-conducted observational study is better than a poorly planned RCT, even if, arguably, observational studies cannot grant us direct epistemic access to causal relations, which is instead possible to have with (carefully planned) experimental methods. This, however, seems to presuppose that scientists are free to choose whatever method they want, but that is not always the case. It is universally recognized today that forcing people to smoke, or to expose them to excessive amount of tar, is not just unfeasible, but deeply unethical. Thus, if we cannot make experiments in such cases, an RCT in this case is simply *not* an option. Instead, in this case, *observational* studies are the only option and a sensible question concerns what type of observational study would deliver better results. A corollary of this position is that it makes little if no sense at all to downgrade an observational study, just because it did not implement the methodology of RCTs, administering a treatment to a test group and not to a control group.

The argument can be pushed even further as to include qualitative studies. The information provided by a case report on *one* patient (or a very small group of patients) is clearly not the same as the information gathered in a large scale cohort study. Yet, this is no *principled* reason to rank it lower; it is instead an empirical matter that rests on the specification of the questions and problems behind the chosen methods. For instance, if the goal is to reconstruct the reasoning that solved a diagnostic problem in a difficult case, a well and carefully written case report may be useful. But if we are trying to establish the population-level impact of a public health intervention, case reports most probably will be of a lesser help.

Thus, using different episodes serves the purpose of illustrating different scientific challenges and, consequently, different philosophical accounts, concepts, or notions to address them. Different episodes do so in a way that any toy example is unable to do: capturing the complexities and subtleties of concepts, forms of reasoning, and of methods in medicine. One virtue of toy example is that they can "distill" the essential properties of a complex problem, and so they enhance philosophical theorizing and debate to the extent that they are used for a specific purpose.

But what we aim to do in this chapter is not *just* assessing the pros and cons of *one* philosophical account with respect to the episodes. Instead, we aim at building a sophisticated philosophical view about medical causation, one that will allow us to analyze specific philosophical or methodological problems, when we encounter them in different episodes. This sophisticated view is presented later in the chapter, when the metaphor of the "causal mosaic" is discussed. Briefly put, the general approach to causation in medicine that we advocate is a *pluralistic* one. The rich range of accounts available in the philosophical literature cannot address all scientific challenges simultaneously—in medicine nor in any other scientific context. Hence, as we argue, a qualified version of causal pluralism is in order. The discussion of each episode of medical causation contains a brief discussion of some key philosophical issues that arise therein. Most of these issues have been discussed, in the philosophy of causality, as candidates for *The-One* theory or account of causality (Reiss (2015, p. 20) refers to these as *straightjacket* theories). While the coming sections provide a descriptive overview of the diversity of causal concepts and accounts involved in medicine, toward the end of the chapter we provide more theoretical arguments in favor of a pluralistic approach for causation in medicine.

Episodes in Medical Causation

Hypertension Treatments: Efficacy and Effectiveness, and the Reference Class Problem

In this episode, we discuss a pair of closely related problems that arise when using current EBM methods in clinical practice. EBM makes a nonempirical claim about applied epistemology in medicine. In essence, this claim is that the best way to aid decision-making about the care of an individual patient is by reference to "current best evidence," which almost always takes the form of a clinical study of some kind. The canonical presentation of this method concerns a clinical question about a patient with epilepsy (Guyatt et al., 1992). The question is as follows: after an isolated, idiopathic seizure, what is the chance of recurrence? This question is answered by referring to a methodologically valid clinical study that studied a group of similar subjects, and reported the overall probability of recurrence at one year, which was found to be between 43 percent and 51 percent. This group probability is then transferred to the individual, meaning that their chance of suffering a subsequent seizure during the first year is also somewhere in the range of 43–51 percent. The intuition is that a methodologically valid clinical study that deals with the disease process or intervention that we are interested in straightforwardly provides evidence that can guide the care of an individual.

In the following section, we discuss two reasons to be somewhat suspicious of this straightforward transition from knowledge of groups to decision-making about an individual that are to be found in the case study of treatment for hypertension. While this is a paradigmatic example of EBM methodology in action in some respects, notably the emphasis given to using large randomized-control clinical studies to gather evidence, we think that it also demonstrates many of the difficulties that might affect inferences from groups to individuals using that evidence.

Efficacy versus Effectiveness

As we suggested earlier, the relationship between individual interventions (such as drug prescription) and knowledge about population outcomes for a drug may be complex. We think that this complexity may arise in part from biological variability in response to medical interventions. We won't defend this claim in a general way, but instead we set out a more specific argument that is (we think) part of this general thesis about variability. We claim that treatment populations, and the individuals in those populations, tend to be unlike trial populations.

It is worth beginning this argument by noting a terminological distinction that suggests that this difference is already well known to clinical trial researchers. Different words are used to refer to the effects of an intervention in a trial, versus the effects of an intervention in the real world. "Efficacy" describes effects in a trial, while "effectiveness" describes effects in populations (Gartlehner et al., 2006). To adopt this medical terminology, we think that part of the difference between efficacy and effectiveness lies in differences between trial and treatment populations.

According to the 2010 Health Survey for England, over 30 percent of adults have high blood pressure (see http://www.hscic.gov.uk/pubs/hse10trends). As roughly half of these adults receive some medical treatment, the resulting number of prescriptions for antihypertensive drugs is very large indeed. Moreover, prescription decisions for high blood pressure are complex. Many different drugs, belonging to different pharmacological families, are available and a very large number of clinical trials, and reviews of those trials, have been performed on these agents. While it is not easy to characterize the 13,603 clinical trials for antihypertensive drugs on human subjects, systematic reviews, and meta-analyses from the past 10 years currently listed by PubMed (August 2015), one source of difference between many of these trials, and many of the clinical decisions that they are intended to guide, concerns comorbidities. As Fortin et al. (2006) argue, most patients in practice have multiple comorbidities, but most subjects in clinical trials do not. In more detail, 54.5 percent of patients in their sample of 424 individuals encountered in practice had hyperlipidemia, and a very large minority had existing heart disease (40.1 percent). While the trials studied by Fortin et al. do not straightforwardly report the number of trial subjects with comorbidities, we note that most trial subjects do not appear to have similar comorbidities (p. 106). This is important, because the presence or absence of other diseases is likely to change the effectiveness of an intervention. For example, hypertension in those with hyperlipidemia carries a much greater risk of adverse cardiovascular outcomes than without. Given that the aim of prescribing antihypertensive treatments is not to reduce blood pressure per se, but to reduce the incidence of these adverse cardiovascular events, it is at least an open question whether treatment with antihypertensives in patients with existing comorbidities has a comparable effect on cardiovascular outcomes to those reported by clinical trials. To illustrate, responses to a particular treatment may be very different in individuals with isolated hypertension compared with individuals with hypertension secondary to renal disease, largely because the mechanisms by which these two kinds of hypertension come about are different.

We should also mention the similar philosophical conversation about external validity—the idea that "the 'same treatment' has the 'same result' in a specific target as it did in the study" (Cartwright and Hardie, 2012, p. 46). While the terminology is different, the underlying issue is the same. Trials are often short on external validity, and we think this occurs because trial populations tend to be unlike treatment populations.

The Reference Class Problem

The reference class problem has a lengthy pedigree in philosophy of science, as it traces back to classical and influential works such as Reichenbach (1949). Simply put, the problem describes a difficulty that affects drawing inferences about individuals from knowledge of groups. Imagine a statistical inference of this kind—say, calculating the probability of my house burning down in the next year. As my house is in Europe, we might look up the overall probability of house fires in Europe, and use this group probability as an estimate of the individual probability of my house burning down. In this case, we have assigned our house to the reference class of houses in Europe. However, this reference class is not the only one to which we might assign my house. We could also have assigned it to the reference class of houses in the United Kingdom, or houses in England, or houses in London, or houses in South London. The difficulty is that each of these reference classes may have a different incidence of house fires. As we can assert that they are all appropriate reference classes, because my house is a member of each, this means that we will end up with different estimates of the individual probability of my house burning down depending on the way that we assign reference class membership.[1]

Given this, how should we select the most appropriate reference class? The bad news is that there appears to be no simple answer to this question—there is no objectively correct reference class to which my house should be assigned. Most attempts to find a solution to the reference class have provided ways of picking out extremely narrow reference classes on the grounds that sufficiently narrow reference classes should contain only identical members. We might term reference classes like this "fully homogeneous." So Wesley Salmon (1989, p. 171), for example, argued that it must be possible to find some reference classes of this kind in nature:

> I maintain, for example, that the class of carbon-14 atoms is objectively homogeneous with respect to the attribute of spontaneous radioactive decay within 5730 years. If our concept does not fit cases of that sort, our explication must be at fault.

Not finding homogeneous reference classes must be, for Salmon, a philosopher's failure, rather than any necessary consequence of ontology. Yet it is very hard to see how such fully homogeneous reference classes might be sought in medicine—even monozygotic twins have different environmental exposures, and so on. The hidden assumption here concerns the pervasiveness of natural kinds as objects of scientific inquiry, and it is one that we are suspicious of (largely because of Dupré, 1993).

Salmon also suggested that, in the absence of fully homogeneous reference classes, we should prefer the most narrow reference class for which reliable statistics are available. Salmon calls this practice the epistemic version of the "reference class rule" (Salmon et al., 1971, p. 43). While this avoids the ontological pitfalls of homogeneous reference classes, it leaves the selection of a particular reference class as a matter of subjective choice. Given the convincing arguments supplied by Hájek (2007), we think that questions regarding the selection of reference classes are most suitably addressed in this epistemic manner. Hájek argues that the reference class problem arises from a fundamental mistake at the roots of contemporary probability theory. While an exhaustive discussion of this argument is beyond the scope of this chapter, Hájek argues that Kolmogorov's definition of conditional probability as "a ratio of unconditional probabilities" (p. 580) is the source of the reference class problem. He argues that the relationship between conditional and unconditional probabilities is the wrong way round. Instead of understanding conditional probabilities as derivative of unconditional ones, we should instead take conditional probabilities as primitive. This would free us from the misleading idea that we can ever generate a fully objective, unconditional, probability for a single event—something that Hájek suggests is at the root of the reference class problem. To illustrate using the example earlier, rather than trying to produce an unconditional probability estimate of the form p(my house burning down next year), we should instead look for an individual conditional probability estimate, such as p(my house burning down | house in the United Kingdom). This explicit statement of what we are conditioning our probability over would then avoid the reference class problem.

However, we still have to select a reference class to which we can assign our event of interest. While, unfortunately, we cannot supply a simple answer as to which that should be, we can outline some of the principles that might be used to guide reference class selection. One example might be to think about the breadth of our reference class. Both broad and narrow reference classes have characteristic advantages and disadvantages, and we can describe these in a general way.

Broad reference classes (like that of houses in the United Kingdom in the example) tend to contain lots of members, and we are more likely to be able to find statistical data that characterizes them well. On the other hand, it might be that our individual is a highly atypical member of this broad class—I might collect fireworks in my house, or something—meaning that the probability of our individual event might reasonably be expected to be very different from that of the broad group. Narrow reference classes (like that of houses in my street) tend to contain fewer members, meaning that our statistical characterization might be less precise. However, these weaker statistics might fit our individual much more closely because an individual is more likely to conform to the typical properties of a narrow reference class as compared to a broad one.

We can find evidence of such a trade-off between different kinds of reference class when we look at contemporary drug policy. The current UK NICE guidance on the treatment of high blood pressure picks out some specific reference classes, and members of these reference classes receive different drugs from nonmembers. Specifically, different prescription practices are advised for hypertension sufferers of different ages, from different ethnic backgrounds, and suffering different comorbidities. The usual first-line treatment for high blood pressure in people under 55 would be an ACE inhibitor (ACEI) or angiotensin receptor blocker (ARB):

1.6.6 Offer people aged under 55 years step 1 antihypertensive treatment with an angiotensin-converting enzyme (ACE) inhibitor or a low-cost angiotensin-II receptor blocker (ARB). (NICE, 2011, p. 17)

However, prescription practices should vary because of age, ethnicity, and other factors:

> 1.6.8 Offer step 1 antihypertensive treatment with a calcium-channel blocker (CCB) to people aged over 55 years and to black people of African or Caribbean family origin of any age. If a CCB is not suitable, for example because of oedema or intolerance, or if there is evidence of heart failure or a high risk of heart failure, offer a thiazide-like diuretic. (p. 17)

The underlying logic is (we think) closely related to Hájek's principle of prioritizing conditional probabilities as a way of drawing the teeth of the reference class problem. Here, several different reference classes are picked out—those under 55 years of age, those over 55 years of age, those of African or Caribbean family origin, and those with other illnesses. This makes explicit the kind of causal reasoning involved. Not "what is the probability of a given drug relieving hypertension," but "what is the probability of this drug relieving hypertension given x, y and z."

Deficiency Diseases: Causation by Omission, Evidence, and Inference

Causation by omission is a worry for most philosophical theories of causation. Why? Largely because absences are (ontologically speaking) just that, absences. Yet causal theories usually feature some commitment to existent objects or events. While the precise commitments vary, most regularity theories are committed to causation as a relation between events (Beebee, 2004). Process theories and mechanisms, on the other hand, understand causation as involving some kind of physical connection between cause and effect (Dowe, 2004; Machamer, Darden, and Craver, 2000). Worries about the difficulty of treating nonexisting things as either relations or as physical connections has produced a variety of accounts that treat causation by absence as something other than causation proper—see the faintly pejorative terminology for absence causation—"fake causation" used by Persson (2002) or "causation*" used by Dowe (2000).

Whatever the reason, causation by absence is troublesome, and usually regarded as an odd or exceptional species of causation. Yet in medicine, absences often participate in causal reasoning. This section will discuss one example of medical causation by absence, which is the case of vitamin D deficiency.

Vitamin D participates in bone mineralization. Its biosynthesis depends on sunlight exposure to the skin. In adults, an absence of sun exposure can lead to the development of osteomalacia, which is a disease of inadequate bone mineralization. In children, vitamin D deficiency causes rickets, which has different clinical manifestations. However, the philosophical analysis in both cases is much the same: *absence* of sunlight causes a disease. Schematically, the mechanism of this disease is as follows. First, persistent lack of sunlight causes reduced cutaneous UV-B exposure. This in turn causes a decrease in the rate of cholecalciferol synthesis, which (over time) can cause osteomalacia.

Here, then, are at least three mechanistic links where an absence causes something to happen. First, an absence of sunlight reduces cutaneous UV-B exposure. Next, reduced UV-B exposure causes a reduction in cholecalciferol synthesis. Finally, the absence of cholecalciferol, over time, causes osteomalacia to develop.

Some philosophers worry about the metaphysics of causation by omission for reasons explained earlier. Yet, others do accept those kinds of causal links, but explain them, for instance, saying that omissions and absences are largely a matter of *language*. For any absence there is something that instead is active or activates, so we could recast the links above using "active" language. This is the strategy adopted by Machamer (2004). In any case, McGrath (2005, p. 125) expresses the general concern elegantly:

DILEMMA: Either there is no causation by omission, or there is far more than common sense says there is.

Diseases due to deficiency are widespread in medicine. Thus, we take side with McGrath's second way: medicine suggests that causation by omission is very common. The challenge for a philosophical theorizing about causation is to make sense of the causal power of omissions and absences, beyond a common sense understanding.

One reason why philosophers find causation by omission tricky is because they want to find worldly causes that make causal claims true. Thus, if we say that vitamin D *deficiency* causes rickets in children, it will be hard to find, in the world, such a thing as a *deficiency*. However, philosophical theorizing about causation is very rich and other accounts allow us to make sense of causal claims about absences and omissions, but we have to change the conceptual framework. Notably, instead of looking for causes, mechanisms, or processes *in the world* we can work at the epistemological level and understand what *evidence* is required to establish causal claims like the one just mentioned and what *inferences* such evidence licenses.

Emphasis on evidence, and specifically about its multifarious character, has been given in the work of Russo and Williamson (2007), Illari (2011), and Clarke et al. (2014). Simply put, this body of work aims to spell out the evidential basis of causal claims (in medicine, but also elsewhere). The thesis, also known as "Russo–Williamson Thesis" (RWT), states that to establish a causal claim we need evidence *that* a cause makes a difference to the occurrence of the effect *and* evidence about *how* a cause produces the effect. This pluralistic view about evidence does not entail that there exist *difference types* of evidence. Instead, RWT offers an understanding of what aspects are important to establish causal knowledge. Moreover, RWT does not imply that difference-making and production are exclusive categories. Quite the contrary is the case. On the one hand, they help each other with establishing causal claims. On the other hand, difference-making considerations are often involved in studying the mechanisms of disease causation and, conversely, considerations about causal production often guide the study of correlation and dependencies. This is explained by Clarke et al. (2014) using the analogy of "reinforced concrete," which is much stronger than concrete and steel *alone*, because these materials are resistant under different types of stress, and *together* they resist better.

Thus, in this conceptual framework, it makes perfect sense to say that vitamin D *deficiency* makes a difference to rickets. The difference it makes may be tracked in population-level correlations, for instance. Then, such claim may be supported by biochemical explanations of the causal pathways that are blocked (or activated) in presence (or absence) of a causal factor such as vitamin D.

Evidential pluralism can also be explained in terms of Susan Haack's view on evidence, which she explains using the metaphor of crosswords. According to Haack (2009), crosswords provide a useful analogy to explain the *structure* of evidence. The way in which we cross words is analogous to the way in which scientists try to find mutual support for their beliefs about the phenomenon under study. The pieces of evidence we put in the "crossword" are not just those pieces of information coming out of lab experiments or randomized studies, but also include a person's experiential evidence. Haack's account clearly has a strong pragmatist flavor, as the way in which we cross the various pieces of evidence does not *just* depend on what the world is like, but also on the interaction of the scientist with the world, on (scientific) language, and on a number of contextual factors.

A pragmatist flavor, although with a slight different emphasis, is also recognizable in Julian Reiss (2015). Simply put, Reiss is interested in what inferences we are (not) allowed to make, depending on the evidence base at our disposal and also on the target of these inferences. An interesting corollary of this view is that the inferences about disease causation licensed by the results of an RCT may not be the same if what is at stake is instead the evaluation of a public health intervention, or the diagnosis of an individual patient.

Interestingly, Reiss argues in favor of this inferentialist view, as it helps regain the broad understanding of (testing) causal relations advocated by Sir Bradford Hill (1965). Hill famously discussed nine *viewpoints*, or aspects, to be considered when analyzing a putative causal relation. Frumkin (2000) summaries them thus:

1. Strength of Association. The stronger the relationship between the independent variable and the dependent variable, the less likely it is that the relationship is due to an extraneous variable.
2. Temporality. It is logically necessary for a cause to precede an effect in time.
3. Consistency. Multiple observations, of an association, with different people under different circumstances and with different measurement instruments increase the credibility of a finding.
4. Theoretical Plausibility. It is easier to accept an association as causal when there is a rational and theoretical basis for such a conclusion.
5. Coherence. A cause-and-effect interpretation for an association is clearest when it does not conflict with what is known about the variables under study and when there are no plausible competing theories or rival hypotheses. In other words, the association must be coherent with other knowledge.
6. Specificity in the causes. In the ideal situation, the effect has only one cause. In other words, showing that an outcome is best predicted by one primary factor adds credibility to a causal claim.
7. Dose–Response Relationship. There should be a direct relationship between the risk factor (i.e., the independent variable) and people's status on the disease variable (i.e., the dependent variable).
8. Experimental Evidence. Any related research that is based on experiments will make a causal inference more plausible.
9. Analogy. Sometimes a commonly accepted phenomenon in one area can be applied to another area.

Reiss correctly points out that, in Hill's account, these viewpoints do not correspond to necessary and sufficient conditions for causality. These are all fallible (yet useful) indicators, rather than strict criteria for causality. This is important because the inferentialist rejects any gold standard for evidence and instead pleads for putting together a "convincing case" for or against a causal claim, on the basis of how different pieces of evidence fit together. According to Reiss, Hill's viewpoints provide useful pragmatic "criteria" that help the inferentialist to come to a judgment about a given causal claim. This is strikingly close to RWT-like arguments, which are nonetheless a bit more specific about the *content* of the (pragmatic) indications given by the viewpoints: viewpoint 1, 3, 7, 8 concern evidence of difference-making or correlation, while viewpoints 2, 4, 5, 8, 9 concern evidence of production or mechanisms.

Ottawa Ankle Rules and Backward Causal Reasoning

The tight relation between causal reasoning, evidence, and inference is recognizable also in other forms of medical reasoning. In the previous section, we highlighted how inferentialist positions à la Reiss are compatible with RWT, with other versions of evidential pluralism such as Haack's, and with Bradford Hill's viewpoints, which remain widely accepted by the medical community. In this section, we highlight another aspect of causal reasoning, that is, its *direction*. While we often reason from causes to effects, in other cases we may also reason from *effects* to causes.

Ankle injuries are common, and can be broadly classified into two groups. The first group are injuries that involve a fracture of one of the bones of the ankle. These injuries are treated by plaster immobilization (and sometimes surgical fixation). The second large group of ankle injuries involves ligaments alone. These are treated more conservatively by rest and appropriate anti-inflammatory drugs. While only about 15 percent of ankle injuries are fractures, the serious consequences of failing to treat them adequately by immobiliza-tion have traditionally led emergency practitioners to adopt a precautionary approach. This has led to the widespread practice of X-raying most ankle inju-ries. Yet this is wasteful and (population-wide) harmful. How then might clini-cians (a) do fewer X-rays while (b) ensuring that ankle fractures are identified and treated appropriately?

The Ottawa ankle rules are a set of rules by which clinicians can make informed decisions about which painful ankles require X-raying, and which do not. They involve reasoning, in a practical way, from effects (in this case symp-toms) to causes (in this case, either fracture or ligamentous injury of the ankle). The basis for this reasoning is that the effects of either fractures or ligamen-tous injuries differ. Specifically, ankle fractures produce a characteristic pat-tern of tenderness (pain evoked by pressing) over the bony parts of the ankle. Additionally, those with ankle fractures experience more pain (and for longer) than those with ligament injuries when standing—in the jargon, they have a protracted inability to weight-bear. This leads to a very simple procedure that can be carried out in the emergency department: the patient is asked to walk four steps, and the ankle is palpated for tenderness over "the bony portions of the lateral and medial malleoli, the navicular, and the proximal fifth metatar-sal" (Mayer, 2009, p. b2901).

Despite their simplicity, the Ottawa ankle rules have surprisingly high pre-dictive power. Using the base-rate of about 15 percent fractures given earlier, the probability of fracture is "less than 1 percent" for a negative result, and "about 22 percent" if positive. In conclusion, "a negative result on applying this rule means an x ray of the ankle is not necessary" (Mayer, 2009, p. b2901). Put another way, this is an excellent example of strong causal reasoning in practice that demonstrates the benefits of adopting a pluralist approach: if all reasoning about cause and effect were forced into the "Does C cause E?" straightjacket (as discussed earlier), the utility of the Ottawa ankle rules would be an anomaly.

Gender Medicine: Confounding and Generic versus Single-case

Yentl is the name of the female protagonist of a play by Isaac Bashevis Singer. She truly is a heroine, as she disguises herself like a man in order to keep studying the Talmud. In the early 1990s, Bernadine Healy (1991) used the term "Yentl syndrome" to indicate a huge gap between genders concerning treatment and diagnosis. She based her claims about gender inequality on data from hospital admission. Healy showed that there exist significant differences in the diagnosis of heart attack for men and women. This is due to the fact that symptoms for the same disease are very different in men and women, due to slightly different physiology. Nearly 30 years later, such differences still exist (Merz and Bairey, 2011). The studies of Healy have been followed up for many other health conditions, and the subfield of "gender medicine" has gradually emerged as a recognized and autonomous area of investigation within medicine (Signani, 2013; Baggio et al., 2013).

The focus on women is perhaps peculiar in that feminist demands for equal treatment in society are now transforming into recognizing important (biological) differences between men and women, these differences being at the base of unequal treatment in health. But the phenomenon is in fact much broader than that. Recent studies show widespread bias in research because it mainly focuses on "WEIRD" people, namely, on individuals coming from countries that are *W*estern, *E*ducated, *I*ndustrialized, *R*ich, and *D*emocratic (Henrich et al., 2010a, b).

These two episodes help us identify further conceptual complexities in medical causation. One such complexity is *heterogeneity* of individuals, discussed in the hypertension section. Gender medicine and studies on WEIRD people point in fact to the problem of correctly specifying the population of reference and, within this population, to specify the most appropriate reference classes. The issue is well known in the social sciences and in the philosophy of causality.

Another is problem is confounding, to be understood more broadly than just in statistical terms. In statistics, confounding variables (C) are variables associated both with the putative outcome (Y) (for instance, a disease) and with its putative cause (X). Because of the association between C and X, the causal effect of X on Y cannot be properly disentangled. The solution is to *control* for confounding variables. But in the case of gender medicine, or of studies on "WEIRD" people, variables like gender, education, socioeconomic status are more than confounders in the statistical sense. They confound the *mechanisms* of disease causation. So in order to understand variations in health and disease, it will not be enough to control for gender, or for different levels of education or socioeconomic status. What looms large is a question about biological uniformity across individuals on the one hand, and about complex biosocial mechanisms on the other hand. This is the idea that humans are sufficiently similar in the relevant respects, thus justifying the generalization of causal claims about disease mechanisms as well as efficacy of treatments. This hypothesis is also at the basis of RCTs, but is sometimes questioned (Victora et al., 2004).

Another problem still is that of "generic versus single-case." One might argue in fact that wrong diagnoses of heart attacks in women (partly) depend on using wrong medical knowledge. The medical sciences aim at building *generic* knowledge about health and disease, which is knowledge that is valid for the whole population. In turn, such knowledge will help in making inferences in the single case, for instance, in diagnosis and prognosis. Gender medicine is pointing to the fact that health and disease (at least *some* aspects of them) may be very different for men and women. This means that we cannot treat *all* individuals alike, but that we must study them separately, and in their specificities.

These specificities may be biological or social. For instance, gender medicine raises the question of how drugs are tested: typically, on male patients in a certain age group, with some average body-mass index, and so on. This, however, ignores the possible effects of drugs on women, who typically have a lower body-mass index and experience hormonal changes every month, during the course of their lives. Just as specificities of women have been neglected, so have those of men. For instance, although much rarer in men than in women, breast cancer does occur in men too. Yet much of what is known and done for men in terms of diagnosis, prognosis and treatment, is extrapolated from studies and treatments for women.

So defining the "correct" population of reference is important not only for building medical knowledge that is valid at the generic level, but also for making inferences concerning individual patients. Relevant causal factors may vary greatly across ethnic groups, men and women, social classes, and so on. Perhaps this variation could be understood as an example of the reference class problem, as discussed earlier.

Asbestos-related Deaths: Social Factors of Disease and Multifactorialism

According to today's knowledge, exposure to asbestos is undoubtedly related to fatal diseases such as asbestosis and lung cancer. Current biomedicine has sound insights about the biochemical mechanisms explaining such diseases— see, for instance, IARC monograph (IARC Working Group, 2012). These issues have been studied extensively in fields such as occupational medicine—the relations among work, work hazards, and health have a long history (Gochfeld, 2005). A paradigmatic example in this respect is asbestos-related deaths close to asbestos factories. Examples abound across different geographical locations. We might mention, for instance, Barking in the United Kingdom (Greenberg, 2003) and Eternit in Italy, for which a memorable sentence was issued in 2009 after a long and difficult trial (Mossano, 2011; Allen and Kazan-Allen, 2012). Many aspects related to latency are, however, still objects of dispute (see, e.g., Terracini et al., 2014; La Vecchia and Boffetta, 2014).

Studies on effects of asbestos exposure help us highlight another dimension of medicine, namely, its interests in understanding health and disease by studying factors *other than* biological. Arguably, in fact, the mechanisms leading to asbestos-related deaths include life style, socioeconomic status, and other social determinants. The argument is not new, and yet it remains controversial (Freese and Lutfey, 2011). For one thing, the inclusion of social factors in the explanation of disease and in public health policy was the very basis of the vision of pioneer healthcare officers during the nineteenth century. Also, social epidemiology has had ups and downs in the past decades, sometimes having to justify why social components of health should be considered at all (for an overview, see Kelly et al., 2014). In recent times, as the literature on the social determinants of health has grown, the idea that social determinants of health act *directly*, rather than via other risk factors, has gained much credibility (see Marmot and Wilkinson, 2005, for example). Yet these social determinants still lack an identified *mechanism*. In fact, while epidemiology has sufficiently proven *that* social factors make a difference to health conditions, a convincing explanation of *how* that is the case is still lacking. The literature, in the "in and out" flutter of fashion, pretty much converged toward the idea that social determinants are *distal*, while biological causes are *proximal*. This gives social determinants a role in establishing difference-making relations, but not mechanisms of disease. These discussions are currently unsettled and it is to be hoped for a genuine integration of sociopsychological approaches and biomedicine to provide broader explanation of health and disease.

For our purposes, these debates are most interesting because they are related to a topic now central in the philosophy of causality: the different characterization, role, and use of "difference-making" and of "mechanisms" in disease causation. These have already been introduced earlier in the deficiency diseases section, but here we can add a further layer of sophistication to the discussion. In fact, a large part of the debate on evidence of mechanisms focused on *biological* mechanism. The question of *how* causes produce their effect is by and large understood in terms of what processes are triggered in our bodies. These processes, in turn, can be described going down to the molecular level.

Yet, episodes like this should at least trigger (or rather, revive) interest in mechanisms that see individuals embedded in the network of social relations. The environment, in fact, is *also* made of our family and peers, the workplace we routinely attend, the infrastructures we have access to, and so on. Thus, an explanation of asbestos-related death should not be limited to the identification of the biochemical processes triggered in our bodies, once exposed to the hazard. Such an explanation should also endeavor to spell out the social, behavioral, or psychological mechanisms involved. In this specific case, for instance, the workplace (Barking, Casale Monferrato) *is* part of the mechanism of exposure, and not just for the workers of asbestos factories. For instance, the wives of workers of the Barking or Eternit factory were also exposed to asbestos fibers because they washed their husbands' coveralls. Or, living near the factory, or downwind, may also have increased exposure. Understanding how these elements enter the mechanisms of disease causation helps identify (precautionary) interventions at a more appropriate level.

Finally, episodes like this point also to problem that is rather ubiquitous in medicine: diseases often have more than one cause. In medicine, and especially in epidemiology, this phenomenon has been labeled as "multifactorialism" (as opposed to *mono*factorialism). Medical theory has long recognized that many diseases may have multiple causes (while acknowledging that others, instead, still admit only one). The most famous epidemiological model developed to account for that is Rothman's causal pies (Rothman, 1976; Rothman et al., 2008). Causal pies display all known factors that play a role in the occurrence of a particular disease. Pie charts, in a sense, visualize contingency tables, but with an important difference: in a pie chart etiological fractions—that is, the components—do not have to sum up to one. This means that we are not looking for the *sum* of the components that make the effect necessary. It is a useful heuristic way of thinking about the multifactorial character of most diseases.

Rothman (1976) made the point that, in many cases, what we call "causes" should instead be understood as *components* of sufficient causes, but that are not themselves sufficient. According to this model, a sufficient cause of a disease is generally not one *single* causal factor, but a complete "causal mechanism." Rothman, to be precise, takes a causal mechanism to be a minimal set of conditions and events that are sufficient for the disease to occur. In this perspective, no specific event condition or characteristic is sufficient, by itself, to produce the disease. So the definition of "cause" does not describe a complete causal mechanism, but only a component of it. It is worth noting that Rothman's use of the term "mechanism" differs from the one discussed earlier, for instance, in relation to RWT. Consider the episode of this section: exposure to asbestos dust is a component of a "bigger" cause that may also include lifestyle (and smoking, dietary habits, etc.), altogether leading to developing lung cancer. To give another example, measles virus is said to be the cause of measles; however, the "complete sufficient cause" of measles also includes lack of immunity to the virus and exposure to the virus.

In this line of reasoning philosophers will readily recognize the "INUS causes" of Mackie (1974). INUS stands for an *I*nsufficient, but *N*onredundant part of an *U*nnecessary but *S*ufficient condition (p. 62). Concepts like INUS or "causal pies" are useful because they allow us to characterize much more precisely the nature of many of the causes that do actually interest us. This can sharpen our reasoning, and thereby have an impact on our practices of inference, prediction, and control. In particular, in adopting a multifactorial view, we are more likely to identify those factors that, though not part of the biological mechanism of disease causation, have an active causal role.

The Causal Mosaic

In previous sections, we showed that medicine is a highly heterogeneous field, where reasoning about causes and effects of health and disease has not a univocal, fixed, or predetermined meaning. Most importantly, causation in medicine amounts to asking a plethora of questions, rather than just one. A straightforward consequence of this analysis of medical practices is that there is not one single causal theory that fits the bill. While pluralism becomes the most plausible candidate, *any* form of pluralism won't do either. In the following, we sketch the main features of a particular form of pluralism. This pluralism draws on the metaphor of building a (causal) "mosaic," where causal theories are not simply ad hoc juxtaposed, but chosen and placed according to how they fare with different types of philosophical questions and with different types of scientific challenges. While a thorough presentation can be found in Illari and Russo (2014), we highlight aspects that are relevant for building a *medical* causal mosaic.

Thinking about causality has a long tradition in philosophy and in science. Some of the discussions carried out in Greek or Medieval thought, or in the development of the scientific method in modern times, may look very different from our current way of thinking about causality. Admittedly, causal thinking had several ups and downs, including vigorous attacks in the early twentieth century due to Ernst Mach in physics, Karl Pearson in statistics, and Bertrand Russell in philosophy. Yet, philosophical thinking did not fade away. Instead, two main strands in philosophical theorizing can be identified since the 1970s and 1980s. One is the counterfactual approach developed mainly by David Lewis (1973, 1983), and the other is the process-tracing, or causal–mechanical, account mainly developed by Wesley Salmon (1984). The past two decades witnessed a steady increase of interest in causal questions, also thanks to the approach based on graphical models as developed by Judea Pearl (2000), Spirtes et al. (1993), and their collaborators. These new, more science-oriented approaches led—more or less directly—to important changes in addressing causal questions (for a discussion, see also Illari et al., 2011; Illari and Russo, 2014).

As far as medicine is concerned, causal thinking has always been central, and this well before Aristotle's doctrine of the four causes or Galenic physiology (for a discussion, see Rabins, 2013), and after (in particular, Rabin discusses medieval conceptions of medical causation, largely neglected in current debates). Arguably, the experimental method of Claude Bernard (1856) started a tradition in medicine that looked for biological causes of health and disease, and nowadays is giving rise to investigations of disease mechanisms at the molecular level. Yet, at the same time, medicine also developed *other* ways of studying health and disease, most prominently epidemiology—which is based on statistical analyses of data—but also narrative medicine—that clearly distances itself from views that "biologize" health and disease.

For one thing, philosophers have being paying increasing attention to the special sciences, for example, economics and other social sciences, biology, or epidemiology. Dedicated discussions about epidemiology and medicine (such as Broadbent, 2013; Howick, 2011) are also part of this heightened specialization of philosophy of science, and notably of philosophy of causality. Consequently, considerable effort was put in trying to formulate questions that are tailored to specific fields, and particularly to the methodological challenges of these fields. This is indeed the rationale behind laying down "episodes" of medical causation discussed earlier, and from these to discuss relevant aspects of causal theories.

In recent years, another question gained ground: how to *use* causal knowledge, namely, what to do once we know (or do not know) causal relations. This happened thanks to work of Donald Gillies (2005), who formulated an "action-oriented theory of causality" and of Nancy Cartwright (2007), who drew philosophers' (as well scientists' and policymakers') attention to very delicate causal issues lingering in policy-making and to the scope of the results of trials. Questions about use are particularly pressing in medicine and public health. This is because we want to use medical knowledge to cure people and save lives. However, *any* medical knowledge won't do here. What is required to diagnose a particular patient carefully differs from what is required to make sound claims about the efficacy of a drug, which is again different from what is required to make sound claims about the efficacy of a public health intervention. Thus, it seems that questions about use cannot be asked in "absolute terms," but need to be specified with respect to the context in which they arise.

A bird's eye view on the vast literature produced in the past decades reveals a sprawling of accounts, concepts, and notions. Causation has been examined in terms of, or in relation to, counterfactuals, mechanisms, probabilities, inference, necessary and sufficient conditions, and many others. Illari and Russo (2014) present these debates and explain how these different accounts can be of help in addressing typical scientific problems about causality, namely, inference, explanation, prediction, control. Illari and Russo conclude, from such diversity and variety of accounts, that it is reasonable to give up on *The One Theory of Causality*. We certainly do not have it as of today; this does not exclude, as a matter of principle, that we will find one theory able to encompass all cases, episodes, and types of causation in the future. While their argument spans philosophy of causality *across* the sciences, this chapter further supported it, making the case *specifically* for medicine.

Even if we agree, prima facie, that there exists a plurality of accounts, concepts, and approaches, we still face the difficulty of making sense of such diversity and variety. How can these accounts coexist together? It is here that the metaphor of a "causal mosaic" proves useful. A mosaic is an image formed of several tiles, possibly different in shape and color. When the tiles are appropriately located one next to the other, an image appears. Each tile participates in the formation of the image, when correctly positioned. Individually, tiles may have beautiful colors or shapes, but they do not have a clearly recognizable meaning. That is to say, the tiles acquire meaning in relation to other tiles, and in the context of the mosaic being built. Philosophical theorizing about causality works just like that. Available accounts of causality all have a role in our understanding of causality. But to see the whole causal picture, we need to place the tiles—the causal accounts—according to how they respond to different philosophical questions (metaphysical, epistemological, semantic, methodological), and according to how they help us with specific scientific challenges (inference, explanation, prediction, control).

Causation in medicine is *one* of the mosaics we might want to build. If we want to understand "medical causation," we have to start with more specific questions. What kind of practice is at stake? What is the specific causal question being asked? What is the underlying philosophical problem or scientific challenge? And so on. Philosophical accounts will help answer such questions by providing an appropriate conceptual framework. Thus, for instance, a theory of evidence based on the mechanism—difference-making distinction—might prove useful to answer questions about drug or treatment efficacy. An account of the levels of causation and of Simpson's paradox might help address the problem of reference classes and of external validity. An approach to causal reasoning might lend support to guidelines for prescribing diagnostic exams such as X-rays. And so on and so forth.

The metaphor is quite telling about philosophical methodology and philosophical practice too. In fact, we clearly do not know in advance what the final causal mosaic may look like and philosophers need to work together, and with scientists, in order to figure out how best to place the tiles. Also, the final picture is clearly dynamic, as the scientific challenges evolves and so does the philosophical theorizing that accompanies it. Last, but not least, causal mosaics may be very idiosyncratic, which should be a reason to foster dialogue and collaboration among philosophers, among scientists, and among those two.

Again, causation in medicine is no exception in this respect. The philosophical community interested in medicine grew significantly in the recent past. We moved from a philosophy of medicine that was by and large populated by questions about ethics, to a much larger group of scholars equally interested in epistemological and methodological questions about medicine. We need to build a *medical* causal mosaic also thinking prospectively in terms of collaborations with ethicists or political philosophers. In fact, the "phil sci" question of how to use medical knowledge easily turns into a moral or political question about whether (and how) we should use such knowledge, or whether we are legitimized in using it, and so on.

We developed the chapter precisely along these ideas, and so ours has been an exercise in building *a* causal mosaic for medical causation, or causation in medicine. What we suggest is *a* reconstruction of how causal questions arise in medicine (broadly construed) and of how to make (philosophical) sense of them. The picture that we lay down reflects some specific philosophical presuppositions and methodology. We espouse the goals and methods of the "Causality in the Sciences" (CitS) approach, which proposes looking at scientific practice in order to select philosophical questions and to "test" them. While scientific practice help philosophical theorizing, philosophical accounts in turn aid scientific practice. CitS advocates in favor of this iterative relation of mutual aid between philosophy and the sciences. It is worth noting that this is very much in line with other approaches, notably those of the developing "Philosophy of Science in Practice" and "History and Philosophy of Science" movements. All look to the practice of science—contemporary or historical—in search of fruitful interactions between the fields of philosophy and of science. CitS also shares much with the philosophy of information, which advocates developing a "timely philosophy," namely, a philosophy that helps address the challenges of science and society *today*.

In sum, we hope that this chapter successfully conveyed the message that causation in medicine is a fertile and growing area of investigation. What we presented here does not even get close to building a full mosaic. But this was not our intention. We wanted instead to propose an approach to *how* one can contribute to building a mosaic of medical causation. This, we maintain, is a task that only the scientific and philosophical communities, together, can achieve.

Acknowledgments

The authors gratefully acknowledge financial support from the Arts and Humanities Research Council via grant AH/M005917/1 ("Evaluating Evidence in Medicine"). An early version of this chapter was presented at the EBM+ project workshop at the University of Kent, Canterbury, in January 2015. We would like to extend our thanks to the workshop participants, especially Jon Williamson, Michael Wilde, Phyllis Illari, and Veli-Pekka Parkkinen, for their thoughtful comments and invaluable input.

Note

1. We are indebted to Connor Cummings, who developed this example in his BSc dissertation at the University College London on reference classes.

References

Allen, D., and Kazan-Allen, L. (2012). *Eternit and the Great Asbestos Trial*. London: The International Ban Asbestos Secretariat. http://www.ibasecretariat.org/eternit-great-asbestos-trial-toc.htm.

Baggio, G., Corsini, A., Floreani, A., Giannini, S., and Zagonel, V. (2013). Gender medicine: A task for the third millennium. *Clinical Chemistry and Laboratory Medicine* 51(4): 713–17. doi: 10.1515/cclm-2012-0849.

Beebee, H. (2004). Causing and nothingness. In *Causation and Counterfactuals*, eds. John Collins, Ned Hall, and L. A. Paul. Cambridge, MA: MIT Press, pp. 291–308.

Bernard, C. ([1856] 1927). *An Introduction to the Study of Experimental Medicine*. New York: Macmillan.

Bradford Hill, A. (1965). The environment of disease: Association or causation? *Proceedings of the Royal Society of Medicine* 58(5): 295–300.

Broadbent, A. (2013). *Philosophy of Epidemiology*. Palgrave Macmillan.

Cartwright, N. (2007). *Hunting Causes and Using Them*. Cambridge: Cambridge University Press.

Cartwright, N., and Hardie, J. (2012). *Evidence-Based Policy: A Practical Guide to Doing It Better*. Oxford: Oxford University Press.

Chang, H. (1999). History and philosophy of science as a continuation of science by other means. *Science & Education* 8(4): 413–25. doi:10.1023/A:1008650325798.

Clarke, B., Gillies, D., Illari, P., Russo, F., and Williamson, J. (2014). Mechanisms and the evidence hierarchy. *Topoi* 33(2): 339–60.

Dowe, P. (2000). *Physical Causation*. Cambridge: Cambridge University Press.

Dowe, P. (2004). Causes are physically connected to their effects: Why preventers and omissions are not causes. In *Contemporary Debates in Philosophy of Science*, eds. Christopher Hitchcock. Oxford: Blackwell, pp. 189–96.

Dupré, J. (1993). *The Disorder of Things: Metaphysical Foundations of the Disunity of Science*. Cambridge, MA: Harvard University Press.

Fortin, M., Dionne, J., Pinho, G., Gignac, J., Almirall, J., and Lapointe, L. (2006). Randomized controlled trials: Do they have external validity for patients with multiple comorbidities? *Annals of Family Medicine* 4(2): 104–108.

Freese, J., and Lutfey, K. (2011). Fundamental causality: Challenges of an animating concept for medical sociology. In *Handbook of the Sociology of Health, Illness, and Healing: A Blueprint for the 21st Century*, eds. Bernice A. Pescosolido, Jack K. Martin, Jane D. McLeod, and Anne Rogers. New York, NY: Springer, pp. 67–81.

Frumkin, H. (2000). *Causation in Medicine*. http://www.aoec.org/CEEM/methods/emory2.html.

Gartlehner, G., Hansen, R. A., Nissman, D., Lohr, K. N., and Carey, T. S. (2006). Criteria for distinguishing effectiveness from efficacy trials in systematic reviews. 12. Agency for Healthcare Research and Quality (US). http://www.ncbi.nlm.nih.gov/books/NBK44029/.

Gillies, D. (2005). An action-related theory of causality. *British Journal for the Philosophy of Science* 56(4): 823–42.

Gochfeld, M. (2005). Chronologic history of occupational medicine. *Journal of Occupational and Environmental Medicine* 47(2): 96–114.

Greenberg, M. (2003). Cape asbestos, barking, health and environment: 1928–1946. *American Journal of Industrial Medicine* 43(2): 109–19.

Guyatt, G., Cairns, J., Churchill, D., Cook, D., Haynes, B., Hirsh, J., Irvine, J., et al. (1992). Evidence-based medicine: A new approach to teaching the practice of medicine. *Journal of the American Medical Association* 268(17): 2420.

Haack, S. (2009). *Evidence and Inquiry: A Pragmatist Reconstruction of Epistemology.* London: Prometheus Books.

Hájek, A. (2007). The reference class problem is your problem too. *Synthese* 156(3): 563–85.

Healy, B. (1991). The Yentl Syndrome. *New England Journal of Medicine* 325(4): 274–76.

Henrich, J., Heine, S., and Norenzayan, A. (2010a). Most people are not WEIRD. *Nature* 466(7302): 29. doi:doi:10.1038/466029a.

Henrich, J., Heine, S., and Norenzayan, A. (2010b). The weirdest people in the world? 139. Rates für Sozial- und Wirtschaftsdaten. http://www.econstor.eu/bitstream/10419/43616/1/626014360.pdf.

Howick, J. H. (2011). *The Philosophy of Evidence-Based Medicine.* John Wiley & Sons.

IARC Working Group. (2012). *Arsenic, Metals, Fibres and Dusts.* IARC. http://monographs.iarc.fr/ENG/Monographs/vol100C/index.php.

Illari, P. (2011). Mechanistic evidence: Disambiguating the Russo–Williamson thesis. *International Studies in the Philosophy of Science* 25(2): 139–57.

Illari, P., and Russo, F. (2014). *Causality: Philosophical Theory Meets Scientific Practice.* Oxford: Oxford University Press.

Illari, P., Russo, F., and Williamson, J. (2011). Why look at causality in the sciences? In *Causality in the Sciences*, eds. Phyllis Illari, Federica Russo, and Jon Williamson. Oxford: Oxford University Press, pp. 3–22.

Jonsen, A. R., and Toulmin, S. (1988). *The Abuse of Casuistry: A History of Moral Reasoning.* Berkeley, CA: University of California Press.

Kelly, M., Kelly, R., and Russo, F. (2014). The integration of social, behavioural, and biological mechanisms in models of pathogenesis. *Perspectives in Biology and Medicine* 57(3): 308–28.

Lewis, D. K. (1973). *Counterfactuals.* Oxford: Blackwell.

Lewis, D. K. (1983). *Philosophical Papers.* Vol. 1. Oxford: Oxford University Press.

Machamer, P. (2004). Activities and causation: The metaphysics and epistemology of mechanisms. *International Studies in the Philosophy of Science* 18(1): 27–39.

Machamer, P., Darden, L., and Craver, C. (2000). Thinking about mechanisms. *Philosophy of Science* 67(1): 1–25.

Mackie, J. L. (1974). *The Cement of the Universe: A Study on Causation.* Oxford: Oxford University Press.

Marmot, M., and Wilkinson, R. (2005). *Social Determinants of Health.* Oxford: Oxford University Press.

Mayer, D. (2009). The injured ankle and foot. *BMJ* 339: b2901.

McGrath, S. (2005). Causation by omission: A dilemma. *Philosophical Studies* 123(1): 125–48.

Merz, C., and Bairey, N. (2011). The Yentl Syndrome is alive and well. *European Heart Journal* 32(11): 1313–15. doi: 10.1093/eurheartj/ehr083.

Mossano, S. (2011). The eternit trial: The verdict is close. *Epidemiologia E Prevensione* 35(3–4): 175–77.

NICE. (2011). Hypertension: Quick reference guide. The National Institute for Health and Care Excellence. www.nice.org.uk.

Pearl, J. (2000). *Causality: Models, Reasoning, and Inference*. Cambridge: Cambridge University Press.

Persson, J. (2002). Cause, effect, and fake causation. *Synthese* 131(1): 129–43.

Rabins, P. V. (2013). *The Why of Things: Causality in Science, Medicine, and Life*. New York, NY: Columbia University Press.

Reichenbach, H. (1949). *The Theory of Probability: An Inquiry into the Logical and Mathematical Foundations of the Calculus of Probability*. University of California Press.

Reiss, J. (2015). *Causation, Evidence, and Inference*. London: Routledge.

Rothman, K. J. (1976). Causes. *American Journal of Epidemiology* 104(6): 587–92.

Rothman, K. J., Greenland, S., and Lash, T. L. (2008). *Modern Epidemiology*. Philadelphia, PA: Wolters Kluwer/Lippincott Williams and Wilkins.

Russo, F. (2009). *Causality and Causal Modelling in the Social Sciences: Measuring Variations*. Methodos Series. New York: Springer.

Russo, F. (2014). What Invariance is and how to test for it. *International Studies in the Philosophy of Science* 28(2): 157–83.

Russo, F., and Williamson, J. (2007). Interpreting causality in the health sciences. *International Studies in Philosophy of Science* 21(2): 157–70.

Salmon, W. C. (1984). *Scientific Explanation and the Causal Structure of the World*. Princeton: Princeton University Press.

Salmon, W. C. (1989). *Four Decades of Scientific Explanation*. Minneapolis, MN: University of Minnesota Press.

Salmon, W. C., Jeffrey, R. C., and Greeno, J. G. (1971). *Statistical Explanation and Statistical Relevance*. Pittsburgh, PA: University of Pittsburgh Press.

Signani, F. (2013). *La Salute Su Misura. Medicina Di Genere Non È Medicina Delle Donne*. Este Edition.

Solomon, M. (2011). Just a paradigm: Evidence-based medicine in epistemological context. *European Journal for Philosophy of Science* 1: 451–66.

Spirtes, P., Glymour, C., and Scheines, R. (1993). *Causation, Prediction, and Search*. Second (2000). Cambridge, MA: MIT Press.

Terracini, B., Mirabelli, D., Magnani, C., Ferrante, D., Barone-Adesi, F., and Bertolotti, M. (2014). A critique to a review on the relationship between asbestos exposure and the risk of mesothelioma. *European Journal of Cancer Prevention* 23(5): 492–94. doi:10.1097/CEJ.0000000000000057.

Vandenbroucke, J. (2009). Commentary: "Smoking and lung cancer"—the embryogenesis of modern epidemiology. *International Journal of Epidemiology* 38(5): 1193–96.

Vecchia, C. La, and Boffetta, P. (2014). A critique of a review on the relationship between asbestos exposure and the risk of mesothelioma: Reply. *European Journal of Cancer Prevention* 23(5): 494–96. doi:10.1097/CEJ.0000000000000051.

Victora, C. G., Habicht, J.-P., and Bryce, J. (2004). Evidence-based public health: Moving beyond randomized trials. *American Journal of Public Health* 94(3): 400–405.

Vineis, P. (2003). Causality in epidemiology. *Social and Preventive Medicine* 48(2): 80–87.

13 Clinical Reasoning and Knowing

Hillel D. Braude

Introduction

Faced with the impossible task of having to define "pornography," Justice Potter Stewart (1964) famously declared that "[p]erhaps I could never succeed in intelligibly doing so. *But I know it when I see it.*" The problem, of course, in having to define "pornography" is that social mores and norms are not fixed, but are constantly shifting. In short, determining how and how much human flesh being revealed constitutes obscenity is an inherently subjective phenomenon. What Justice Stewart observed in relation to pornography also applies, perhaps surprisingly, to the attempt to define clinical reasoning (CR) and its relation to explicit knowing.

CR is notoriously difficult to define. Despite the ubiquity of references to CR in the medical literature, there exist very few formal attempts to define it. An online search of Medline from 1946 to January 15, 2015, using the term "clinical reasoning" in the title elicited 648 references. Of these, only two actually attempted to define CR. The authors of both articles remarked that their research was motivated by the present lack of any consensual definition of CR in the literature (Cote and St-Cyr Tribble, 2012; Durning et al., 2013). The authors of the remaining 646 articles presumably had a tacit conception of CR in their minds, or else attempted to define it through referring to its presumed components without a formal definition. However, this lack of a clear definition of CR is an important indicator that its fundamental epistemic components are not yet well understood.

In an analysis of metacognition Joëlle Proust (2013, pp. 2–3) remarks that "[p]articularly when a definition is still only partly understood, a definition should help us to refer to it without incorporating a given theory as part of its meaning." The same holds true for the attempt to define CR. Until we are clearer about its meaning, any definition should avoid slipping in an implicit theoretical bias. Indeed, as will become clear in this chapter, it is precisely the complex relation between theory and practice that makes it so difficult to present a concise, universally applicable definition of CR.

Consider the influential definition of CR as a particular form of cognition applied to evaluating and managing a patient's medical problem provided by Barrows and Tamblyn (1980). This definition accords with the dominant hypothetico-deductive model of CR. According to this model, a clinician begins by creating working hypotheses, inferred from the patient's presenting symptoms. These hypotheses are then gradually refined through the process of elimination until the most compelling hypothesis is chosen that best accounts for the chief clinical diagnosis (Barrows and Feltovich, 1987). The hypothetico-deductive approach to CR is singular in being strictly cognitive, and thereby only accounting for explicit analytic inferences. It does not account for tacit forms of knowing as an essential, if not inalienable, aspect of CR. Yet, despite the cognitivist critique, proponents of CR in terms of tacit knowing and intuition persistently present an alternative model of clinical rationality. From this perspective, this definition of CR cannot, therefore, be considered conclusive.[1]

The psychological analysis of CR using the tools of cognitive science over the past few decades has certainly contributed to an increased understanding of the cognitive processes involved in clinical decision-making. At the same time, as I shall argue in this chapter, CR is more than a process of cognition. First, because CR incorporates metacognition, requiring further introspection and analytic reflection. Second, CR is a form of intersubjective consciousness that needs to be addressed phenomenologically (Braude, 2012a, 2013). Finally, CR also incorporates an implicit call for moral action for the good of another person that requires the clinician to evaluate between technical means and ends. These fundamental aspects of CR situates it as a form of Aristotelian practical wisdom or *phronesis*. Additionally, *phronesis* is able to contain the tension between an inferential or analytic mode of discursive thinking and a nondiscursive or intuitive mode. *Phronesis* also incorporates the nondualistic relation between the body and mind within CR that is lacking in its modern cognitive definition. If pornography pertains to the uncovering of the human flesh, CR refers to the revealing of dimensions of the relation between the body and the mind through the experience of a patient's illness in relation with her physician and other caregivers.

In this chapter, I shall consider the relation between CR and knowing in relation to explicit cognition, metacognition, tacit knowing, and clinician subjectivity. Additionally, this analysis will emphasize the role of nonanalytic processes associated with intuition in CR. The fundamental question that I address is whether the literature on metacognition refers to another level of cognition, or instead introduces or points toward a mental event or act of consciousness that is qualitatively different from cognition. I argue that modeling CR on *phronesis* reveals the fundamental embeddedness of CR in human life, integrating biological life processes with clinical reflection.

Alvan Feinstein on Clinical Judgment

I begin this chapter by focusing on the work of the late physician Alvan Feinstein. Despite the passing years since the publication of his classic work on *Clinical Judgment*,[2] Feinstein's contribution to the epistemology of clinical medicine is exemplary for his elegant synthesis of explicit and tacit knowing in CR. Feinstein devoted his career to exploring and delineating the nature of CR in a manner that remains true to the clinical context.[3] In *Clinical Judgment* Feinstein (1967, p. 53) makes the following intriguing point:

> His human sensory organs give a clinician the power to make many observations of which no inanimate instrument is capable, and his human mind enables him to make constant scientific improvements in the way he performs his observations and interpretations. The clinician cannot begin to improve these functions, however, until he recognizes himself as a unique and powerful piece of scientific equipment. He can then contemplate and, if necessary, revise the fundamental aspects of what he does and how he thinks when he collects the human data for which he is the main and often the only, perceptual apparatus.

Feinstein emphasizes here the idea that the human sensory capabilities of the clinician provides the most powerful instrument for clinical judgment.

In highlighting the importance of physician subjectivity for clinical interaction, Feinstein is not simply referring, for example, to the well-known placebo effect of the personality of the clinician for patient well-being, but rather to a rational sensibility that is essential for effective CR and that resists abstraction into computational methodology. It is important to remember that Feinstein himself did not consider the art of medicine as a mystical practice, but as a process that could be quantified while respecting the epistemic constraints on explicit knowing provided by the clinical context. One consequence of this approach is to move away from a notion of CR based on the temporally static pathological correlate of disease. Following on from Feinstein, Eric Cassell (2015, pp. 22) has noted that "[c]linicians and clinical medicine require an alternative definition of sickness that does not diminish the importance of pathophysiology and the effects of disease but encompasses the impact of sickness on the patient's life and the impress of the patient in the sickness."

Tacit Knowing

The emphasis on individual variability in the clinical context renders Feinstein's epistemology of medicine compatible with theories of CR modelled on tacit knowing. As Michael Polanyi (1962, 1966) emphasized, tacit knowing forms a subterranean dimension upon which all of our explicit knowing is constructed. It refers to knowledge that functions at the periphery of attention and makes explicit knowledge possible. Stephen Henry (2010), who has championed the application of tacit knowing to CR, argues that there are two features of tacit knowing especially relevant to clinical medicine. First, explicit knowledge could not exist without prior existence of a "tacit background." For example, tacit knowing occurs when a physician who is explicitly listening to a patient's story is simultaneously aware, but in a qualitatively different way, of the patient's tone of voice, facial expression, and choice of words. Moreover, these tacit particulars are crucial to informing the physicians' processes of clinical judgment. Second, the mechanism of how "tacit particulars give rise to explicit knowledge cannot be fully captured in formal models or discrete steps; the relationship is ultimately inarticulable" (p. 293).

These two features are particularly interesting because they establish what appears to be a paradox of rationality. On the one hand, tacit knowing is essential for explicit rational forms of knowledge, most notably scientific knowing. On the other hand, since the tacit foundations of explicit knowing are essentially nonanalytic, it implies that the sense of rationality associated with tacit knowing is grounded on that which resists explicit analysis. Clinical medicine is particularly axiomatic for the application of tacit knowing, since it is characterized by uncertainty. As Henry observes, medical practice is inherently uncertain, not only because we can never have complete clinical information, but also because of this dimension of tacit knowing that resists full analysis and articulation.

For Polanyi (1946, 1962, 1997), tacit knowing is synonymous with practical intuition. It functions through integrating particulars derived from the level of subsidiary awareness with focal or explicit awareness (Wilczak, 1973). In Feinstein's model, effective CR works through a combination of intuitive and explicit processes directed toward the particular individual patient and unique clinical context. Clinical intuition is essential for mediating between first-order observations and subsequent inferential levels. For Feinstein (1977, p. 529), clinical decisions do not reflect decontextualized universal judgments, but are influenced by factors such as "pathophysiological changes, psychosocial factors and support, personal preferences of patients, and strategies for giving comfort and reassurance."[4]

Decision Analysis

The analysis of CR in terms of tacit knowing is often contrasted with the hypothetico-deductive model. In fact, these two approaches toward CR represent two different structures of rationality. The ever-expanding work in cognitive science on decision-making provides a powerful means of evaluating these two approaches. However, until fairly recently, cognitive science has been used primarily as a means to support the hypothetico deductive model and to critique the intuitive support of CR. In the following paragraphs, I shall review this approach and describe the recent attempt to unify tacit and explicit knowing in CR through cognitive science.

In the nearly four decades since Feinstein's work has been published there have been many studies on the cognitive processes involved in clinical reasoning. The most influential approach has developed from applying the tools of decision analysis, pioneered by psychologists Daniel Kahneman and Amos Tversky (1974). Central to their approach is the related concepts of "biases" and "heuristics." A bias can be defined as a *deviation* from a normatively correct answer (Gigerenzer et al., 1989, p. 227). A heuristic can be defined as a principle of cognition in everyday reasoning that reduces the "complex task of assessing probabilities and predicting values to simpler judgmental operations" (Kahneman and Tversky, 1974, p. 1124). Kahneman and Tversky's strategy in their classic paper was to identify biases in judgment that are associated with heuristics in decision-making under uncertainty. This approach is associated with the cognitive science conception of rationality, evaluating behavior in terms of how closely it adheres to or departs from the optimum prescribed by a particular normative model (Stanovich, 2011). For the most part, the application of decision analysis to medicine has demonstrated the inherent fallibility of even expert clinicians (Elstein, 2000, 2009).

The classic biases singled out by Kahneman and Tversky relate to inaccurate assessment of probabilities. These include the representative bias, the availability bias, and the anchoring bias. As Round (2001, p. 113) summarizes, "The representativeness bias is a subjective judgment of the extent to which an event in question is similar in essential properties to its parent population (Kahneman and Tversky, 1972). In other words, the bias overestimates the similarity between people or events and gives undue weight to small samples." The "availability bias suggests there is a tendency to attribute too much weight to 'easily available' information, or to an event which is easily remembered because of particularly salient features (Detmer et al., 1978); an example is overestimation" (Round, 2001, p. 113). "The anchoring bias occurs when people are asked to estimate the probability of an event. The initial probability is placed at too extreme a figure and insufficient adjustment is made for subsequent information (Hogarth, 1980)" (p. 113).

Medicine has provided a preeminent context for the application of clinical decision analysis. For example, citing the representative heuristic Balla, Elstein, and Christensen (1989, p. 580) provide the following clinical case where ignoring the base rates of tuberculosis in the population might lead the clinician to an erroneous diagnosis:

When presented with yellow cerebrospinal fluid obtained at a lumbar puncture in a patient with a headache a clinician may diagnose subarachnoid hemorrhage even in the absence of an accurate history of abrupt onset of symptoms. The decision maker thinks primarily of yellow fluid as equivalent to the presence of blood, though less commonly it could also be related to raised protein concentrations due to other causes, such as tuberculous meningitis. Judgment is made by perceived likeness to something well known to the decision maker even if the basis for this is otherwise wrong. In this instance the lack of the abrupt onset headache and the knowledge that tuberculous meningitis is common in the locality would indicate that a subarachnoid bleed would be a less likely diagnosis.

The number of potential heuristics and biases are legion and are continuing to grow. The expansion of neuroscience to include studying the influences of affect on cognition has also resulted in affective biases being considered as sources precluding optimal human judgment and decision-making in medicine. For example, the framing bias refers to the impact on how the affective presentation of an issue impacts the choices made by decision-makers (Round, 2001). Pat Croskerry (2008; Croskerry et al., 2008), who has championed applying the tools of cognitive science to examine our inherent cognitive biases involved in clinical reasoning, cites more than forty different kinds of cognitive and affective biases that may contribute to impaired clinical judgment.

In summary, the cognitive impediments affecting effective clinical decision-making relate to the structure of cognition, the psychological ego defenses of the decision-maker, as well as the neurophysiological state of the decision-maker at the moment of decision. For example, sleep deprivation is a major source for potentially impaired decision-making (Croskerry, 2014). Common to all of these biases are the fact that they are all cognitive, and yet their influence and impact is unknown to the decision-maker at the time of the decision.

Croskerry (2014) has proposed a methodology of "critical thinking" or "cognitive debiasing" in order for clinicians to overcome preconceptual predisposition to cognitive biases in clinical reasoning. He defines "critical thinking" as "the ability to be in control of one's thinking … to consciously examine the elements of one's reasoning, or that of another, and evaluate that reasoning against universal intellectual standards—clarity, accuracy, precision, relevance, depth, breadth, and logic. It also involves the structural examination of sources of information" (p. 13). The succession of stages involved in cognitive debiasing include moving from a state of lack of awareness of a particular bias, to awareness, to the ability to detect the bias, to considering a change, to initiating strategies for change, to the accomplishment of change, and finally to the maintenance of the change in the future (Croskerry et al., 2013). One of the key strategies involved is metacognition, referring to the "deliberate disengagement or decoupling from intuitive judgments and engagement in analytical processes to verify initial impressions" (p. ii67).

As emphasized in this chapter, theories of CR based on tacit knowing and eradication of cognitive biases represent two approaches toward rationality in medicine. The cognitive science approach considers rationality in terms of evaluating the proximity of results of decisions in terms of degrees of distance from the optimum (Stanovich, 2011). Accordingly, clinicians are often found wanting in scientific rationality. Cognitive debiasing is intended to restore this clinical rationality through reflection on and eradication of the tendency toward cognitive biases. On the other hand, theories of tacit knowing propose a model of clinical rationality that is derived from the clinical context, and the actual practice of treating individuals. Rationality is broadened to include unconscious processes as essential for human cognition. For example, particular patient preferences might depart from rational treatment norms, but taking them into account is an essential component of good medical practice.

While these two models of rationality seem poles apart, there is one important point of connection between them. Both models posit the notion that unconscious processes of cognition play an important role in CR. According to tacit knowing these processes inform all levels of CR. Indeed, CR according to this model is unthinkable without the prior foundation of tacit knowing. Meta-reflection on these processes provides a means of rendering them more explicit, and in connecting between the levels of focal and subsidiary awareness. Thus, not all subsidiary knowledge will be available for explicit analysis, but the task of the clinician is to bring as much to the fore as is possible. While the hypothetico-deductive model of CR has a much narrower sense of rationality, it is similar to the tacit knowing model, at least as articulated by Croskerry, in acknowledging the presence of unconscious processes of cognition. However, in contrast with tacit-knowing, the cognitive science definition of rationality has no place to account for decision-making that departs from statistical norms. The purpose of cognitive debiasing is to proximate clinical decision-making as closely to these statistical norms and decision-making rules as possible. Both models are "ameliorative" in the sense that they consider it possible for clinicians to improve CR through reflection; however, they present radically different notions of clinical rationality.

Dual-process Theory

This tale of the dichotomy between tacit knowing and hypothetico-deductive reasoning does not end here. Heralding the end of the long stalemate between these approaches, theorists are beginning to find creative ways for reconciling these two approaches. The most promising breakthrough in terms of reconciling these two approaches is in terms of applying the dual-process theory (DPT) brain function to CR (Marcum, 2012). According to this theory cognitive function is characterized by two systems or processes—Type 1 and Type 2—reflecting different evolutionary structures of brain development.[5] As described by Stanovich (2011), Type 1 processing is defined by its autonomy from input from higher-level cortical control. Other correlated features include rapid execution, the ability to avoid overloading central processing capacity, and the tendency to operate in parallel without involving Type 2 processing. In contrast, Type 2 processing operates largely in series, and is relatively slow and computationally expensive. Additionally, Type 2 processing is often language-based, associating it with explicit analytic inferential cognition. Type 1 processing is often associated with emotional regulation and the reliance on heuristics. A key function of Type 2 processing is to override Type 1 processing, associated with intuitions and other inherent tendencies toward irrationality understood in the cognitive science definition of degrees of distance from the optimum. In the instance of conflict between the two systems, it is assumed that a person is better served by overriding Type 1 processing, since Type 2 processing is "more attuned to the person's needs as a coherent organism" (p. 23).

The model of DPT appears to present a very convenient and increasingly accepted model of cognitive function with which to reconcile tacit and explicit knowing in CR. Marcum (2012) has proposed an "integrated model" in which processes of CR are initiated through type 1 non-analytic processes. Accordingly, following clinical examination a clinician will form an initial diagnostic impression, largely through pattern recognition and other forms of tacit or intuitive knowing. This initial diagnostic hypothesis will result in a clinical decision provided there is adequate clinical evidence in support of it based on previous clinical experience. This clinical process will, therefore, integrate Type 1 noninferential and Type 2 inferential processes. If for whatever clinical reason no obvious clinical decision can be made, especially if there is a conflict between Type 1 and 2 processes, then Type 2 analytic processes will intervene and predominate in order to attain the most thoughtfully reflective clinical decision. In developing this "integrated approach," Marcum suggests that combining analytic and nonanalytic processes is necessary in order to reduce the likelihood of errors in clinical judgment.

While this "integrated approach" does reconcile tacit and explicit forms of knowing in CR, it still carries over the prejudice from cognitive science against tacit knowing as inherently error-prone, if not irrational. Croskerry (2009) identifies several loci in the integrated model where the diagnostic process could break down and fail: first, the pattern associated with the initial pattern might be misidentified. Second, the overlearning that occurs through repeated processing in Type 2 and allows the response to default to Type 1 might occur prematurely. Third, the surveillance/monitoring performance of Type 2 over Type

1 may become compromised for a variety of reasons. Fourth, there are many instances in which Type 1 processes override Type 2 reasoning in medical practice. What is most noteworthy about this list is that while Type 1 processes are generally reliable where they occur smoothly, essentially all cognitive clinical decision-making errors occur through a fault or reversion to Type 1 processing. This also applies to errors associated with Type 2 processing. When Type 2 processes become so habitual as to preclude reflection, they essentially become a form of error prone Type 1 processing. While the integrated model represents a large step in terms of reconciling intuitive and explicit knowing in CR, it still does so in terms of the predominant cognitive science conception of rationality. The gap still exists in terms of reconciling the cognitive science approach, with a model of CR that acknowledges uncertainty and individual variability as an inherent component of the clinical context.

The integrated approach rests on the central mediating concept of metacognition. Metacognition generally refers to the kind of processes involved in thinking about one's own thinking. It may also refer to the activity of monitoring and controlling one's own cognitive activity (Proust, 2013). Stanovich (2011) refers to this additional layer of cognitive processing as "reflection." According to Marcum (2012), metacognition provides the capacity to think about both analytic and nonanalytic cognitive processes at a higher level of reflection. This capacity provides a cognitive mechanism to monitor CR and "ultimately to normalize a clinical decision" (p. 954). Marcum observes that "[m]etacognition monitors CR operations and ultimately validates or rejects, through its regulatory or controlling function, a diagnostic or therapeutic decision. In addition, it allows the clinician to evaluate the process by which the decision was made and whether that process can be utilized in future CR" (p. 957). In summary, metacognition is essential for the feed-forward and feed-back processes involved in mediating between Type 1 and Type 2 processes in the process of CR. Without the capacity for metacognition, there would be no way of linking these two cognitive structures and processes in any meaningful way. While the DPT is not an essential building block for the theory of metacognition, at a speculative level DPT and metacognition may be considered to be complementary or even analogous concepts. Proust (2010, p. 996) notes that "noetic feelings" referring to the "subjective, emotional correlates of subpersonal features" might be related to System 1 activation. The metacognitive role of System 2 "might be to provide corrective inferences about one's current abilities, based on conceptual knowledge about mental facts" (p. 996). While a form of metacognition appears indispensable to explain the application of DPT in the practical world, for which CR is exemplary, DPT is not indispensable for the theoretical validity of metacognition. Reflecting deeper on the nature of metacognition in relation with CR provides a window into defining more precisely the role of cognition in CR, as well as the limits of its conceptualization in terms of cognition alone.

Thus, a sustained philosophical analysis of metacognition is essential to understand the epistemology of cognitive structures and processes in CR.

Metacognition and Neurobiology of Decision-making

Proust (2013, p. 1) defines "metacognition" as a "set of capacities through which an operational cognitive system is evaluated or represented by another in a context sensitive way." This definition is intended to be theoretically neutral as far as possible, because the definition of "metacognition" among theorists of cognitive science is still contested. On the one hand, the "inclusivist" position argues that metacognition involves the capacity to attribute mental states to oneself, as well as to others.[6] This approach considers the "meta" in metacognition to be a form of monitoring that is causally related to a mental event as a form of representational knowing. On the other hand, the "exclusivist" position that Proust espouses considers metacognition to be a competence for self-evaluation that is based, at least in part, on nonanalytic knowledge (pp. 3–4). According to Proust's view, metacognition is a form of self-evaluation containing a set of functional features that are independent of those associated with the self-attribution of mental states. Proust bases her defense of the exclusivist conception of metacognition on three main claims. First, she argues that mental and ordinary actions do not possess the same basic normative structure. Second, metacognition conceived as self-evaluation of one's mental properties is a constitutive ingredient of every mental action, but is not part of ordinary basic actions. Third, metacognition is not unique to humans, but is also instantiated in "speechless speeches," as evidenced by nonhuman primates (p. 5). For example, Rhesus monkeys are able to evaluate their ability to discriminate different visual stimuli (Proust, 2010). It has been demonstrated that monkeys like humans can learn complex reasoning involving probabilistic cues (Yang and Shadlen, 2007). This last point is important, because it is Proust's primary aim to demonstrate that metacognition is not solely to be understood in terms of analytic representational knowing. Hence, the importance of noetic feelings for her theory of metacognition. As Proust (2010, p. 8) writes, "the reflexive structure of command and monitoring, and the intervention of epistemic feelings, allow an agent to conduct mental actions on the basis of nonconceptual contents."

Why is this important for the present analysis of CR? While Proust considers the possibility that "noetic feelings" might be associated with Type 1 cognitive processes, she does not argue that metacognitive self-evaluation subsumes these feelings into forms of representational knowing. Rather, metacognition is characterized by the monitoring of mental events through nonconceptual reflexes and contents. Yet, the application of DPT to CR is premised on making Type 1 processes accountable to Type 2 forms of explicit cognition. Thus, while the integrated approach presents an advance in the literature of CR, by ceding an important place to tacit knowing, it still does so in explicit representational terms. The self-evaluative conception of metacognition provides an alternative model that grants equal status to noetic feelings as essential components of the natural kind features that constitute metacognition. A theory of CR that takes seriously this theory of metacognition needs also to grant a more privileged role to forms of tacit knowing. This implies revising the conception of rationality that is used in developing or critiquing a theory of CR. First and foremost, this definition of rationality needs to incorporate the essential temporal uncertainty that is part and parcel of the clinical encounter.

Even though Proust presents a theoretical framework for metacognition, it receives empirical support from recent neurobiological research of decision-making, which is metonymic for aspects of cognition tractable to experimental neuroscience (Shadlen and Kiani, 2013). The approach pioneered by Bill Newsome and Michael Shadlen, which investigates probabilistic decision-making at the level of individual neurons in primates, provides an insight or "window" into human cognition that is of direct relevance for understanding the role and limitations of cognition in a theory of CR (Shadlen and Kiani, 2013). Decision-making at the level of the individual neuron provides parallels with personal decision-making studied by neuropsychology. The probabilistic reasoning of individuals critiqued by decision analysis is premised, though not paralleled, on the probabilistic decision-making at the neuronal level. For example, the field of signal detection theory (SDT) proposes that the "raw representation of evidence gives rise to a 'decision variable' (DV), upon which the brain applies a 'decision rule' to say yes/no, more/less, or category A/B" (p. 792). Additionally, as Shadlen and Kiani note,

> [e]vidence accumulation creates a map linking a DV and the probability that a decision made on the basis of the DV will be correct. The brain appears to have implicit knowledge of this mental architecture, which it then uses to assign a sense of certainty or confidence about the decision. (p. 793)

The DV incorporates signals related to value, time, and prior probability, which "must be 'read out' by neurons that sense thresholds, calculate certainty, and trigger the next step, be it a movement or another decision" (p. 797).

Some important points arise from this neural model of decision-making that bear directly on metacognition. First, different brain modules can operate using "parallel intentional architecture" on the same information, even with divergent results (Shadlen et al., 2008; Shadlen and Kiani, 2013). Second, integrating different neural networks allows processing on an extended time scale that enables the brain of the individual decision-maker to be liberated from the immediacy of sensory events (Shadlen and Kiani, 2013). Long integration time permits the achievement of insights and decisions that would otherwise be unobtainable. Finally, the outcome of a decision might not in fact be an action, but rather the initiation of another decision process. There is a freedom or flexibility inherent to the neural architecture of decision-making that links with sensory information, motor activity, and probabilistic reasoning that while dependent on the determinism of neural activity, also enables a certain "freedom from immediacy." This integrated theory of the brain provides the implicit possibility for metacognition in the sense of the capacity of the brain to "make decisions about decisions about decisions" (p. 800). Moreover, nonconscious cognitive processing is an essential foundation for explicit knowing as well as other behavioral decisions. What may be too little evidence to pass the threshold of conscious awareness may provide sufficient information for subsequent decisions and behavior. In summary, the neurobiological research of decision-making presents scientific support for Proust's self-evaluative theory of metacognition, and demonstrates that there is no simple divide between tacit and explicit knowing. A theory of CR that wishes to incorporate the relation between Type 1 and Type 2 cognitive processes needs likewise to acknowledge the inherent rationality of subliminal cuing, and other preconscious nonanalytic cognitive processes.

Modelling Clinical Reasoning on Phronesis

The neurobiological research on decision-making in primates in relation to metacognition indicates that there is no direct transformation of processes of tacit knowing into explicit cognition. This presents a scientific explanation of what proponents of tacit knowing in medicine have known all along from their clinical experience. Tacit knowing in medicine, for example, as evidenced in the work of Feinstein, represents a form of knowing that includes components that are inferential, but resist explication in the light of day, and processes that are truly prereflective. Marcum's "integrated theory" does not sufficiently take cognizance of this unconscious substrate of CR. Indeed, it is questionable whether conceiving of CR purely in terms of cognition does not limit CR to a form of instrumental rationality. The fundamental question that arises is whether the literature on metacognition refers to another level of cognition, or else instead introduces or points toward a mental event or act of consciousness that is qualitatively different from cognition. Proust (2013) has demonstrated that metacognition cannot be conceived in terms of representation of oneself, analogous to the representation of the mind of another. Similarly, CR presents an intersubjective relation—between the consciousness of doctor and patient—that at times resists abstraction into analyzable components. What then is the fitting conceptual container for this relation? As others and I have argued, conceiving CR as a kind of practical wisdom modeled on Aristotelian *phronesis* provides the most fitting model to depict what good clinicians do when they interact with patients (Pellegrino and Thomasma, 1981; Gatens Robinson, 1986; Widdershoven-Heerding, 1987; Beresford, 1996; McGee, 1996; Montgomery, 2000; Braude, 2012b; Cassell, 2015).

In the *Nicomachean Ethics* Aristotle lists *phronesis* (φρονησις) as one of the intellectual virtues alongside philosophic wisdom, or *sophia* (σοφια), and understanding, or *nous* (νους) (1925, 1103a6). Aristotle notes that practical reasoning requires means of verification that are appropriate for the subject matter at hand.

> For it is the mark of an educated man to look for precision in each class of things just so far as the nature of the subject admits; it is evidently equally foolish to accept probable reasoning from a mathematician and to demand from a rhetorician scientific proofs. (1094b)

Through his understanding of *phronesis*, Aristotle inverts a deep prejudice against privileging theoretical abstraction in Platonic idealism; recognizing that there are simply some domains of human endeavor that resist analytic abstraction but are embodied in the person possessing practical wisdom. As Aristotle writes:

> Regarding *practical wisdom* we shall get at the truth by considering who are the persons we credit with it. Now it is thought to be the mark of a man of practical wisdom to be able to deliberate well about what is good and expedient for himself, not in some particular respect, e.g. about what sorts of thing conduce to health or to strength, but about what sorts of thing conduce to the good life in general. This is shown by the fact that we credit men with practical wisdom in some particular respect when they have calculated well with a view to some good end which is one of those that are not the object of any art. It follows that in the general sense also the man who is capable of deliberating has practical wisdom. Now no one deliberates about things that are invariable, nor about things that it is impossible for him to do. Therefore, since scientific knowledge involves demonstration, but there is no demonstration of things whose first principles are variable (for all such things might actually be otherwise), and since it is impossible to deliberate about things that are of necessity, practical wisdom cannot be scientific knowledge nor art; not science because that which can be done is capable of being otherwise, not art because action and making are different kinds of thing. The remaining alternative, then, is that it is a true and reasoned state

of capacity to act with regard to the things that are good or bad for man. (1140a)

Unpacking the role of *phronesis* in relation to CR merits a much longer study than what can be provided here. Arguably, the most important quality of *phronesis* is its integrative function, in linking different forms of knowing. For Aristotle *phronesis* is distinct from other virtues in being both moral and intellectual. As Edmund Pellegrino and David Thomasma (1981) note, *phronesis* has a vital integrative role in linking the intellectual virtues, such as science (*episteme*), art (*techné*), and intuitive wisdom (*nous*), with the moral virtues such as temperance and courage. Additionally, *phronesis* provides a means of balancing the relation between means and ends by enabling "us to discern which means are most appropriate to the good in particular circumstances" (p. 21). I have argued previously that *phronesis* is a particularly useful model for clinical reasoning because it allows for the possibility of linking and integrating different cognitive processes according to the context, and need of the moment. Different forms of cognition, such as affect, emotion, executive attention, rational cognition, and intuition, may all constitute practical wisdom. Additionally, *phronesis* links the moral, ontological, and epistemological components of clinical medicine into a single framework. Thus, "Modelling clinical reasoning on *phronesis* succeeds in providing a means of integrating the different cognitive components of clinical reasoning, while maintaining respect for the gestalt of clinical reasoning as a particular form of conscious experience" (Braude, 2012a, pp. 947–48).

Phronesis is analogous to metacognition in providing the means to reflect on our human decisions. Yet, it does so without relying on a narrow cognitive rationality that evaluates decisions solely in terms of categories of explicit knowing and representation. Moreover, the integrative function of *phronesis* does more than provide a means of reflecting on our intentions, thoughts, and actions. According to Croskerry (2013), diagnoses and treatment plans are the two major products of clinical decision-making. Yet, CR as a form of *phronesis* does much more than this in expanding CR from a predominantly disease centered approach to include patient subjectivity and clinical experience. This "narrative thinking" that is increasingly considered to be a necessary core skill for clinicians applies both to the patient's personal story over time, as well as the physiological processes associated with the natural history of a particular disease (Cassell, 2015).

In his recent book on *The Nature of Clinical Medicine*, Eric Cassell refers to at least twelve themes that narrative thinking about a particular clinical case should reveal. This list includes:

1. The chain of events that led to the present state.
2. The diagnosis.

3. The causative factors in the illness.
4. Causality in the scientific sense.
5. The patient's purpose and goals and the impairments of function that interfere with their fulfillment.
6. The meanings that the patient has attached to what is happening, or has not occurred.
7. The attitude and emotional reaction of the patient to what has happened.
8. The patient's values.
9. The role that the patient's personality, life, medical history, and personal characteristics play in the illness and its projected outcome.
10. The pace of the disease process or the pathophysiology.
11. The relation of the patient and the doctor.
12. The doctor's relationship with other doctors and the institution. (p. 93)

This list includes reviewing the cognitive biases that might impair the cognitive function of a clinician, yet also highlights the fact that clinical wisdom cannot be adequately contained or explained through cognitive critique alone. The individual patient and the individual clinician and the relationship between them is greater than the sum of its cognitive parts.

Shadlen and Kiani (2013) suggest that the same basic machinery at the single level of the cell may give rise to human narrativity. Furthermore, they suggest that the translation from the outcome of one neural decision to the "engagement" of another circuit provides the basis of subjectivity and narrative. *Phronesis* and metacognition appear to be analogous concepts. Yet, metacognition strictly speaking only refers to the ability to critique and reflect on one's own cognitions. I suggest that the intrasubjective and intersubjective capacity for engagement that is inherent within the concept of metacognition and exemplary in clinical interaction can only be fully understood in relation to *phronesis*. In this sense, *phronesis* is not simply a theoretical concept, but points to a form of lived biological event that cannot be wholly contained in cognition.

This claim is justified through an analysis of the relation between CR as a form of *phronesis* and two forms of human activity and knowing—*poiesis* and *praxis*. These terms were already described by Plato and reconfigured by Aristotle. *Poiesis* refers to any human activity that results in a product external to the human activity itself. The act of making associated with crafts (*techné*) is associated, therefore, with *poiesis*. *Praxis*, on the other hand, is a form of practical activity that is intended to further human well-being or the good, and is not associated with any particular end product external to the act. *Phronesis* is a particularly curious form of knowing, since it is characterized by possessing both these forms of knowing. *Phronesis* demonstrates this dual quality by being concerned with both technical issues and intermediary steps toward the end of action.

In the light of the previous discussion, it is not surprising, therefore, that Aristotle uses the metaphor of medicine as exemplary for the dual nature of *phronesis*. In the *Nicomachean Ethics* (1925), Aristotle cites medicine as a form of practical wisdom whose end is the health of the individual. "Just as medicine does not govern health, but is for the sake of health" (1145a 11). Medicine is an exemplary form of practical wisdom, since in determining what is best for a particular individual technical know-how is necessary but not sufficient. Medicine as a form of practical wisdom resembles *poiesis* in requiring technical expertise to achieve the ends of clinical action. At the same time, this knowledge can never be divorced from the self-knowing associated with *phronesis*, and the inherent temporality of human action.[7]

Medicine is also exemplary for *phronesis* because of the inherent uncertainty associated with medical knowing. This uncertainty, as was mentioned before, derives from the tacit component of CR that resists fully explicit knowing. More fundamentally, this variability is associated with the biological substrate of human temporal life. In dealing with human beings, in their full complexity, and not simply with static disease entities modeled on pathological correlation, clinicians come into close contact with the human life-world. Of all the interpreters of Aristotle, Martin Heidegger (2003) comes close to this understanding in interpreting *phronesis* as a kind of *circumspection about human life* concerned both with technical issues and intermediary steps within its phenomenological horizon as well as the end of action. In this sense, *phronesis* is more than a particular form of cognition, but an instantiation of human-beingness. CR is a particularly privileged form of *phronetic* knowing. It certainly performs an integrative function in integrating different kinds of understanding, tacit and explicit. The analysis of CR uncovers the biological substrate of the human condition, and links human cognition with its underlying cellular machinery. At the same time, the attempt to define CR reveals the chains of interpretation and meaning connecting cellular life and the conscious ability to reflect on these connections through subjective consciousness, metacognition, and narrativity. A comprehensive theory of CR needs to account for this relation between its constitutive parts, while respecting the sum of the whole as it manifests in lived experience of clinical interaction.

Notes

1. My epistemological approach in this chapter arises from the consideration that the lack of conceptual clarity around CR arises from its inherent complexity. Thus, the term CR covers over conceptual tensions between different processes of cognition as well as dichotomies arising from the mind–body relation. For example, the tension between cognition and affect, between explicit and tacit knowing, and between medicine as a technique and as a form of care or discipline of the self.

2. The term "clinical judgment" generally refers to the conclusion of a process of "clinical reasoning." However, in his emphasis on processes involved in clinical decision-making, there is no practical distinction between Feinstein's use of the term "clinical judgment" and what I refer in this chapter to as "clinical reasoning."

3. Feinstein (1967) devoted his academic medical career to applying mathematical concepts to develop a bottom up epistemology of clinical reasoning that developed from the medical context and the treatment of individuals. He was particularly fond of the use of Boolean algebra and Venn diagrams as a "sublime intellectual mechanism for describing the procedures of clinical reasoning" (p. 159). However, the particular mathematical and epidemiological methodologies Feinstein advocated in his attempt to establish a science of CR is secondary to his fundamental insight that clinical judgment depends "not on a knowledge of causes, mechanisms, or names for disease, but on a knowledge of patients" (p. 12). These mathematical and epidemiological tools are valuable in the manner that they provide explicit quantification of clinical data. The moment they become the ends themselves, rather than the means of rendering medicine more scientific, they are no longer justifiably a component of CR, but another unrelated discipline or human endeavor.

4. I have argued elsewhere that clinical intuition "unites different elements such as deductive knowledge, information from observation, past experience with groups of individuals, as well as statistical information" (Braude, 2009, p. 193).

5. In accord with Stanovich, I will henceforth refer to these cognitive phenomena primarily in terms of Type 1 and Type 2 processes rather than systems.

6. See Proust (2013) for a full list of influential theorists who defend the self-attributive view.

7. This analysis of *phronesis* and *techné* in relation *praxis* and *poiesis* is reliant on the distinction emphasized by Martin Heidegger (2003). See also the related discussion on *phronesis* by H. G. Gadamer (1975) and Robert Bernasconi (1989). As Gadamer (1975) and Bernasconi (1989) discuss, it is a deep question whether and how Aristotelian *phronesis* is guided by theoretical understanding. In my own interpretation of *phronesis* (Braude, 2012b) I claim that Aristotle did posit an important role for intuition (*nous*) in his conception of *phronesis*.

References

Aristotle. (1925). *Nicomachean Ethics*, W. D. Ross, trans. Oxford: Clarendon Press.

Balla J., Elstein A. S., and Christensen C. (1989). Obstacles to acceptance of clinical decision analysis. *British Medical Journal* 298(6673): 579–82.

Barrows, H. S., and Feltovich, P. J. (1987). The Clinical reasoning process. *Medical Education* 21: 86–91.

Barrows, H. S., and Tamblyn, R. M. (1980). *Problem Based Learning: An Approach to Medical Education*. New York: Springer.

Beresford, E. B. (1996). Can phronesis save the life of medical ethics? *Theoretical Medicine* 17: 209–24.

Bernasconi, R. (1989). Heidegger's destruction of phronesis. *The Southern Journal of Philosophy* XXVIII(S1): 127–47.

Braude, H. D. (2009). Clinical intuition versus statistics: Different modes of tacit knowledge in clinical epidemiology and evidence-based medicine. *Theoretical Medicine and Bioethics* 30(3): 181–98.

Braude, H. D. (2012a). Conciliating cognition and consciousness: The perceptual foundations of clinical reasoning. *Journal of Evaluation in Clinical Practice* 18: 945–50.

Braude, H. D. (2012b). *Intuition in Medicine: A Philosophical Defense of Clinical Reasoning*. Chicago: The University of Chicago Press.

Braude, H. D. (2013). Human all too human reasoning: Comparing clinical and phenomenological intuition. *The Journal of Medicine and Philosophy* 38(2): 173–89.

Cassell, E. (2015). *The Nature of Clinical Medicine: The Return of the Clinician*. Oxford: Oxford University Press.

Cote S., and St-Cyr Tribble, D. (2012). Clinical reasoning in nursing, concept analysis. [French], *Recherche en Soins Infirmiers* 111: 13–21.

Croskerry P. (2008). Cognitive and affective dispositions to respond. In *Patient Safety in Emergency Medicine*, eds. P. Croskerry, K. Cosby, S. Schenkel, and R. Wears. Philadelphia: Lippincott, Williams and Wilkins, pp. 219–27.

Croskerry, P. (2009). Clinical cognition and diagnostic error: Applications of a dual process model of reasoning. *Advances in Health Science Education* 14: 27–35.

Croskerry, P. (2013). 'From mindless to mindful practice—Cognitive bias and clinical decision making. *The New England Journal of Medicine* 368(286): 2445–48.

Croskerry, P. (2014). Clinical reasoning: How can we teach it? Dalhousie University, Faculty of Medicine Summer Institute, June 5–7, 2014. http://medicine.dal.ca/content/dam/dalhousie/pdf/faculty/medicine/departments/core-units/cpd/P_Croskerry_CR_Can%20We%20Teach%20It.pdf (accessed January 21, 2015).

Croskerry, P., Abbass, A., and Wu, A. (2008). How doctors feel: Affective issues in patient safety. *Lancet* 372: 1205–206.

Croskerry, P., Singhal, G., and Mamede, S. (2013). Cognitive debiasing 2: Impediments to and strategies for change. *BMJ Quality and Safety* 22: ii65–ii72.

Detmer, D., Fryback, D. G., and Gassner, K. (1978). Heuristics and biases in medical decision making. *Journal of Medical Education* 53: 682–83.

Durning, S. J., Artino, A. R., Jr, Schuwirth, L., and van der Vleuten, C. (2013). Clarifying assumptions to enhance our understanding and assessment of clinical reasoning. *Academic Medicine* 88(4): 442–48.

Elstein, A. S. (2000). Clinical problem solving and decision psychology. *Academic Medicine* 75(10): S134–36.

Elstein, A. S. (2009). Thinking about diagnostic thinking: A 30 year perspective. *Advances in Health Sciences Education* 14: 7–18.

Feinstein, A. R. (1967). *Clinical Judgment*. Baltimore, MA: Williams Wilkins.

Feinstein, A. R. (1977). *Clinical Biostatistics*. Saint Louis: C.V. Mosby.

Gadamer, H. G. (1975). *Truth and Method*. New York: Seabury Press.

Gatens Robinson, E. (1986). Clinical judgement and the rationality of the human sciences. *Journal of Medicine and Philosophy* 11: 167–78.

Gigerenzer, G., Swijtink, Z., Porter, T., Beatty, J., and Kruger, L. (1989). *The Empire of Chance: How Probability Changes Science and Everyday Life*. Cambridge: Cambridge University Press.

Heidegger, M. (2003). *Plato's Sophist*, R. Rojcewicz and A. Schuwer, trans. Bloomington and Indianapolis: Indiana University Press.

Henry, S. G. (2010). Polanyi's tacit knowing and the relevance of epistemology to clinical medicine. *Journal of Evaluation in Clinical Practice* 16(2): 292–97.

Hogarth, J. M. (1980). Judgement, drug monitoring, and decision aids. In *Monitoring for Drug Safety*, ed. W. H. W. Lancaster: MTP Press.

Kahneman, D., and Tversky, A. (1972). Subjective probability: A judgement of representativeness. *Cognitive Psychology* 12(4): 430–54.

Kahneman, D., and Tversky, A. (1974). Judgment under uncertainty: Heuristics and biases. *Science* 185: 1124–31.

Marcum, J. A. (2012). An integrated model of clinical reasoning: Dual-process theory of cognition and metacognition. *Journal of Evaluation in Clinical Practice* 18: 954–61.

McGee, G. (1996). Phronesis in clinical ethics. *Theoretical Medicine* 17(4): 317–28.

Montgomery, K. (2000). *Phronesis* and the misdescription of medicine. In *Bioethics: Ancient Themes in Contemporary Issues,* eds. M. G. Kuczewski and R. P. Cambridge, Massachusetts/London, England: The MIT Press, pp. 57–66.

Pellegrino, E., and Thomasma, D. C. (1981). *A Philosophical Basis of Medical Practice.* Oxford: Oxford University Press.

Polanyi, M. (1946). *Science, Faith and Society.* London: Oxford University Press.

Polanyi, M. (1962). *Personal Knowledge: Towards a Post-Critical Philosophy.* London: Routledge and Kegan Paul.

Polanyi, M. (1966). *The Tacit Dimension.* Garden City, NY: Doubleday & Company.

Polanyi, M. (1997). Creative imagination. In *Society, Economics & Philosophy: Selected Papers of Michael Polanyi,* ed. R. T. Allen. New Brunswick: Transaction Publishers, pp. 249–66.

Proust, J. (2010). Metacognition. *Philosophy Compass* 5: 989–98.

Proust, J. (2013). *The Philosophy of Metacognition: Mental Agency and Self-Awareness.* Oxford: Oxford University Press.

Round, A. (2001). Introduction to clinical reasoning. *Journal of Evaluation in Clinical Practice* 7(2): 109–17.

Shadlen, M. N., and Kiani, R. (2013). Decision making as a window on cognition. *Neuron* 80: 791–806.

Shadlen, M. N., Kiani, R., Hanks, T. D., and Churchland, A. K. (2008). Neurobiology of decision making: An intentional framework. In *Better Than Conscious? Decision Making, the Human Mind and Implications for Institutions,* eds. C. Engel and W. Singer. Cambridge: The MIT Press, pp. 71–102.

Stanovich, K. E. (2011). *Rationality and the Reflective Mind.* New York: Oxford University Press.

Stewart, P. (Justice) (1964), 378 U.S., 197.

Widdershoven-Heerding, I. (1987). Medicine as a form of practical understanding. *Theoretical Medicine* 8: 179–85.

Wilczak, P. F. (1973). *Faith, Motive, and Community: An Interpretation of the Philosophy of Michael Polanyi.* Divinity School: The University of Chicago.

Yang, T., and Shadlen, M. N. (2007). Probabilistic reasoning by neurons. *Nature* 447: 1075–89.

14 New Directions in Philosophy of Medicine

Jacob Stegenga, Ashley Graham Kennedy, Şerife Tekin, Saana Jukola, and Robyn Bluhm

Introduction

As we have seen from the previous chapters, philosophy of medicine is a dynamic area of research, raising, and seeking to answer, a plethora of metaphysical, practical, and moral questions in medicine. Such questions are of importance not just for their intrinsic philosophical interest, but also because they have implications for medical research, practice, and policy. Recent work in philosophy of medicine has addressed such questions as the appropriate evidence base for medicine, the nature and definition of "health" and of "disease," and the relative contributions of scientific research and patients' experiences to an understanding of medical questions.

The purpose of this chapter is to describe what we see as several important new directions for philosophy of medicine. This recent work (i) takes existing discussions in important and promising new directions, (ii) identifies areas that have not received sufficient and deserved attention to date, and/or (iii) brings together philosophy of medicine with other areas of philosophy (including bioethics, philosophy of psychiatry, and social epistemology). To this end, the next part focuses on what we call the "epistemological turn" in recent work in the philosophy of medicine; the third part addresses new developments in medical research that raise interesting questions for philosophy of medicine; the fourth part is a discussion of philosophical issues within the practice of diagnosis; the fifth part focuses on the recent developments in psychiatric classification and scientific and ethical issues therein, and the final part focuses on the objectivity of medical research.

The Epistemological Turn

Some of the best scholarship in philosophy of medicine in the past two decades has been about the epistemology of medical research. This is a welcome development after a period in which much good work in philosophy of medicine was focused on conceptual topics, most notably analyses of health and disease, or normative topics, especially ethical issues that arise in medical practice. Philosophers such as John Worrall, Nancy Cartwright, Alex Broadbent, Kirstin Borgerson, Phyllis Illari, and Jeremy Howick have been at the forefront of this turn to epistemology in the philosophy of medicine. Two of the most prominent topics in the epistemological turn were the epistemic merits of randomized controlled trials (RCTs) and the role of mechanisms in grounding various sorts of causal claims. Here we describe four ways in which present and future work in the philosophy of medicine has been and will continue to develop this turn toward epistemology.

Some of the central epistemological debates in philosophy of medicine have been about the epistemic status of RCTs and systematic reviews. RCTs are considered to be one of the pillars of the evidence-based medicine (EBM) movement, and systematic reviews are also placed at the top of EBM evidence hierarchies. However, both have recently been the targets of philosophical criticism (Worrall, 2002, 2007; Borgerson, 2009; Stegenga, 2011). Other philosophers suggest that knowledge of mechanisms can aid in making causal inferences, while theoreticians in the EBM movement tend to hold that reasoning from mechanisms is too often unreliable (Howick, 2011a; Russo and Williamson, 2007). These EBM methodological principles and their associated philosophical critiques have tended to articulate epistemological merits and vices at a rather coarse grain: is randomization necessary to support reliably causal hypotheses in medicine? Is meta-analysis the platinum standard of evidence? Is knowledge of mechanisms necessary to infer causation or to warrant extrapolation? Such questions could be fruitfully addressed at a finer grain.

An example of a fine-grained approach to methodology is the assessment of particular details of RCTs rather than arguing about the merits of randomization generally. Likewise, McClimans (2013) investigates the various measurement instruments employed in RCTs, thereby unpacking details about RCTs left unanalyzed when the merits of RCTs simpliciter are debated. Similarly, rather than argue about the merits of meta-analysis tout court, as Stegenga (2011) does, one could articulate the ways in which meta-analyses can be better or worse. Or, to take another example, rather than arguing whether knowledge of mechanisms is necessary for causal inferences in medicine, one could attempt to formulate precisely how mechanisms can aid in causal inferences and extrapolation from experimental populations to target populations. Steel (2007), for example, argues that "comparative process tracing" of mechanisms can aid in extrapolating causal knowledge.

Another example of fine-grained approaches in the epistemological turn is evidence hierarchies. Arguments for and against the standard evidence hierarchies have recently been articulated (Howick, 2011b; Stegenga, 2014). But

Osimani (forthcoming) argues that different kinds of hypotheses, such as hypotheses about harms of medical interventions, require different kinds of evidence compared to hypotheses about benefits of medical interventions; thus, general arguments about the justification of EBM evidence hierarchies might be too coarse-grained. Indeed, changing the metaphor, Bluhm (2005) argues that evidence hierarchies should be replaced by evidence networks, to take into account the rich information that various types of studies in clinical research can provide. One final example is the ways in which recent trial designs attempt to take into account some of the complexities of clinical practice. In short, a fine-grained analysis of the methodological details of medical research is on the forefront of the epistemological turn in philosophy of medicine.

The second aspect of the epistemological turn in philosophy of medicine involves articulating the intersection between social, ethical, and methodological aspects of medical research. An example of such a concern of present (and future) work in philosophy of medicine is to articulate the methodological and social conditions under which many of the problems of medical research are possible. For example (Jukola, 2015; see also the end of this chapter), argues that a compelling way to understand the shortcomings of meta-analysis requires not just an examination of the methodological details of meta-analysis, but also an examination of the social context in which this technique is employed. As another example, De Melo-Martin and Intemann (2011) argue for a feminist approach to understanding problems with contemporary biomedical research. A different sort of interest regarding the relationship between social, ethical, and methodological aspects of medical research investigates the influence that social or ethical values can have on the production and interpretation of evidence. In a widely discussed paper, Douglas (2000) argues for the central role of values in scientific reasoning, and this thesis is especially prominent in medical research. For example, Kennedy (2013) argues that ethics and evidence are "intertwined" in the practice of differential diagnosis. As another example, Tekin (2014) argues that psychiatric nosology is "at the crossroads of science and ethics."

In the past decade, there have been many proclamations of a thesis that one could call "medical nihilism." Various versions of medical nihilism emphasize the lack of reproducibility of many high-profile research findings in medicine, the nefarious activities of medical scientists associated with pharmaceutical companies, and perhaps most troubling, the low effectiveness of the vast majority of recent pharmaceuticals. Contributors to this literature include prominent physicians, epidemiologists, and journalists. Recent examples include books by Marcia Angell (2004), Moynihan and Cassels (2005), Carl Elliott (2010), Ben Goldacre (2012), and Peter Gøtzsche (2013), and articles by epidemiologists such as John Ioannidis, Lisa Bero, Peter Jüni, and Jan Vandenbroucke. A third task for present philosophy of medicine in the epistemological turn is to assess just how deep and troubling the thesis of medical nihilism is. Stegenga (forthcoming), for example, argues that medical nihilism is a compelling thesis for much of recent medicine.

Medical nihilism is motivated, in part, by noting problems with the sociopolitical nexus in which medical research takes place. A fourth set of concerns for present and future philosophy of medicine in the epistemological turn is to address questions such as: How should medical research be modulated given the recent work on epistemology of such research? Who should pay for medical research? What kinds of projects should be prioritized by funders of medical research? Should the results and products of medical research be protected by intellectual property laws? As an example of recent work in this domain, Brown (2008) argues that medical research should be socialized and the results of medical research should not be protected by patent laws. A broadly similar proposal is suggested by Reiss (2010). The epistemological turn has uncovered numerous epistemological problems with contemporary medical research, and such problems call for normative guidance.

In what follows, we discuss some of these elements of the epistemological turn in the philosophy of medicine in more detail, including issues related to evidence hierarchies, extrapolation, diagnosis, the construction of psychiatric categories, and the pursuit of objectivity in medical research.

Beyond RCTs and Meta-analyses

In addition to these recent developments in philosophy of medicine, there are a number of developments in medical research itself that should be of interest to philosophers. As noted earlier, much of the work being done on philosophical questions raised by clinical research has examined RCTs. This is in large part due to the influence of EBM and, in particular, to its "hierarchy of evidence," which stipulates that the best quality evidence comes from RCTs and systematic reviews of RCTs. The rationale behind the hierarchy of evidence is that designs higher on the hierarchy have greater internal validity and more precision in their estimates of outcomes than those lower on the hierarchy. Yet, as critics of EBM have pointed out, this precision may come at the cost of generalizability. First, because many RCTs have strict inclusion and exclusion criteria, many of the patients who might be treated with a drug in clinical practice would not have qualified for participation in the trial that tested that drug. Second, because RCTs compare average outcomes in the treatment and the control groups for a study, they give little information about differences in outcomes among the patients in the study. Meta-analyses exacerbate this problem, since they usually average the (average) results across studies to get a more precise estimate of outcomes.

While EBM itself has not tended to acknowledge the gravity of these problems, there have been a number of recent trends in medical research that have attempted to address the issue of variable treatment outcomes, either by conducting research in a setting that more closely resembles clinical practice or by studying outcomes specifically in groups of patients who have a particular demographic or physiological characteristic. This section surveys several of these trends and outlines their potential interest for philosophers of medicine.

Research Generalizability and Clinical Care

RCTs with strict inclusion and exclusion criteria tend to be so-called explanatory trials, which aim to provide evidence that an intervention causes an outcome of interest by showing that, in carefully controlled, "ideal" conditions, a therapeutic intervention provides better outcomes than a placebo control (Thorpe et al., 2009). The strength of these trials is that they are considered to provide evidence that the experimental intervention causes the outcomes(s) being measured; this is because the trial is designed to ensure that, as far as possible, the only difference between the treatment and the control groups is that the treatment group receives the intervention being tested. An efficient way to show differences between study groups is to minimize variability *within* groups. To achieve this, explanatory studies have strict inclusion and exclusion criteria; for example, limiting eligibility to a narrow age range and enrolling only patients with no comorbid conditions, who are not taking concomitant medications. As a result of these decisions about study eligibility, subjects who qualify for participation in explanatory trials are different in important respects from typical patients who are treated in clinical practice. It is therefore not clear how well causal relationships between treatment and outcome observed in subjects enrolled in explanatory studies might hold up in other kinds of patients.

Because of this, greater attention is now being paid to research that is more closely integrated with clinical practice. In a 2007 workshop report, the US Institute of Medicine called for the development of a "learning healthcare system," defined as a system of healthcare "in which knowledge generation is so embedded into the core of the practice of medicine that it is a natural outgrowth and product of the healthcare delivery process and leads to continual improvement in care." Although the workshop addressed a broad range of issues, one key point made was that RCTs are not sufficient to inform clinical practice, in part because of the concerns about generalizability noted earlier.

Learning healthcare systems would conduct a variety of kinds of research, including long-term observational studies and studies using administrative databases and patient records. They would still conduct RCTs, but these studies would tend to be pragmatic rather than explanatory; that is, they would be designed to reflect the conditions in which an intervention is used in practice, rather than an idealized test environment. Pragmatic trials, for example, tend to enroll a broader range of patients than explanatory trials, as well as to involve physicians working in a wider variety of care settings. They may also, unlike explanatory trials, allow variability in treatment protocol.

While some studies that take a more pragmatic approach to research design are RCTs, others may examine outcomes in the context of actual clinical practice, for example, examining patient records or using nonrandomized designs to follow patients who receive an intervention of interest. Thorpe et al. (2009) categorize these as pragmatic features; they have developed a tool that characterizes study designs along a number of dimensions to determine whether they are more explanatory or more pragmatic in design, or even whether those studies are RCTs.

This spectrum of research designs raises interesting epistemological and ethical questions for philosophers of medicine. For example, work in research ethics has traditionally taken it to be the case that a sharp distinction can be made between research and clinical practice, but this can no longer be assumed. For example, according to Thorpe et al. (2009), one pragmatic feature a study could have is tracking patient outcomes over the long term using healthcare records (which is something generally done in the context of clinical practice) rather than using the kind of formal follow-up that is the norm in clinical research. Philosophers of medicine may also be interested in elucidating the strengths and weaknesses of different kinds of studies, building on the body of work that examines the epistemology of EBM. Work in this area will also have implications for research ethics, as it challenges the traditional research/practice distinction that is the foundation of the Belmont Report (United States, 1978; see also Largent et al., 2011; Kass et al., 2012).

Tracking Outcomes within Specific Patient Groups

A number of other developments in clinical research are related to the second problem identified with respect to RCTs, that is, the fact that RCTs tend to look only at average outcomes in the treatment and in the control groups. We briefly survey three of these developments here: gender medicine, "basket trials," and the US National Institutes of Mental Health's Research Domain Criteria (RDoC). These examples come from different areas of medicine and also differ in the kind of characteristics they use to "sort" patients into relevantly similar groups. While these examples are not concerned directly with treatment outcomes, they do aim ultimately to improve health interventions by ensuring that they target only groups of patients in which there is a higher-than-average chance of benefit. One reason for this broad development in clinical research is that most new drugs being developed have very low treatment effects (a problem that has contributed to the medical nihilism mentioned earlier); the hope is that particular groups of patients might experience better results.

Gender medicine (also known as gender-specific medicine) has developed in order to understand better the effects of sex and gender differences on health.[1] This includes "prevention, clinical signs, therapeutic approach, prognosis, psychological and social impact" (Baggio et al., 2013). As with anything that focuses on differences between women and men, gender medicine includes not only biological dimensions but also social and political dimensions. Traditionally, clinical research has been conducted mainly on men, on the grounds that women's hormone cycles present a serious confounding factor that complicates the interpretation of data. In 1982, Rebecca Dresser pointed out that medical research was conducted almost entirely on white men, and she argued that the near exclusion of other demographic groups was both ethically and epistemologically problematic. With regard to women in particular, she noted that in addition to the resulting lack of knowledge of diseases that affect only women (e.g., uterine cancer), women and men can have physiological differences that influence both the manifestations of disease and response to treatment. Currently, in the United States, the NIH requires studies to enroll participants from different demographic groups, so that study samples are more representative of the population. There is disagreement, however, about the epistemological value of analyzing treatment outcomes in different subgroups of participants in an RCT; gender medicine takes a clear stance on this issue by recommending that potential outcome differences between women and men be examined.

Another attempt to develop more clinically useful groupings of patients comes from oncology research. "Basket trials" are designed to provide quick information about the efficacy of drugs in groups of patients who have a specific, usually rare, mutation—regardless of the histology of the tumors. These studies build on evidence that, even in trials of therapies that do not appear to be effective in treating cancer, a small number of patients may respond to the therapy, sometimes quite dramatically. These patients were found to have similar mutations, suggesting that new treatments may target specific genetic markers (Lynch et al., 2004). Trials that utilize these findings enroll patients who have a particular mutation, and then group patients with the same kind of cancer into smaller "baskets" within the bigger trial. In some cases treatments are effective across different cancer types, although in others the picture is more complicated. For example, vemurfenib has been approved for treatment of melanoma, in which a mutation called *BRAF* V600E is fairly common. The drug is not effective in treating colorectal cancer associated with this mutation, but may be effective for metastatic papillary thyroid cancer (Willyard, 2013). More recently, it has been suggested that, based on the molecular mechanisms involved, vemurfenib may be effective for treatment of colorectal cancer when used as part of a combination therapy (Prahallad et al., 2012). This work suggests that understanding the relationship between tumor type and mutation type may be important. Although advocates believe that basket trials have the promise to revolutionize cancer treatment, it should be noted that the available evidence is still very scant.

The most radical attempt to find new ways of grouping patients is the RDoC project, which aims to replace current, symptom-based diagnostic categories—and, by extension, prognostic and treatment categories—with new diagnostic groups that are rooted in genetics, behavioral sciences, and, especially, neuroscience.[2] The RDoC framework consists of a matrix, in which the rows represent constructs that are "the fundamental unit of analysis" in the National Institutes of Mental Health (NIMH) framework and which describe specific dimensions of psychological functioning, such as reward learning, cognitive performance monitoring, and attachment formation and maintenance. The columns of the matrix reflect units or levels of analysis (e.g., genes, cells, neural circuits, self-reports) and the cells of the matrix contain information about which specific genes (etc.) have been shown to be relevant to the construct. The NIMH notes explicitly that this may entail that patients with different diagnoses (according to the current system), but similar functional impairments related to a construct, may end up qualifying for the same research study. Similarly, using constructs as the basic categorization may entail that among patients with the same diagnosis, only some will be eligible for a study that examines a particular construct.

The NIMH notes that the RDoC project is still in its preliminary stages, and very much open to revision (including the possible addition of new constructs). It also notes that the true test of the framework as a whole and of particular constructs is their clinical usefulness: "the critical test is how well the new molecular and neurobiological parameters predict prognosis and treatment" (Insel et al., 2010). At the same time, it is clear that the NIMH is betting that the biological approach is the best way to achieve progress in psychiatry and to overcome the limitations of the current symptom-based approach. "If we assume that the clinical syndromes based on subjective symptoms are unique and unitary disorders, we undercut the power of biology to identify illnesses linked to pathophysiology and we limit the development of more specific treatments" (National Institutes of Mental Health, RDoC website).

Initiatives like RDoC, basket trials, and gender medicine raise philosophically interesting questions about the establishment of prognostic (and, particularly in the case of RDoC, of diagnostic) groups. For example, they may inform the debates in philosophy of medicine about the role of knowledge of mechanisms in clinical research and in patient care, which may ideally take the "fine-grained" approach to medical epistemology we have described earlier.

Diagnosis

Compared with discussions of clinical research on treatments, which has also been the primary focus of the previous sections of this chapter, there is less philosophical work on diagnosis. This represents a significant research gap, as diagnosis is of pivotal importance in medical practice, and as such is the starting point of the clinical encounter. Before treatment or prognostic evaluation of a patient can begin, there must be at least a working diagnosis. If a clinician does not begin the clinical encounter by working to obtain an accurate diagnosis, then subsequent treatments prescribed for the patient are likely to fail, and prognoses to be inaccurate. In light of the important role of diagnosis in medical practice, it might seem somewhat surprising that the philosophy of medicine literature on diagnosis is sparse. A recent survey, for example, found that of the 627 articles published over a 10-year span in the two main philosophy of medicine journals, *Journal of Medicine and Philosophy* and *Theoretical Medicine and Bioethics*, only 4 included a discussion of diagnosis (Stempsey, 2008). Addressing this research gap is another new area in which philosophers of medicine are beginning to work. There are many issues in diagnosis and diagnostics that have as yet to benefit from philosophical attention. In the next section, we note a few of them and then examine one in detail: the question of how to evaluate the medical worth of a diagnostic test.

Philosophical Questions in Diagnostic Practice

Philosophical questions in diagnostic practice can be roughly divided between those that concern diagnostic *reasoning* and those that concern *diagnostics* (tests and procedures that are used in the process of medical diagnosis). In the first category, there are questions of whether there is a logic of diagnosis, and if so, whether this logic is computable, and whether the diagnostic reasoning process is generalizable.

In the second category, which we examine more closely here, the questions concern the diagnostic tests and procedures themselves, and how they should be evaluated. In the first instance, diagnostic tests need to be evaluated for accuracy. However, even once a diagnostic test is determined to be relatively accurate, the question of whether it is valuable remains. In order to answer this question, one needs at least a working theory of what counts as valuable in the medical context. Thus the process of determining the medical worth of a diagnostic test has both epistemic and ethical components.

Diagnostic Accuracy and Patient Outcomes

Before we can determine whether a diagnostic test is valuable, we must first determine whether the test is accurate. Currently, there is discussion in the medical literature[3] about the best way to determine diagnostic accuracy. While, as we have seen, RCTs are considered by the EBM movement to be the gold standard for determining both *treatment* and *prevention* efficacy, until recently they have not been used to determine test accuracy. However, RCTs are now being used, for example, to determine whether one diagnostic test is more accurate (i.e., more sensitive and specific) than another. This can be done, for instance, to test the comparative accuracy of a new, or lesser used, diagnostic test against the currently accepted clinical reference standard (the test that is deemed to be the most reliable available test for diagnosing a given condition).[4] For example, one might be interested in determining the comparative accuracy of duplex ultrasonography versus angiography (the clinical reference standard) for diagnosing arterial stenosis in patients presenting with cervical bruit. As the sensitivity and specificity of diagnostic tests such as these can vary across population subgroups, the two tests must be evaluated in comparable groups, one of which is randomized to receive the older test, and the other of which is randomized to receive the newer test. Or, the trial could be designed so that the same group receives both tests (Bossuyt et al., 2006).

Once a diagnostic test's degree of accuracy is determined, that is, once it is found to provide reliable information about the condition in question, it must still be determined whether the test is worth using. Even when a diagnostic is accurate, this does not guarantee that it might improve patient outcomes. In fact, the information gained from diagnostic testing alone never has a direct impact on patient outcomes (although it can have positive or negative indirect effects, see, for instance, Cournoyea and Kennedy (2014))—only diagnostic, treatment, and preventative *decisions* made subsequent to obtaining test results have this kind of impact. Thus while the result (accurate or inaccurate) of a diagnostic test might in turn lead to a decision that has an impact on the patient, the information generated by the test alone does not have this power. Some have argued that, because of this, we ought not only to be concerned with determining test accuracy, but also with finding out whether performing a test ultimately improves the lives of patients. In order to determine this, we need to know whether a given diagnostic test is a good predictor, not only of the condition it is intended to diagnose, but also of treatment outcomes for this condition. This information can, at least in theory, be determined via clinical trial evaluation. However, just how to design a trial that reliably provides this information is not immediately straightforward. The reason for this is that, unlike in the case of treatment trials,[5] in the case of trials of the impact of a diagnostic on patient outcomes, the evaluation is not of the test alone, but rather of the way in which the test guides treatment decisions that will in turn affect the patient. Thus, a trial of the impact of a diagnostic test on patient outcomes is really a trial of the *test plus treatment* (and perhaps also of cost, impact of the information gained on the patient, etc.). In other words, while we can test the accuracy of one diagnostic against the accuracy of another, this, in itself, does not constitute a measure of the effect of the test on a patient.

Various ways have been suggested for designing trials that might yield reliable information about the way that diagnostic tests affect patients. One central concern in designing these trials is the decision of when or where to randomize. Different quantities might be measured depending upon whether one decides to randomize before the decision is made to perform the test being evaluated (in which case it would not be possible to distinguish between treatment versus prognostic value of the test), versus after deciding to perform the test but prior to test result (in which case the test results would not need to be revealed to investigators or participants), versus after receiving the test result, and then randomizing to treatment (for instance, only those who test positive for the condition in question, in which case investigators and trial participants would know the test results). In designing a test plus treatment trial in order to determine the effect of a diagnostic on patient outcomes, one must first decide exactly what is to be measured before deciding upon when to randomize the trial.

Diagnostics and Medical Value

Related to the question of the relationship between an accurate diagnostic and patient impact is the question of whether a diagnostic test or procedure can be considered valuable when it has no direct effect on patient outcome. For example, one might ask whether an accurate diagnostic test for an untreatable disease has any medical worth.[6] This question is, at least in part, an ethical one, and is currently debated within the medical community. While it has been established that many patients do want to know what is wrong with them, even when a treatment for their illness or condition is not available, clinicians are divided over whether an accurate test for an untreatable disease should ever be performed (Lijmer and Bossuyt, 2009). To resolve this issue depends upon how we understand value in the medical context—for example, whether we believe that value is tied inextricably to patient outcomes or whether we believe that a test that provides knowledge is valuable even when it does not lead to improved patient health. Some clinicians have explicitly argued that what makes a test valuable *for the patient* is not its degree of correspondence with the truth—that is, they argue that diagnostic value is not in accurate diagnosis alone, but in whether that diagnosis, and subsequent treatment, can prevent the patient from suffering (Lijmer and Bossuyt, 2009). The argument is that patients undergoing a diagnostic test for arterial stenosis, for example, are not interested simply in knowing whether they have the condition, but in whether treating the condition might prevent a cerebrovascular episode.

The above issue cannot be addressed solely by an analysis of diagnostic accuracy. Instead, both the test's predictive and prognostic value must be evaluated as well. But this is an example of a condition that *is* treatable, and one might argue that while it is clear that in such a case the patient would be interested not only in a diagnosis but also in a treatment for the condition diagnosed, in other cases the patient's interests might not be as clear. Consider, for instance, the question of whether a predictive genetic test for Huntington's disease has medical worth. The test can be given to a healthy person with a family history of the disease and then allows the person to know whether he or she will develop the disease in the future. The test is very accurate; however, since there is no currently available treatment for Huntington's disease, it is arguable whether it has any medical value. On the one hand, one might argue that there is value in simply knowing one's future health fate. On the other hand, one could argue that since medicine is an applied practice that aims at improving patient health, and that, further, operates under limited resources, it would be a waste of both time and monetary resources to perform a test that will not in any way improve the health outcome of the patient. Thus, a determination of the worth of a diagnostic test is complex and depends not only on a determination of accuracy, but also on an estimation of the resulting value of performing the test, and this estimation may differ depending on how one analyzes value.

In summary, diagnostic reasoning and testing is a new area of research within the field of philosophy of medicine, and the questions to be analyzed in this area are both varied and complex, in many cases containing both epistemic and ethical, as well as theoretical and applied, components.

New Directions in Philosophy of Psychiatry

In contrast to other areas of philosophy of medicine, questions about diagnosis have been of central concern in the philosophy of psychiatry. More generally, the relationship between philosophy of psychiatry and philosophy of medicine is not as close as it perhaps should be. This state of affairs may reflect the general relationship between psychiatry and the rest of medicine. There is an ongoing debate about whether, why, and to what extent psychiatry is distinct from medicine. Some people argue that psychiatry is conceptually no different than other branches of medicine (Guze, 1992), though they may acknowledge that our relatively poor understanding of the pathophysiology of mental illness entails that, in practice, psychiatry faces distinct challenges. Others argue that psychiatry is, and will always be, importantly different than other areas of medicine (Laing, 1985). We believe that there could be a productive exchange of ideas between philosophy of psychiatry and philosophy of medicine; however, this discussion is beyond the scope of the chapter. Here, we will focus on questions relevant to psychiatric diagnosis.

Mental illness is an urgent and growing public health problem, contributing to the global burden of disease throughout the world. Vast deficiencies in mental healthcare across the globe are matched by ongoing controversy over the nature, causes, and best treatments for disorders such as schizophrenia and depression. Mental disorder, its nature, its research, and its care have been of interest not only to philosophers who are concerned about the nature of the mind, and in the scientific explanation of complex human phenomena, such as mental disorders, but also to philosophers of medicine and ethicists who focus on issues relevant to the development of effective and ethical treatment of mental disorders (Gupta, 2014).

The goal of this section is to outline the issues concerning the scientific and ethical issues surrounding the psychiatric classification systems, as they have become the focus of increased controversy leading to and following the publication of the fifth edition of the Diagnostic and Statistical Manual of Mental Disorders (DSM-5) (American Psychiatric Association, 2013). The DSM-5 offers the standard criteria for classification of mental disorders. It is designed for pragmatic use across a variety of settings to accomplish a plethora of tasks: to facilitate clinical treatment; to develop educational programs about mental illness; to provide clear criteria of eligibility for various administrative and policy related purposes, including the determination of insurance coverage and disability aid; and to further scientific research into mental disorder etiology, psychopharmacology, and forensics. One core concern that stems from the multiplicity of the purposes assigned to the DSM-5 is its questionable capacity in fully fulfilling these roles. This concern, which is getting stronger following the publication of the DSM-5, focuses on its usefulness in the clinical context during the diagnosis and treatment of mental disorders, and utility for advancing research on the etiology of mental disorders. With respect to clinical use, we highlight the problems associated with its symptom-based approach to classifying mental disorders. For instance, this feature has led to the removal of the bereavement exclusion criterion from the major depression category, allowing complicated grief to be diagnosed as depression on the grounds that grief related distress and depression are manifest through the same symptoms. We then turn to research related limitations of the DSM-5. Here we also review

RDoC, the alternative schema for psychiatric research created by the NIMH, as an alternative to the DSM-5 for research purposes.

A core concern about the fitness of the DSM-5 for clinical purposes is the descriptive approach to mental disorder classifications, in which mental disorders are individuated through symptoms and signs, as opposed to focusing on the individual's experience as a complex and multidimensional person (Sadler, 2005; Radden, 2009; Tekin, 2015; Tekin and Mosko, 2015). The symptom-based classification of mental disorders was adopted in the DSM-III (1980) and guided both the DSM-IV (1994) and the recently published DSM-5 (2013). The development of this approach was an expression of psychiatry's move toward an evidence-based scientific framework, away from the etiological approaches of the DSM-I (1952) and the DSM-II (1968). These earlier approaches relied on empirically undefended theoretical assumptions about the workings of the mind, rather than outwardly observable disease correlates. Mental disorders, also called "reactions" in these manuals, were represented in relation to the causal factors thought to underlie them (American Psychiatric Association, 1952). These causal factors were described in the framework of psychoanalysis and taken either to be a dysfunction in the brain or a general difficulty in adaptation to environmental stressors due to unresolved sexual conflicts of childhood.

In the DSM-III, a descriptive approach replaced this framework because clusters of symptoms and signs, by virtue of their observability and measurability, were thought to facilitate objective scientific research and reliable clinical diagnosis. A scientifically valid category of mental disorder requires external validators, such as symptoms and signs, not simply theories (Robins and Guze, 1970). Thus, symptom and sign clusters were resourceful constructs for scientists whose goal was to investigate better the neurological and genetic underpinnings of mental illness. The proponents of the descriptive approach have first come up with a broad list of signs and symptoms individuating mental disorders, knowing that these are only abstractions and that they do not capture the full complexity of mental disorders. The hope was that as psychiatry progressed symptoms and signs would be better delineated and more refined categories might be developed. However, this did not happen; rather the characterization of mental disorders as symptom clusters remained. The categories have departed further from the complex and real experiences of individuals with mental disorders.

One significant disadvantage of operationalizing a symptom-based approach is that the symptom clusters fail to represent certain complexities involved in mental disorder, which are neither immediately observable nor readily measurable. In a mental disorder experience, the individual's relationship with herself, her physical environment, and her social environment is strained or severed, adding many layers of complexities to mental disorders. These include the developmental trajectory of mental disorder in the individual from childhood to adulthood; the individual's particular life history; interpersonal relationships; biological and environmental risk factors; gender, race, and socioeconomic status; the first-person-specific dimension of the symptoms, such as what the individual hears when she hears voices; and the meaning the individual ascribes to these elements of life in her sociocultural context. DSM-5 categories, by virtue of highlighting symptoms, abstract (or bracket) the self-related and context-specific aspects with mental disorders. By saying little about how the disorder experience is integrated into the patient's life, the categories are simply a "repertoire of behavior" (Radden, 2009). Such neglect of the complexity of the experiences of those with mental disorders has jeopardized the DSM-5's project as an effective tool for clinical diagnosis and treatment.

These worries are escalated with the DSM-5's removal of the bereavement exclusion criterion from the depression category, which allows an individual experiencing complicated grief to be diagnosed as having depression. The argument for this change is as follows: since there are significant overlaps between symptoms and signs of depression and the experiences of those experiencing complicated grief, and science, there is no scientific evidence for characterizing bereavement related distress and depression as distinct conditions; hence, whatever treatment helps the latter might also help the former (Zisook and Kendler, 2007; Zisook et al., 2001). Those arguing against the change insist that the cited evidence base is slim and that there are significant differences between complicated grief and depression (Horwitz and Wakefield, 2007; Wakefield and First, 2012; Kleinman, 2012; Frances, 2013; Wakefield, 2015). Concerns have also been raised about the clinical efficacy of this change, with the argument that folding complicated grief into depression does not facilitate the development of psychotherapeutic approaches to address complicated grief clinically (Tekin, 2015; Tekin and Mosko, 2015).

The DSM-5 has also not satisfied those interested in developing a psychiatric taxonomy system that advances research in psychiatry. Just before the publication of the DSM-5 in 2013, the NIMH abandoned the DSM-5 for research purposes (Insel and Lieberman, 2013). The argument put forward was that the DSM-5 categories are not sufficient for research purposes because they lack validity, and that a diagnostic system aiming to scrutinize mental illness should more directly reflect modern neuroscience, as "mental illness will be best understood as disorders of brain structure and function that implicate specific domains of cognition, emotion, and behavior" (Insel and Lieberman, 2013).

As an alternative to the DSM-5, the NIMH announced the RDoC project, which attempts to create a new conceptual framework to describe psychiatric research. RDoC brings together the resources provided by various basic sciences, including genetics and neuroscience. It lays out a model of basic psychological capacities that are believed to uncover the biological mechanisms underlying psychopathology. Instead of organizing psychopathology into DSM-5 categories like schizophrenia and major depressive disorder, the RDoC explicates psychopathology in terms of basic psychological processes (e.g., declarative memory, perception) and their underlying biological mechanisms.

Insel and Lieberman (2013) provide three fundamental tenets of the RDoC. First, RDoC is a diagnostic approach based on biology, not on observable signs and symptoms. Second, it takes mental disorders to be biological disorders involving brain circuitry that implicate the specific domains of cognition, emotion, or behavior. It is expected that scientists can better identify and investigate the circuits implicated in mental illness as neuroscience and genetics advance. Third, the mapping of the cognitive, circuit, and genetic aspects of mental disorders can yield new and better targets for treatment.

The success of RDoC as a useful guide for research remains to be determined, as the NIMH task force works to complete the project. Skeptics question the ability of RDoC to rescue psychiatry from its crisis, suggesting that it would fail to increase validity as it is grounded on assumptions about how the brain works rather than on actual scientific facts about the complex mechanisms by which the brain operates (Hoffman and Zachar, in press). Some critics have suggested that the primacy of neuroscientific and genetic research in psychopathology continues an unfortunate trend that ignores the crucial role of the phenomenology of mental illness, and this may have negative implications for treatment (Graham and Flanagan, 2013). Finally, some critics worry that the developers of the RDoC are making the same mistake as those who were instrumental in developing the symptom-based criteria for mental disorders. As discussed earlier, the proponents of the descriptive approach characterized mental disorders through a list of signs and symptoms, knowing that these are only abstractions and that they do not capture the full complexity of mental disorders. However, as the DSM project evolved, they dropped the recognition that such characterizations are abstractions, leaving the categories of mental disorders further away from the true complexities of mental disorders. Similarly, the worry is that the RDoC's proposed molecular and neurobiological mental disorder parameters, which are expected to be better identified and investigated as neuroscience and genetics develop, may be uncritically accepted as the true targets of research (Bluhm, in press), leading to disorientation in the field of psychiatric research.

Objectivity and Medical Research

A final area that we want to highlight as an important new direction in philosophy of medicine is that of the objectivity of medical research. We noted earlier that philosophy of medicine is beginning to take account of the relationship between medical research and the broader social context within which it occurs. The social context of medical research, in part, helps to constitute the objectivity of medical research and, in part, serves to threaten that very objectivity.

As a discipline whose results often bear direct social relevance, medical research attracts considerable interest among the general public. For instance, 58 percent of Americans say they are interested in new medical discoveries (National Science Foundation, 2014) and, according to the Welcome trust monitor report (2013), 75 percent of adults in the United Kingdom reported being curious about medical research. Media reports on new cures, clinical guidelines, and possible health threats may influence the behavior of the members of the public. Scandals such as the ones related to the link between the painkiller Vioxx and cardiovascular events (Biddle, 2007) and selective serotonin reuptake inhibitors and suicidal ideation (Healy, 2012) have raised doubts about the trustworthiness of medical research and the integrity of scientists working in the field. Similarly, the recent outbreaks of vaccine-preventable diseases—such as measles, whooping cough, and polio—have been associated with the rise of the antivaccine movement and the distrust of established medical expertise (Poland and Jacobson, 2011). The public's reactions to these events show that one of the most important current challenges for the community of medical scientists is securing the public's trust in its research. One of the conditions for maintaining trust in science is that research is conducted in a way that is thought to be objective. Thus, searching for the means that best support objectivity is a central assignment for medical scientists and philosophers of medicine.

Commercial interests have been associated with many of the scandals that have threatened the apparent trustworthiness of medical science, since industry-funded drug trials report favorable results for company products when compared to trials funded by independent agencies (Lundh et al., 2012). Furthermore, reports of secrecy and dubious practices in medical research, particularly in the development of new drugs, have started to emerge (Sismondo, 2008). Biomedical research is a highly commercialized field. In 2012, 58 percent of research in the United States was funded by private sources (Moses et al., 2015). Consequently, critics have argued that the objectivity of the discipline is being compromised. Yet, it is not self-evident what actually is called for when objectivity of research is demanded.

Traditionally the objectivity of research has been associated with the integrity of individual scientists: objectivity is a trait that researchers need to cultivate in themselves.[7] According to this understanding, researchers should be on guard against their own biases and withdraw from assignments that might involve conflicts of interests that could undermine their impartiality (Shamoo and Resnik, 2009). However, studies on implicit biases have shown that individuals are not very good at recognizing their own biases (Uhlman and Cohen, 2007). Furthermore, even when individuals do their best not to let their preferences influence their reasoning, human actions tend to be affected by extraneous factors. For example, even small gifts can have an impact on the prescribing practices of physicians (Katz et al., 2003). Thus, it seems that relying on individuals' integrity is not enough to ensure that research results are unbiased. Because of this, when the grounds for conducting objective medical research are investigated, the perspective has to be shifted from evaluating the attitudes of individuals to examining practices and methods that would best ensure unbiased outcomes.

Which methods best promote the objectivity of research have been a debated issue in philosophy of science. The controversies are partly rooted in the intrinsic complexity of the concept of objectivity. As recent historical and philosophical analyses have suggested, objectivity is a multifaceted concept, and its different meanings can be used for promoting diverse practices. For example, Porter (1995) and Daston and Galison (2010) have traced the transformations of the concept and its different meanings through several centuries. According to these scholars, different virtues have been attached to objectivity. Daston and Galison (2010), for example, describe how the ideal of mechanical objectivity encouraged atlas makers in the late nineteenth and early twentieth centuries to find ways of depicting nature without the interference of human judgment and interpretation, even if it happened at the expense of describing the details of the object of interest. They detail how bacterial cultures and other objects could be illustrated using photography in a way that apparently had not been affected by subjective interpretations, but earlier methods of depicting nature, such as the drawings of expert artists, were better at portraying spatial depth and color. Thus, the photographs had less diagnostic utility than drawings, despite the fact that the latter were always influenced by the subjectivity of the artists. Similarly, Porter (1995) shows how in the discipline of accounting, portraying the object of interest in a quantified form has been used as a means of guarding the line of business from outsiders' accusations of corruption. What is common in these descriptions of the use of the term "objectivity" is that pursuing certain practices that are labeled objective or that ensure objectivity is a way of trying to build trust—both between the members of the communities following these practices and among outsiders.

Achieving objectivity is thought to require removing detrimental subjectivity, and the biases associated with it, from the process, and thereby improving the trustworthiness of results (cf. Daston and Galison, 2010, pp. 373–74). According to Douglas (2004, p. 454), the "implicit call to trust" is still common in the diverse ways in which the term "objective" is used today. She has specified eight different senses of objectivity that can be used to refer to outcomes of different kinds of processes. Due to the complexity of the term, it is possible to praise a method for producing objective results or denounce it as biased— depending on which of the senses of objectivity is chosen as the ideal to follow.

Because of the rhetorical force behind stating something to be objective, these choices can influence methodologies and have bearings on philosophical discussions concerning medical research.

Douglas's analysis can be used to evaluate the discussions concerning the objectivity of medical research as it elucidates the fact that not all senses of objectivity are applicable in every context. For example, one way of trying to constrain subjectivity and avoid biased results is to aim at making individual judgments redundant by establishing guidelines and procedures that give detailed instructions on how to carry out research. Douglas (2004, pp. 461–62) calls this ideal "procedural objectivity." This understanding of objectivity has led to discussions over the use of meta-analyses in amalgamating evidence. Stegenga (2011) has argued that meta-analysis falls short of being the platinum standard of evidence: despite the communally accepted guidelines, performing a meta-analysis necessarily involves numerous judgments on the analyst's part, which, in turn, opens the door for individual biases and subjective preferences and, thus, mitigates the method's objectivity. Stegenga's analysis demonstrates why following the ideal of disposing of the need for individual judgments fails in a context where the reliability of medical knowledge is sought: it is practically impossible.

In addition, focusing on the way in which studies and analyses are conducted, that is, on the "internal" processes of scientific inquiry, overlooks an important area that influences science, namely, the impact an institutional context of research has on knowledge production. For example, Young et al. (2008) worry that medical science may be biased by the current publication practices, which encourage researchers to pursue projects that are likely to be accepted by the most prestigious journals. Publication bias—studies showing positive results are published more often than studies with negative results—is perhaps the most significant bias affecting medical publishing, which systematically biases the literature (Godlee and Dickersin, 2003). Brown (2010), in turn, has argued that the funding structure in the field of biomedicine, that is, the prevalence of industry funding and the pressure to produce commercially applicable results, is creating lacunae in published literature. If the available funding guides research toward searching for only certain types of explanations for phenomena and the interests that motivate planning research in this way are not in line with generally accepted goals of research, then it might be the case that the outcomes of research regarded in their entirety have been biased. In other words, medical research is not objective. For instance, if funding is available only for those studies on mental illnesses that may produce patentable outcomes, important features of the phenomena may be left unstudied (Musschenga et al., 2010).

According to critics who urge taking notice of practices related to the allocation of funding and dissemination of results, focusing on individual studies and assessing only their internal quality leaves invisible certain features of research activities that may systematically bias scientific knowledge. In the context of medical research, this is particularly worrisome. According to the principles of EBM, the results of meta-analyses and other systematic reviews trump individual studies, and treatment guidelines are usually based on amalgamated evidence (Howick, 2011b). Because of this, the objectivity of medical research should be evaluated by using a concept of objectivity that accommodates the possibility of systematic biases that are caused by factors not belonging to the internal stages of research.

According to a traditional understanding, practices that take place in the context of discovery, that is, when research questions and hypotheses are developed, do not have an influence on the objectivity of knowledge production because through rigorous testing any possible biases can be removed in the so-called context of justification. In the light of recent empirical studies on the pharmaceutical industry (Sismondo, 2008) and philosophical analyses (Brown, 2010), however, this assumption should be questioned. Contrary to the traditional understanding of the distinction between the contexts of discovery and justification, testing of claims may not weed out all biases. The objectivity and trustworthiness of medical research can be severely compromised because of publication bias or problematic practices that occur in the phases of the allocation of resources, which fall on the discovery side of the discovery-justification distinction. If the way of framing research questions and projects results in a skewed understanding of the object of interest, it is possible to talk about the violation of objectivity (Brown, 2010). Consequently, the objectivity of medical research has to be examined from a perspective that takes notice of a wider spectrum of practices and factors than is traditionally considered.

A viable candidate for a new perspective on the aforementioned issues comes from social epistemology. Social epistemological theories have highlighted the importance that the institutional context of inquiry has for the reliability of produced information. For example, Longino (1990, 2002) has argued that the objectivity of research is dependent on the institutional and social context in which inquiry takes place and because of this, instead of exclusively evaluating individual scientists or single studies, those who are interested in addressing biases should pay attention to the organizational structure of science. Likewise, Biddle (2007) has argued that epistemic problems of biomedical research should be addressed with institutional arrangements.

In sum, different understandings of objectivity direct our attention to assessing diverse features of scientific practice. In the light of recent analyses that have disclosed problematic practices related to current biomedical research, it seems that those ideals of objectivity that are applicable for assessing individual scientists or particular methods for testing hypotheses are insufficient for capturing which factors may bias the eventual results. Because of this, it is essential to develop analyses of objectivity further that examine how conditions for this virtue are constituted at the level of research communities.

Conclusion

Philosophy of medicine has developed greatly over the past decade or so, with a new focus on epistemological questions (and their relationship with ethical questions). This chapter has identified several areas in which new and interesting philosophical questions are being addressed, and it has described how this research is beginning to build on and expand philosophical research on medicine, medical research, and the social context in which these activities are conducted.

Notes

1. See also chapter 10 of this volume for a discussion of gender medicine.
2. Here we discuss RDoC further, placing it in the larger context of discussions in philosophy of psychiatry. We focus only on RDoC as an attempt to develop ways of categorizing patients, which are intended to result in improved care.
3. See, for example, Bossuyt et al. (2000, 2006); and Ferrante di Rufano et al. (2012).
4. As with the debate regarding the epistemic merits of RCTs with respect to assessing the efficacy of therapeutic interventions, the requirement that comparative accuracy of diagnostic tests be assessed with RCTs is debatable—though we do not articulate the debate here.
5. RCTs of therapeutic treatments are subject to well-known epistemic and ethical problems of their own. However, as these issues have been elsewhere addressed in the philosophy of medicine literature, we will not discuss them here.
6. In such cases, a test might have a negative effect on patient outcomes, perhaps due to the intervention of the test, the cost, the anxiety from information gained, and so on. On the other hand, it might have a positive effect. Some studies (Lijmer and Bossuyt, 2009, for example) show that patients want to know what is wrong with them even when there isn't the possibility of doing anything about it.
7. See, for example, Smith (2004) for a defense of a view according to which the objectivity of science can be reduced to individuals.

References

American Psychiatric Association. (1952) *Diagnostic and Statistical Manual: Mental Disorders*, 1st edition. Washington, DC: American Psychiatric Association.
American Psychiatric Association. (1968) *Diagnostic and Statistical Manual of Mental Disorders*, 2nd edition. Washington, DC: American Psychiatric Association.
American Psychiatric Association. (1980) *Diagnostic and Statistical Manual: Mental Disorders*, 3rd edition. Washington, DC: American Psychiatric Association.

American Psychiatric Association. (1994) *Diagnostic and Statistical Manual of Mental Disorders*, 4th edition. Washington, DC: American Psychiatric Association.

American Psychiatric Association. (2013), *Diagnostic and Statistical Manual: Mental Disorders*, 5th edition. Washington, DC: American Psychiatric Association.

Angell, M. (2004), *The Truth about the Drug Companies: How They Deceive Us and What to Do about It*. New York: Random House.

Baggio, G., Corsini, A., Floreani, A., Giannini, S., and Zagonel, V. (2013). Gender medicine: A task for the third millennium. *Clinical Chemistry and Laboratory Medicine* 51(4): 713–27.

Biddle, J. (2007). Lessons from the Vioxx debacle: What the privatization of science can teach us about social epistemology. *Social Epistemology* 21(1): 21–39.

Bluhm, R. (2005). From hierarchy to network: A richer view of evidence for evidence-based medicine. *Perspectives in Biology and Medicine* 48(4): 535–47. doi:10.1353/pbm.2005.0082.

Bluhm, R. (in press). Evidence-based medicine, biological psychiatry, and the role of science in medicine. In *Extraordinary Science: Responding to the Current Crisis in Psychiatric Research*, eds. Jeffrey Poland and Şerife Tekin. Cambridge, MA: MIT University Press.

Borgerson, K. (2009). Valuing evidence: Bias and the evidence hierarchy of evidence-based medicine. *Perspectives in Biology and Medicine* 52(2): 218–33. doi:10.1353/pbm.0.0086.

Bossuyt, P. M., Irwig, L., Craig, J., and Glasziou, P. (2006). Comparative accuracy: Assessing new tests against existing diagnostic pathways. *British Medical Journal* 332: 389–92.

Bossuyt, P., Lijmer, J., and Mol, B. (2000). Randomized comparisons of medical tests: Sometimes invalid, not always efficient. *Lancet* 356: 1844–47.

Brown, J. (2008). The community of science®. In *The Challenge of the Social and the Pressure of Practice: Science and Values Revisited*, eds. M. Carrier, D. Howard, and J. Kourany. Pittsburgh: University of Pittsburgh Press.

Brown, J. (2010). One-shot science. In *The Commercialization of Academic Research*, ed. H. Radder. Pittsburgh: Pittsburgh University Press, pp. 90–109.

Brozek, J. L. Akl. E. A., Jaeschke, R., Lang D. M., Bossuyt, P., Glasziou, P., Helfland, M., Ueffing, E., Alonso-Coello, P., Meerpohl, J., Phillips, B., Horvath, A. R., Bousquet, J., Guyatt, G. H., Schünemann, H. J., and GRADE Working Group. (2009). The GRADE approach to grading quality of evidence about diagnostic tests and strategies. *Allergy* 64: 1109–16.

Cournoyea, M., and Kennedy, A. (2014). Causal explanatory pluralism and medically unexplained physical symptoms. *Journal of Evaluation in Clinical Practice* 20(6): 928–33.

Daston, L., and Galison, P. (2010). *Objectivity*. New York: Zone Books.

De Melo-Martin, I., and Intemann, K. (2011). Feminist resources for biomedical research: Lessons from the HPV vaccines. *Hypatia* 26(1): 79–101. doi:10.1111/j.1527-2001.2010.01144.x.

Douglas, H. (2000). Inductive risk and values in science. *Philosophy of Science* 67(4): 559–79.

Douglas, H. (2004). The irreducible complexity of objectivity. *Synthese* 138: 453–73.

Dresser, R. (1982). Wanted: Single, white male for medical research. *Hastings Center Report*, 22(1): 24–29.

Elliott, C. (2010). *White Coat, Black Hat: Adventures on the Dark Side of Medicine*. Boston: Beacon Press.

Ferrante di Rufano L., Hyde, C. J., McCaffrey, K. J., Bossuyt, P. M. M., and Deeks, J. J. (2012). Assessing the value of diagnostic tests: A framework for designing and evaluating trials. *British Medical Journal* 344.

Frances, A. (2013). Last plea to DSM-5: Save grief from the drug companies. *Huffington Post*, January 7.

Godlee, F., and Dickersin, K. (2003). Bias, subjectivity, chance, and conflict of interest in editorial decisions. In *Peer review in Health Sciences*, 2nd edition, eds. F. Godlee and T. Jefferson. London: BMJ Publishing, pp. 91–117.

Goldacre, B. (2012). *Bad Pharma: How Drug Companies Mislead Doctors and Harm Patients*. New York: HarperCollins.

Gøtzsche, P. (2013). *Deadly Medicines and Organized Crime*. London: Radcliffe Publishing.

Graham, G., and Flanagan, O. (2013). Psychiatry and the brain. Oxford University Press blog; August 1. https://blog.oup.com/2013/08/psychiatry-brain-dsm-5-rdoc/.

Gupta, M. (2014). *Is Evidence-Based Psychiatry Ethical?* Oxford: Oxford University Press.

Guze, S. B. (1992). *Why Psychiatry Is a Branch of Medicine*. New York: Oxford University Press.

Healy, D. (2012). *Pharmageddon*. Berkeley: University of California Press.

Hoffman, G., and Zachar, P. (in press). RDoC's metaphysical assumptions: Problems and promises. In *Extraordinary Science: Responding to the Current Crisis in Psychiatric Research*, eds. Jeffrey Poland and Şerife Tekin. Cambridge MA: MIT University Press.

Horwitz, A. V., and Wakefield, J. C. (2007). *The Loss of Sadness: How Psychiatry Transformed Normal Sadness into Depressive Disorder*. New York: Oxford University Press.

Howick, J. (2011a). Exposing the vanities—and a qualified defense—of mechanistic reasoning in health care decision making. *Philosophy of Science* 78(5): 926–40.

Howick, J. (2011b). *The Philosophy of Evidence-Based Medicine*. Chichester UK: Wiley-Blackwell, BMJ Books.

Insel, T., and Lieberman, J. A., (2013). DSM-5 and RDoC: Shared Interests. http://www.nimh.nih.gov/news/science-news/2013/dsm-5-and-rdoc-shared-interests.shtml.

Insel, T., Cuthbert, B., Garvey, M., Heinssen, R., Pine, D. S., Quinn, K., Sanislow, C., and Wang, P. (2010). Research Domain Criteria (RDoC): Toward a new classification framework for research on mental disorders. *American Journal of Psychiatry* 167(7): 748–51.

Institute of Medicine. (2007). IOM roundtable on evidence-based medicine. In *The Learning Healthcare System: Workshop Summary*, eds. L. Olsen, D. Aisner, and J. M. McGinnis. Washington, DC: National Academies Press.

Jukola, S. (2015). Meta-analysis, ideals of objectivity, and the reliability of medical knowledge. *Science and Technology Studies* 28(3): 101–120.

Kass, N. E., Faden, R. R., Goodman, S. N., Provenost, P., Tunis, S., and Beauchamp, T. L. (2013). The research-treatment distinction: A problematic approach for determining which activities should have ethical oversight. *Hastings Center Report* 43(1): S4–S15.

Katz, D., Caplan, A., and Mertz, J. (2003). All gifts large and small. Toward an understanding of the ethics of pharmaceutical industry gift-giving. *American Journal of Bioethics* 3(3): 39–46.

Kennedy, A. G. (2013). Differential diagnosis and the suspension of judgment. *Journal of Medicine and Philosophy* 38(5): 487–500. doi: 10.1093/jmp/jht043.

Kleinman, A. (2012). The art of medicine: Culture, bereavement, psychiatry. *Lancet* 379(9816): 608–609.

Laing, R. D. (1985). *Wisdom, Madness and Folly: The Making of a Psychiatrist 1927–1957*. London: Macmillan.

Largent, E. A., Joffe, S., and Miller, F. G. (2011). Can research and care be ethically integrated? *Hastings Center Report* 41(4): 37–46.

Lijmer, J., and Bossuyt, P. (2009). Various randomized designs can be used to evaluate medical tests. *Journal of Clinical Epidemiology* 62: 364–73.

Longino, H. (1990). *Science as Social Knowledge*. Princeton: Princeton University Press.

Longino, H. (2002). *The Fate of Knowledge*. Princeton: Princeton University Press.

Lundh, A., Sismondo, S., Lexchin, J., Busuioc, O. A., and Bero, L. (2012). Industry sponsorship and research outcome, Cochrane Database of Systematic Reviews 2012, Issue 12. Art. No: MR000033. doi: 10.1002/14651858.MR000033.pub2.

Lynch, T. J., Bell, D. W., Sordella, R., Gurubhagavatula, S., Okimoto, R. A., Brannigan, B. W., Harris, P. L., Haserlat, S. M., Supko, J. G., Haluska, F. G., Louis, D. N., Christiani, D. C., Settleman, J., and Haber, D. A. (2004). Activating mutations in the epidermal growth factor receptor underlying responsiveness of non-small-cell lung cancer to gefitinib. *NEJM* 350: 2129–39.

McClimans, L. (2013). The role of measurement in establishing evidence. *Journal of Medicine and Philosophy* 38(5): 520–38.

Moses, H., III, Matheson, D. M. Cairns-Smith, S, George, B. P., Palisch, C., and Dorsey, E. (2015). The anatomy of medical research: US and international comparisons. *JAMA* 313(2): 174–89. doi:10.1001/jama.2014.15939.

Moynihan, R., and Cassels, A. (2005). *Selling Sickness: How the World's Biggest Pharmaceutical Companies Are Turning Us All into Patients*. Vancouver: Greystone Books.

Musschenga, A., van der Steen, W., and Ho, V. (2010). The business of drug research: A mixed blessing. In *The Commodification of Academic Science*, ed. H. Radder. Pittsburgh: Pittsburgh University Press, pp. 110–31.

National Institutes of Mental Health. NIMH Research Domain Criteria (RDoC), available at http://www.nimh.nih.gov/research-priorities/rdoc/nimh-research-domain-criteria-rdoc.shtml (accessed March 12, 2015).

National Science Foundation. (2014). *Science and Engineering Indicators 2014*. Arlington: VA (NSB 14-01).

Osimani, B. (forthcoming). Hunting side effects and explaining them: Should we reverse evidence hierarchies upside down? *Topoi*.

Poland, G., and Jacobson, R. (2011). The age-old struggle against antivaccinationists. *New England Journal of Medicine* 364(2): 97–99.

Porter, T. (1995). *Trust in Numbers*. Princeton: Princeton University Press.

Prahallad, A., Sun, C., Huang, S., Di Nicolantonio, F., Salazar, R., Zecchin, D., Beijersbergen, R. L., Bardelli, A., and Bernards, R. (2012). Unresponsiveness of colon cancer to BRAF(V600E) inhibition through feedback activation of EGFR. *Nature* 483(7387): 100–103.

Radden, J. (2009). *Moody Minds Distempered: Essays on Melancholy and Depression*. New York: Oxford University Press.

Reiss, J. (2010). In favour of a Millian proposal to reform biomedical research. *Synthese* 177(3): 427–47. doi: 10.1007/s11229-010-9790-7.

Robins, E., and Guze, S. B. (1970). Establishment of diagnostic validity in psychiatric illness: Its application to schizophrenia. *American Journal of Psychiatry* 126(7): 983–87.

Russo, F., and Williamson, J. (2007). Interpreting causality in the health sciences. *International Studies in the Philosophy of Science* 21: 157–70.

Sadler, J. (2005). *Values and Psychiatric Diagnosis*. Oxford: Oxford University Press.

Shamoo, A., and Resnik, D. (2009). *Responsible Conduct of Research*, 2nd edition. Oxford: Oxford University Press.

Sismondo, S. (2008). How pharmaceutical industry funding affects trial outcomes: Causal structures and responses. *Social Science and Medicine* 66(9): 1909–14.

Smith, T. (2004). "Social" objectivity and the objectivity of values. In *Science, Values, and Objectivity*, eds. P. Machamer, and G. Wolters. Pittsburgh: Pittsburgh University Press, pp. 143–71.

Steel, D. (2007). *Across the Boundaries: Extrapolation in Biology and the Social Sciences*. New York: Oxford University Press.

Stegenga, J. (2011). Is meta-analysis the platinum standard? *Studies in the History and Philosophy of Biological and Biomedical Sciences* 42: 497–507.

Stegenga, J. (2014). Down with the hierarchies. *Topoi* 33(2): 313–22. doi:10.1007/s11245-013-9189-4.

Stegenga, J. (forthcoming). *Medical Nihilism*. Oxford: Oxford University Press.

Stempsey, W. (2008) Philosophy of medicine is what philosophers of medicine do. *Perspectives in Biology and Medicine* 51(3): 379–91.

Tekin, Ş. (2014). Psychiatric taxonomy: At the crossroads of science and ethics. *Journal of Medical Ethics* 40(8): 513–14. doi:10.1136/medethics-2014-102339.

Tekin, Ş. (2015). Against hyponarrating grief: Incompatible research and treatment interests in the DSM-5. In *The Psychiatric Babel: Assessing the DSM-5,* eds. P. Singy and S. Demazeux.

Tekin, Ş., and Mosko, M. (2015). Hyponarrativity and context-specific limitations of the DSM-5. *Public Affairs Quarterly* 29(1): 109–45.

Thorpe, K. E., Zwarenstein, M., Oxman, A. D., Treweek, S., Furberg, C. D., Altman, D. G., Tunis, S., Bergel, E., Harvey, I. Magid, D. J., and Chalkidou, K. (2009). A pragmatic-explanatory continuum indicator summary (PRECIS): A tool to help trial designers. *Journal of Clinical Epidemiology* 62(5): 646–75.

Uhlmann, E., and Cohen, G. (2007). "I think therefore it's true": Effects of self-perceived objectivity on hiring discrimination. *Organizational Behavior and Human Decision Processes* 104: 207–23.

United States. (1978). *The Belmont Report: Ethical Principles and Guidelines for the Protection of Human Subjects of Research.* Bethesda, MD: The Commission.

Wakefield, J. C. (2015). The loss of grief: Science and pseudoscience in the debate over DSM-5's elimination of the bereavement exclusion. In *The Psychiatric Babel: Assessing the DSM-5,* eds. P. Singy and S. Demazeux. *History, Philosophy and the Theory of the Life Sciences* Series. Springer Press.

Wakefield, J. C., and First, M. B. (2012). Validity of the bereavement exclusion to major depression: Does the empirical evidence support the proposal to eliminate the exclusion in DSM-5?, *World Psychiatry* 11: 3–10.

Wellcome trust. (2013). *Welcome trust monitor wave 2. Tracking public opinions science, biomedical research and science education.* Retrieved from http://www.wellcome. ac.uk/stellent/groups/corporatesite/@msh_grants/documents/web_document/wtp053113.pdf.

Willyard, C. (2013). "Basket studies" will hold intricate data for cancer drug approvals. *Nature Medicine* 19(6): 655.

Worrall, J. (2002). What evidence in evidence-based medicine? *Philosophy of Science* 69: S316–S330.

Worrall, J. (2007). Why there's no cause to randomize. *British Journal for the Philosophy of Science* 58(3): 451–88.

Young, N., Ioannidis, J., and Al-Ubaydli, O. (2008). Why current publication practices may distort science. *PloS Medicine* 5(10): e201. doi:10.1371/journal.pmed.0050201.

Zisook, S., and Kendler, K. S. (2007). Is bereavement-related depression different than non- bereavement-related depression? *Psychological Medicine* 37: 779–94.

Zisook, S., Shuchter, S. R., Pedrelli, P., Sable, J., and Deaciuc, S. C. (2001). Bupropion sustained release for bereavement: Results of an open trial. *Journal of Clinical Psychiatry* 62: 227–30.

Part III

Research Resources

Glossary of Key Terms

As for any discipline, contemporary philosophy of medicine has a unique set of terms; but, it also shares a number of terms with ancillary disciplines. The goal of this glossary is twofold: to include as many salient terms as possible and to provide sufficient working definitions of them. Also, references to relevant literature are cited to provide additional resources.

Absolutism: the belief in unconditional and nonrelative principles or standards for knowing or acting—often contrasted to relativism. Kraus, M. (2011). *Dialogues on Relativism, Absolutism, and Beyond: Four Days in India*. Lanham, MD: Roman & Littlefield. Jackson, F., and Smith, M. (2006). Absolutist moral theories and uncertainty. *Journal of Philosophy* 103(6): 267–83.

Analysis/Analytical: a judgment entailed from premises with respect to formal or logical reasoning—often contrasted to synthesis/synthetic. Beaney, M. (2014). Analysis. In: E. N. Zalta, ed. *Stanford Encyclopedia of Philosophy*. http://plato.stanford.edu/archives/spr2015/entries/analysis/.

Analytical (Logic of) medicine: an approach to medical knowledge and practice that utilizes conceptual and logical analysis. Schaffner, K. F., ed. (1985). *Logic of Discovery and Diagnosis in Medicine*. Berkeley, CA: University of California Press. Sadegh-Zadeh, K. (2015). *Handbook of Analytic Philosophy of Medicine*, 2nd edition. New York: Springer.

Autonomy: the capacity or right for self-determination. Dryden, J. (2015). Autonomy. In: *Internet Encyclopedia of Philosophy*. http://www.iep.utm.edu/autonomy/.

Beneficence: to promote another's welfare or good—often contrasted to maleficence. Shelp, E. E., ed. (1982). *Beneficence and Health Care*. Dordrecht: Reidel. Beauchamp, T. (2013). The principle of beneficence in applied ethics. In: E. N. Zalta, ed. *Stanford Encyclopedia of Philosophy*. http://plato.stanford.edu/archives/win2013/entries/principle-beneficence/. Kinsinger, F. S. (2009). Beneficence and the professional's moral imperative. *Journal of Chiropractic Humanities* 16: 44–46.

Biomarker: a measurable substance that indicates disease incidence and clinical outcome. Strimbu, K., and Tavel, J. A. (2010). What are biomarkers? *Current Opinion in HIV and AIDS* 5(6): 463–66. http://doi.org/10.1097/COH.0b013e32833ed177.

Biopsychosocial model: a model of healthcare introduced by George Engels that incorporates the biological, psychological, and social factors into patient care. Engel, G. L. (1977). The need for a new medical model: A challenge for biomedicine. *Science* 196: 129–36.

Causation: the agency involved in producing an effect—includes the principle of causality that every effect has a cause. Blackburn, S. (2005). *Oxford Dictionary of Philosophy*, 2nd edition, p. 57. New York: Oxford University Press.

Clinical expertise: the expert opinion resulting from a clinician's education and experience. Haynes, R. B., Devereaux, P. J., and Guyatt, G. H. (2002). Clinical expertise in the era of evidence-based medicine and patient choice. *Evidence Based Medicine* 7(2): 36–38.

Clinical judgment: a conclusion in terms of diagnosis, prognosis, or therapy drawn from critically thinking about clinical evidence. Kienle, G. S., and Kiene, H. (2011). Clinical judgment and the medical profession. *Journal of Evaluation in Clinical Practice* 17(4): 621–27.

Cognition: the mental faculties involved in the acquisition of knowledge through perceiving and conceiving. Reed, S. (2013). *Cognition: Theories and Application*, 9th edition. Belmont, CA: Wadsworth.

Cognitive bias: errors in judgment attributable to cognitive limitations or prejudices. Wilke, A., and Mata, R. (2012). Cognitive bias. In: V. S. Ramachandran, ed. *The Encyclopedia of Human Behavior*, 2nd edition, volume 1, pp. 531–35. London: Academic Press.

Cohort study: a longitudinal study in which one or more groups are followed in terms of outcomes. Levin, K. A. (2006). Study design IV: Cohort studies. *Evidence-Based Dentistry* 7(2): 51–52.

Consciousness: the ability to perceive or to be aware of either mental or physical phenomena. Velmans, M. (2009). How to define consciousness—and how not to define consciousness. *Journal of Consciousness Studies* 16(5): 139–56.

Counterfactual: a conditional statement expressing what would have happened had circumstances been different. Marshall, G. (2009). Conterfactual. In: J. Scott and G. Marshall, eds. *A Dictionary of Sociology*, 3rd edition, p. 137. Oxford: Oxford University Press.

Critical reasoning/thinking: the cognitive faculty or skill of evaluating evidence and forming an argument in order to make a reasonable judgment. Butterworth, J., and Thwaites, G. (2013). *Thinking Skills: Critical Thinking and Problem Solving*, 2nd edition. New York: Cambridge University Press.

Cure: to restore biological, physiological, or mental functioning or to relieve symptoms associated with disease or disorder. Weintraub, P. (2009). Metaphysical medicine: The murky meaning of cure. *Psychology Today*, https://www.psychologytoday.com/blog/emerging-diseases/200902/meta-physical-medicine-the-murky-meaning-cure. Marcum, J. A. (2011). Medical cure and progress: The case of type 1 diabetes. *Perspectives in Biology and Medicine* 54(2): 176–88.

Diagnosis: the determination of a pathological condition through examination of clinical symptoms and evidence. Ahlzén, R. (2010). Diagnosis: An introduction. In: R. Ahlzén, M. Evans, P. Louhiala et al., eds. *Medical Humanities Companion: Diagnosis*, volume 2, pp. 11–27. Oxford: Radcliffe Publishing.

Diagnostic reasoning: the cognitive and inference processes, including assessing and evaluating clinical evidence, involved in arriving at a diagnosis or differential diagnosis. Lawson, A. E., and Daniel, E. S. (2011). Inferences of clinical reasoning and diagnostic error. *Journal of Biomedical Informatics* 44(3): 402–12.

Dignity: the condition or state of having value or worth either intrinsically or extrinsically. Blackburn, S. (2005). *Oxford Dictionary of Philosophy*, 2nd edition, p. 100. New York: Oxford University Press. Düwell, M., Braarvig, J., Brownsword, R., et al., eds. (2014). *Cambridge Handbook of Human Dignity: Interdisciplinary Perspectives*. New York: Cambridge University Press.

Disease: a pathological dysfunction of the body. Scully, J. L. (2004). What is disease? *EMBO Reports* 5(7): 650–53. Boyd, K. M. (2000). Disease, illness, sickness, health, healing, and wholeness: Exploring some elusive concepts. *Medical Humanities* 26: 9–17. Ereshefsky, M. (2009). Defining "health" and "disease." *Studies in History and Philosophy of Biological and Biomedical Science* 40(3): 221–27.

Dual process theory of cognition: the theory that cognition is composed of two systems, the first intuitive and the second logical. Evans, J. St. B. T., and Stanovich, K. E. (2013). Dual-process theories of higher cognition. *Perspectives on Psychological Science* 8(3): 223–41.

Dualism: the belief that there are two separate and often opposing realities, such as mind–body—often contrasted to monism. Robinson, H. (2012). Dualism. In: E. N. Zalta, ed. *Stanford Encyclopedia of Philosophy*. http://plato. stanford.edu/archives/win2012/entries/dualism/.

Efficient cause: that which brings about or initiates an effect. Schmaltz, T. M., ed. (2014). *Efficient Causation: A History*. New York: Oxford University Press.

Embodiment: the experience of the lived body within the world. Williams, S. (2004). Embodiment. In: J. Gabe, M. Bury, and M. A. Elston, eds. *Key Concepts in Medical Sociology*, pp. 73–76. London: SAGE.

Empiricism: the belief in experience for justifying knowledge—often contrasted to rationalism. Meyers, R. G. (2014). *Understanding Empiricism*. New York: Routledge. Markie, P. (2013). Rationalism vs. empiricism. In: E.N. Zalta, ed. *Stanford Encyclopedia of Philosophy*. http://plato.stanford.edu/ archives/sum2015/entries/rationalism-empiricism/.

Enlightenment: a Western European movement beginning in the seventeenth century that privileged reason and individualism over religious scholasticism, with one of its greatest achievements being the Scientific Revolution. Fitzpatrick, M., Jones, P., Knellwolf, C., et al., eds. (2004). *The Enlightenment World*. London: Routledge.

Epidemiology: *Dictionary of Epidemiology* defines it as, "The study of the distribution and determinants of health-related states or events in specified populations, and the application of this study to the control of health problems." Last, J. M., ed. (2001). *Dictionary of Epidemiology*, 4th ed., p. 62. New York: Oxford University Press.

Epigenetics: the modification in gene expression as the result of factors, particularly environmental, other than changes in DNA nucleotide sequence. Berger, S. L., Kouzarides, T., Shiekhattar, R., et al. (2009). An operational definition of epigenetics. *Genes & Development* 23: 781–83. Tost, J. (2008). *Epigenetics*. Norfolk, UK: Caister Academic Press.

Epistemological pluralism/relativism: the multiple contexts or systems by which to know and does not privilege one context or system of knowing over another. Boghossian, P. (2006). *Fear of Knowledge: Against Relativism and Constructivism*. Oxford: Clarendon Press. Kalderon, M. E. (2009). Epistemic relativism. *Philosophical Review* 118(2): 225–40. Seidel, M. (2014). *Epistemic Relativism: A Constructive Critique*. New York: Palgrave Macmillan.

Epistemological turn: a shift, beginning during the Enlightenment, from metaphysical issues to emphasis on issues concerning the discovery and justification of knowledge. Northoff, G. (2004). *Philosophy of the Brain: The Brain Problem*. Philadelphia, PA: John Benjamins Publishing.

Epistemology: the study of knowledge as justified true belief in terms of its scope and validity. Steup, M. (2005). Epistemology. In: E. N. Zalta, ed. *Stanford Encyclopedia of Philosophy*. http://plato.stanford.edu/archives/spr2014/entries/epistemology/. Truncellito, D. A. (2007). Epistemology. In: *Internet Encyclopedia of Philosophy*. http://www.iep.utm.edu/epistemo/.

Evidence: the data or observations from formal investigation in the sciences. Achinstein, P. (2001). *Book of Evidence*. New York: Oxford University Press. Goldenberg, M. J. (2006). On evidence and evidence-based medicine: Lessons from the philosophy of science. *Social Science & Medicine* 62(11): 2621–32.

Evidence hierarchy: ranking clinical evidence in terms of pyramidal levels, with low quality evidence from pathophysiological mechanism or expert opinion occupying the bottom of the pyramid, followed by unfiltered evidence from observational and cohort studies and randomized clinical trials forming the mid-levels, and culminating in filtered evidence from systematic reviews and meta-analysis. Grondin, S. C., and Schieman, C. (2011). Evidence-based medicine: Levels of evidence and evaluation systems. In: M. K. Ferguson, ed. (2014). *Difficult Decisions in Thoracic Surgery: An Evidence-Based Approach*, pp. 13–22. New York: Springer.

Evidence network: rather than ranking evidence based on hierarchies, evidence is ranked in terms of interrelationships or network relationships among population-based studies, laboratory research, and randomized controlled trials. Bluhm, R. (2005). From hierarchy to network: A richer view of evidence for evidence-based medicine. *Perspectives in Biology and Medicine* 48(4): 535–47.

Evidence-based medicine: David Sackett and colleagues provide the most widely quoted definition: "Evidence based medicine is the conscientious, explicit, and judicious use of current best evidence in making decisions about the care of individual patients." Sackett, D. L., Rosenberg, W. M., Gray, J. A., et al. (1996). Evidence based medicine: What it is and what it isn't. *British Medical Journal* 312(7023): 71–72. Howick, J. H. (2011). *The Philosophy of Evidence-Based Medicine*. Oxford: Wiley-Blackwell.

Evolutionary medicine: an approach to medicine that utilizes Darwinian evolutionary theory. Stearns, S. C. (2012). Evolutionary medicine: Its scope, interest and potential. *Proceedings of the Royal Society of London B: Biological Sciences* 279(1746): 4305–21. Pearlman, R. (2013). *Evolution and Medicine*. New York: Oxford University Press.

Existentialism: an approach to human existence that emphasizes human freedom and responsibility. Crowell, S. (2015). Existentialism. In: E. N. Zalta, ed. *Stanford Encyclopedia of Philosophy*. http://plato.stanford.edu/archives/spr2015/entries/existentialism/. Burnham, D. (2011). Existentialism. In: *Internet Encyclopedia of Philosophy*. http://www.iep.utm.edu/existent/.

Explanation: a statement or set of statements that accounts or gives reason for a phenomenon. Achinstein, P. (1983). *The Nature of Explanation*. New York: Oxford University Press. Achinstein, P. (2010). *Evidence, Explanation, and Realism: Essays in Philosophy of Science*. New York: Oxford University Press.

Explicit knowledge: knowledge that can be articulated or transmitted through tangible means—often contrasted to tacit knowledge. Collins, H. (2010). *Tacit and Explicit Knowledge*. Chicago, IL: University of Chicago Press.

Fact: a statement whose veracity or truthfulness reflects a judgment process concerning evidence. Fleck, L. (1979). *Genesis and Development of a Scientific Fact*. Chicago, IL: University of Chicago Press. Latour, B., and Woolgar, S. (1986). *Laboratory Life: The Construction of Scientific Facts*. Princeton, NJ: Princeton University Press.

Final/teleological cause: that for which an effect is brought about, that is, its purpose. Leunissen, M. (2010). *Explanation and Teleology in Aristotle's Science of Nature*. New York: Cambridge University Press.

Formal cause: that about which an effect is brought about, that is, its form. Sokolowski, R. (1995). Formal and material causality in science. *American Catholic Philosophical Quarterly* 69: 57–67. Ferejohn, M. T. (2013). *Formal*

Causes: Definition, Explanation, and Primacy in Socratic and Aristotelian Thought. New York: Oxford University Press.

Foundationalism: the epistemological position that knowing is based on certain and noninferential principles and evidence. Fumerton, R. (2000). Foundationalist theories of epistemic justification. In: E. N. Zalta, ed. *Stanford Encyclopedia of Philosophy.* http://plato.stanford.edu/archives/sum2010/entries/justep-foundational/.

Fragmentation: a state of being broken into constitutive parts or components—often contrasted to wholeness. Bohm, D. (1971). Fragmentation in science and in society. *Science Teacher* 38(1): 10–15. Bohm, D. (1976). *Fragmentation and Wholeness.* Jerusalem: Van Leer Jerusalem Foundation. Stich, S. (1993). *The Fragmentation of Reason: Preface to a Pragmatic Theory of Cognitive Evaluation.* Cambridge, MA: MIT Press.

Gender: The World Health Organization offers the following definition: "the socially constructed characteristics of women and men—such as norms, roles and relationships of and between groups of women and men." WHO: http://www.who.int/gender-equity-rights/knowledge/glossary/en/. Esplen, E., and Jolly, S. (2006). *Gender and Sex: A Sample of Definitions.* BRODGE: http://www.iwtc.org/ideas/15_definitions.pdf.

Gender medicine: healthcare that focuses on a specific gender, often to the exclusion of another gender. Schenck-Gustafsson, K., DeCola, P. R., Pfaff, D. W., et al., eds. (2012). *Handbook of Clinical Gender Medicine.* Basel: Karger. Kuhlmann, E., and Annandale, E., eds. (2012), *The Palgrave Handbook of Gender and Healthcare*, 2nd edition. New York: Palgrave Macmillan. Miller, V. M., Rice, M., Schiebinger, L., et al. (2013) Embedding concepts of sex and gender health difference into medical curricula. *Journal of Women's Health* 22(3): 194–202.

Genetics: the study of genes and their expression in living organisms. Hartl, D. L. (2014). *Essential Genetics: A Genomic Perspective*, 6th edition. Burlington, MA: Jones & Bartlett.

Genomic medicine: utilizing genomic information to care for patients clinically. NHGRI (2012) Definition of "Genomic Medicine": https://www.genome.gov/pages/About/NACHGR/Sept2012AgendaDocuments/Genomic_Medicine_Definition_080112_RChisolm.pdf. Kumar, D., and Eng, C., eds. (2015). *Genomic Medicine: Principles and Practices*, 2nd edition. New York: Oxford University Press.

Genomics: the study of an organism's set of genes and their expression both developmentally and evolutionarily. Hartl, D. L. (2014). *Essential Genetics: A Genomic Perspective*, 6th edition. Burlington, MA: Jones & Bartlett.

Healing: to make whole, to relieve the suffering associated with illness, and to find meaning in illness. Egnew, T. R. (2005). The meaning of healing: Transcending suffering. *Annals of Family Medicine* 3(3): 255–62. Boyd, K. M.

(2000). Disease, illness, sickness, health, healing, and wholeness: Exploring some elusive concepts. *Medical Humanities* 26: 9–17.

Health: World Health Organization defines it as "a state of complete physical, mental and social well-being and not merely the absence of disease or infirmity." WHO: www.who.int/governance/eb/who_constitution_en.pdf. Ahmed, P. I., and Coelho, G. V., eds. (1979). *Toward a New Definition of Health: Psychological Dimensions.* New York: Plenum Press. Boyd, K. M. (2000). Disease, illness, sickness, health, healing, and wholeness: Exploring some elusive concepts. *Medical Humanities* 26: 9–17. Ereshefsky, M. (2009). Defining "health" and "disease." *Studies in History and Philosophy of Biological and Biomedical Science* 40(3): 221–27.

Hermeneutics: the exegetical process of interpretation, especially of literary texts. Ramberg, B., and Gjesdal, K. (2005). Hermeneutics. In: E. N. Zalta, ed. *Stanford Encyclopedia of Philosophy.* http://plato.stanford.edu/archives/win2014/entries/hermeneutics/.

Heuristic: the rules of thumb or mental shortcuts to facilitate problem solving or other cognitive activities. Ippoliti, E., ed. (2015). *Heuristic Reasoning.* New York: Springer. Sunstein, C. R. (2005). Moral heuristics. *Behavioral and Brain Sciences* 28: 531–73.

Historicism: the belief that just as natural laws govern natural phenomena so historical laws govern human affairs. Hamilton, P. (2003). *Historicism.* New York: Routledge. Ryn, C. G. (1998). Defining historicism. *Humanitas* 11(2): 86. http://www.nhinet.org/humsub/ryn11-2.htm.

Holism: the property of the whole is greater than the sum of the individual properties of its parts. Smuts, J. (1926). *Holism and Evolution.* London: Macmillan. Esfeld, M., ed. (2001). *Holism in Philosophy of Mind and Philosophy of Physics.* Dordrecht: Kluwer.

Human Genome Project: an international project to map and sequence, both physically and functionally, the human genome, along with genomes from other selected species. Lee, T. F. (1991). *The Human Genome Project: Cracking the Genetic Code of Life.* New York: Springer. Murray, T. H., Rothstein, M. A., Murray, Jr., R. F., eds. (1996). *The Human Genome Project and the Future of Health Care.* Bloomington, IN: Indiana University Press. Salem, R. M., and Rodriguez-Murillo, L. (2013). Human genome project. In: M. D. Gellman and J. R. Turner, ed. *Encyclopedia of Behavioral Medicine*, pp. 1003–1004. New York: Springer.

Humanism: the belief in the adequacy of human agency without religious faith in supreme agency. Law, S. (2011). *Humanism: A Very Short Introduction.* New York: Oxford University Press. Fowler, J. (1999). *Humanism: Beliefs and Practices.* Brighton, UK: Sussex Academic Press.

Idealism: the belief that reality is mind-dependent—often contrasted to realism. Guyer, P., and Horstmann, R.-P. (2015). Idealism. In: E. N. Zalta, ed. *Stanford Encyclopedia of Philosophy*. http://plato.stanford.edu/archives/fall2015/entries/idealism/.

Illness: the impact of pathology on a person's daily life. Boyd, K. M. (2000). Disease, illness, sickness, health, healing, and wholeness: Exploring some elusive concepts. *Medical Humanities* 26: 9–17. Conrad, P., and Barker, K. K. (2010). The social construction of illness: Key insights and policy implications. *Journal of Health and Social Behavior* 51(S): S67–S79.

Integrative medicine: an approach to healthcare that includes the patient as a whole. Boon, H., Verhoef, M., O'Hara, D., et al. (2004). Integrative healthcare: Arriving at a working definition. *Alternative Therapies in Health and Medicine* 10(5): 48–56. Rakel, D., ed. (2012). *Integrative Medicine*, 3rd edition. Philadelphia: Elsevier.

Intuition: the cognitive faculty of immediate apprehension or understanding. Osbeck, L. M., and Held, B. S., eds. (2014). *Rational Intuition: Philosophical Roots, Scientific Investigations*. New York: Cambridge University Press. Cholle, F. P. (2011). What is intuition, and how do we use it? *Psychology Today*, https://www.psychologytoday.com/blog/the-intuitive-compass/201108/what-is-intuition-and-how-do-we-use-it. Sadler-Smith, E. (2008). *Inside Intuition*. New York: Routledge.

Life-world: a person's experience of daily living. Schutz, A., and Luckmann, T. (1979). *The Structures of the Life-World*, volume 1. Evanston, IL: Northwestern University Press. Galvin, K., and Todres, L. (2013). *Caring and Well-Being: A Lifeworld Approach*. London: Routledge.

Maleficence: doing harm—often contrasted to beneficence. Miles, M. (2003). *Inroads: Paths in Ancient and Modern Western Philosophy*. Toronto: University of Toronto Press.

Material cause: that from which an effect is constituted. Sokolowski, R. (19955). Formal and material causality in science. *American Catholic Philosophical Quarterly* 69: 57–67.

Mechanism: a series of causal events. Machamer, P., Darden, L., and Craver, C. F. (2000). Thinking about mechanisms. *Philosophy of Science* 67(1): 1–25. Bunge, M. (2004). How does it work? The search for explanatory mechanisms. *Philosophy of the Social Sciences* 34(2): 182–210.

Mechanistic reasoning: a rational process involved in linking a series of causal events. Howick, J. (2011). Exposing the vanities—and a qualified defense—of mechanistic reasoning in health care decision making. *Philosophy of Science* 78(5): 926–40. Russ, R. S., Scherr, R. E., Hammer, D., et al. (2008). Recognizing mechanistic reasoning in student scientific inquiry: A framework for discourse analysis developed from philosophy of science. *Science Education* 92(3): 499–525.

Medical humanism: the inclusion of the human condition into medicine, especially clinical practice—often contrasted to medical scientism. Vannatta, J.,

Schleifer, R., and Crow, S. (2005). *Medicine and Humanistic Understanding: The Significance of Literature for Medical Practices.* Philadelphia, PA: University of Pennsylvania Press. Bishop, J. P. (2008). Rejecting medical humanism: Medical humanities and the metaphysics of medicine. *Journal of Medical Humanities* 29(1): 15–25. Shapiro, J., Coulehan, J., Wear, D., et al. (2009). Medical humanities and their discontents: Definitions, critiques, and implications. *Academic Medicine* 84(2): 192–98.

Medical (therapeutic) nihilism: the belief in the ineffectiveness of medicine and/or therapy and that medicine often does more harm than good. Mukherjee, S. (2015). *The Laws of Medicine: Field Notes from an Uncertain Science.* New York: Simon & Schuster. Herman, J. Therapeutic nihilism? *Israel Journal of Medical Sciences* 32(304): 259–64.

Medical pluralism: the diversity of approaches to the nature and practice of medicine, whether Western medical specialties and/or complementary and alternative medicine. Tilburt, J. C., and Miller, F. G. (2007). Responding to medical pluralism in practice: A principled ethical approach. *Journal of the American Board of Family Medicine* 20(5): 489–94. Jutte, R., ed. (2013). *Medical Pluralism: Past—Present—Future.* Stuttgart: Franz Steiner.

Medical scientism: medical practice based on the biomedical sciences—often contrasted to medial humanism. Loughlin, M., Lewith, G., and Falkenberg, T. (2013). Science, practice and mythology: A definition and examination of the implications of scientism in medicine. *Health Care Analysis* 21(2): 130–45. Pigliucci, M. (2015). Scientism and pseudoscience: A philosophical commentary. *Journal of Bioethical Inquiry* 12(4): 569–75. McCormick, J. (2001). Scientific medicine—fact or fiction? The contribution of science to medicine. *Occasional Paper, Royal College of General Practitioners* 80: 3–6.

Metacognition: the awareness and capacity to understand one's cognitive or thought processes. Dunlosky, J., and Metcalfe, J. (2009). *Metacognition.* London: SAGE. Proust, J. (2013). *The Philosophy of Metacognition: Mental Agency and Self-Awareness.* New York: Oxford University Press.

Metaphysics: the domain of philosophy that investigates existence. van Inwagen, P., and Sullivan, M. (2014). Metaphysics. In: E. N. Zalta, ed. *Stanford Encyclopedia of Philosophy.* http://plato.stanford.edu/archives/spr2015/entries/metaphysics/.

Methodology: a set of procedures for investigation and of rules for analysis. World Health Organization (2001). *Health Research Methodology: A Guide for Training in Research Methods,* 2nd edition. Manila: World Health Organization. Brink, H., van der Walt, C., and van Rensburg, G. (2006). *Fundamentals of Research Methodology for Health Care Professionals.* Cape Town: JUTA.

Molecular biology: the study of living processes and mechanisms at the macromolecular level. Rosenberg, A. (2001). Philosophy of molecular biology. eLS: http://onlinelibrary.wiley.com/doi/10.1038/npg.els.0003448/pdf. Sarkar,

S. (2005). *Molecular Models of Life: Philosophical Papers on Molecular Biology.* Cambridge, MA: MIT Press. Morange, M. (2000). *A History of Molecular Biology.* Cambridge, MA: Harvard University Press.

Molecular medicine: the diagnosis and treatment of disease at the molecular level. Trent, R. J. (2012). *Molecular Medicine: Genomics to Personalized Healthcare,* 4th edition. Amsterdam: Elsevier. Boniolo, G., and Nathan, M. J. (2017). *Philosophy of Molecular Medicine: Foundational Issues in Research and Practice.* Taylor & Francis.

Monism: the belief in reality's unity—often contrasted to dualism. Schaffer, J. (2014). Monism. In: E. N. Zalta, ed. *Stanford Encyclopedia of Philosophy.* http://plato.stanford.edu/archives/sum2015/entries/monism/.

Multifactorial: the result of numerous factors or causes. Sham, P. C., and Bishop, D. T., eds. (2000). *Analysis of Multifactorial Diseases.* Oxford: BIOS. Broadbent, A. (2013). Multifactorialism and beyond. In: *Philosophy of Epidemiology,* pp. 145–61. New York: Palgrave Macmillan.

Nanotechnology: the manipulation of matter at the nano (<100 nanometers) scale. Nouailhat, A. (2006). *An Introduction to Nanoscience and Nanotechnology.* London: ISTE. Allhof, F., Lin, P., and Moore, D. (2010). *What Is Nanotechnology and Why Does It Matter? From Science to Ethics.* Oxford: Wiley-Blackwell.

Narrative: a spoken or written story or account of events. Altman, R. (2008). *A Theory of Narrative.* New York: Columbia University Press.

Narrative medicine: an approach to clinical practice that includes the patient's illness story. Mehl-Madrona, L. (2007). *Narrative Medicine: The Use of History and Story in the Healing Process.* Rochester, VT: Bear & Company. Marini, M. G. (2016). *Narrative Medicine: Bridging the Gap between Evidence-Based Care and Medical Humanities.* New York: Springer.

Natural selection: the notion that organisms better adapted to the environment leave or produce more offspring. Brandon, R. (2008). Natural selection. In: E. N. Zalta, ed. *Stanford Encyclopedia of Philosophy.* http://plato.stanford.edu/archives/spr2014/entries/natural-selection/. Munz, P. (1993). *Philosophical Darwinism: On the Origins of Knowledge by Means of Natural Selection.* London: Routledge.

Naturalism: the belief that mind-independent or natural causes are responsible for reality—often contrasted to normativism. Papineau, D. (2015). Naturalism. In: E. N. Zalta, ed. *Stanford Encyclopedia of Philosophy.* http://plato.stanford.edu/archives/fall2015/entries/naturalism/. Jacobs, J. (2009). Naturalism. In: *Internet Encyclopedia of Philosophy.* http://www.iep.utm.edu/naturali/.

Normativism: the belief that mind-dependent or social norms are responsible for reality—often contrasted to naturalism. Turner, S. (2013). The argument of explaining the normative. *RIS* 71(1): 192–94. Maël, L. (2013). Defining disease beyond conceptual analysis: An analysis of conceptual analysis in philosophy of medicine. *Theoretical Medicine and Bioethics* 34(4): 309–25. Hamilton, R. P. (2010). The concept of health: Beyond normativism and naturalism. *Journal of Evaluation in Clinical Practice* 16(2): 323–29.

Objectivity: the belief that judgments can be made independent of subjective perspective—often contrasted to subjectivity. Mulder, D. H. (2004). Objectivity. In: *Internet Encyclopedia of Philosophy*. http://www.iep.utm.edu/objectiv/. Daston, L., and Galison, P. (2010). *Objectivity*. New York: Zone Books.

Observational study: a study in which observations are made under uncontrolled conditions—often contrasted to randomized controlled trial. Hackshaw, A. (2015). *A Concise Guide to Observational Studies in Healthcare*. Oxford: Wiley-Blackwell. Rosenbaum, P. R. (2002). *Observational Studies*. New York: Springer.

Ontology: the metaphysical study of the nature of being. Hofweber, T. (2014). Logic and ontology. In: E. N. Zalta, ed. *Stanford Encyclopedia of Philosophy*. http://plato.stanford.edu/archives/fall2014/entries/logic-ontology/. Poli, R., and Seibt, J., eds. (2010). *Theory and Application of Ontology: Philosophical Perspectives*. New York: Springer.

Patient-centered medicine: Institute of Medicine defines it as "care that is respectful of and responsive to individual patient preferences, needs, and values, and ensuring that patient values guide all clinical decisions." Institute of Medicine. (2001). *Crossing the Quality Chasm: A New Health System for the 21st Century*. Washington, DC: National Academy of Science. Bardes, C. L. (2012). Defining "patient-centered medicine." *New England Journal of Medicine* 366(9): 782–83.

People-centered public health: an approach to healthcare that includes all the stakeholders of the healthcare system, from lay volunteers to public policy. De Maeseneer, J., van Weel, C., Daeren, L., et al. (2012). From "patient" to "person" to "people": The need for integrated, people centered health care. *International Journal of Person Centered Medicine* 2(3): 601–14. South, J., White, J., and Gamsu, M. (2013). *People-Centered Public Health*. Bristol, UK: Polity Press. Biehl, J., and Petryna, A., eds. (2013). *When People Come First: Critical Studies in Global Health*. Princeton, NJ: Princeton University Press.

Person-centered medicine: an approach to healthcare that focuses on the personhood of those involved in therapeutic relationships. Mezzich, J. E., Snaedal, J., van Weel, C., et al. (2011). Introduction to person-centred medicine: From concepts to practice. *Journal of Evaluation in Clinical Practice* 17: 330–32. Miles, A. (2012). Person-centered medicine—at the intersection of science, ethics and humanism. *International Journal of Person Centered Medicine* 2(3): 329–33.

Personalism: a philosophical movement in the early twentieth century that emphasized the importance of the person in understanding self and reality. Williams, T. D., and Bengtsson, J. O. (2013). Personalism. In: E. N. Zalta, ed. *Stanford Encyclopedia of Philosophy.* http://plato.stanford.edu/archives/ spr2014/entries/personalism/. Buford, T. O. (2011). Personalism. In: *Internet Encyclopedia of Philosophy.* http://www.iep.utm.edu/personal/.

Personalized medicine: utilization of patient's genetic profile to diagnose disease and to determine prognosis and treatment. Redekop, W. K., and Mladsi, D. (2013). The faces of personalized medicine: A framework for understanding its meaning and scope. *Values in Health* 16: S4–S9. Garassino, M. (2013). *What Is Personalized Medicine?* Viganello-Lugano: ESMO Press. Jain, K. K. (2015). *Textbook of Personalized Medicine,* 2nd edition. New York: Humana Press.

Personhood: the state of being a person. Merrill, S. B. (1998). *Defining Personhood: Toward the Ethics of Quality in Clinical Care.* Amsterdam: Rodopi. Farah, M. J., and Heberlein, A. S. (2007). Personhood and neuroscience: Naturalizing or nihilating? *American Journal of Bioethics* 7(1): 37–48.

Phenomenology: the study of intentional human consciousness as experienced through first-person viewpoint. Smith, D. W. (2013). Phenomenology. In: E. N. Zalta, ed. *Stanford Encyclopedia of Philosophy.* http://plato.stanford.edu/archives/win2013/entries/phenomenology/. White, D. E. (2009). Phenomenology. In: *Internet Encyclopedia of Philosophy.* http://www.iep.utm.edu/phenom/.

Phronesis: the epistemic virtue of practical wisdom or prudence. Russell, D. C. (2009). *Practical Intelligence and the Virtues.* Oxford: Clarendon Press. Tyreman, S. (2000). Promoting critical thinking in health care: Phronesis and criticality. *Medicine, Health Care, and Philosophy* 3(2): 117–24.

Placebo: intervention used either as a control for clinical trials (placebo control) or as a therapeutic effect due to patient's perception (placebo effect). Moerman, D. E. (2002). *Meaning, Medicine, and the "Placebo Effect."* Cambridge: Cambridge University Press. Benedetti, F., Enck, P., Frisaldi, E., et al., eds. (2014). *Placebo.* New York: Springer. Shapiro, A. K. (1964). A historic and heuristic definition of the placebo. *Psychiatry* 27(1): 52–58.

Pluralism: the belief in a diversity of methods to investigate phenomena and of causes to explain them. Kellert, S. H., Longino, H. E., and Waters, C. K., eds. (2006). *Scientific Pluralism.* Minneapolis, MN: University of Minnesota Press. Brody, B. (2003). *Taking Issue: Pluralism and Casuistry in Bioethics.* Washington, DC: Georgetown University Press.

Positivism: the belief that statements can be rationally and empirically justified without recourse to metaphysics. Alexander, J. C. (2014). *Positivism, Presupposition and Current Controversies.* London: Routledge. Creath, R. (2011). Logical empiricism. In: E. N. Zalta, ed. *Stanford Encyclopedia of Philosophy.* http://plato.stanford.edu/archives/spr2014/entries/logical-empiricism/.

Presupposition: an assumption upon which a proposition or question is based. Blome-Tillman, M. (2014). *Knowledge and Presuppositions.* New York: Oxford University Press. Beaver, D. I., and Geurts, B. (2011). Presupposition. In: E. N.

Zalta, ed. *Stanford Encyclopedia of Philosophy*. http://plato.stanford.edu/ archives/win2014/entries/presupposition/. Alexander, J. C. (2014). *Positivism, Presupposition and Current Controversies*. London: Routledge.

Prognosis: to presage or predict a disease's course or outcome. Rizzi, D. A. (1993). Medical prognosis—some fundamentals. *Theoretical Medicine* 14(4): 365–75. Gospodarowicz, M., Mackillop, W., O'Sullivan, B., et al. (2001). Prognostic factors in clinical decision making. *Cancer* 91(S8): 1688–95.

Randomized controlled trial: a trial in which observations are made under randomized and controlled conditions—often contrasted to observational or cohort study. Machin, D., and Fayers, P. M. (2010). *Randomized Clinical Trials: Design, Practice and Reporting*. Oxford: Wiley-Blackwell. Hannan, E. L. (2008). Randomized clinical trials and observational studies: Guidelines for assessing respective strengths and limitations. *JACC: Cardiovascular Interventions* 1(3): 211–17. Christ, T. W. (2014). Scientific-based research and randomized controlled trials, the "gold" standard? Alternative paradigms and mixed methodologies. *Qualitative Inquiry* 20(1): 72–80.

Rationalism: the belief in reason for the justification of knowledge—often contrasted to empiricism. Nelson, A., ed. (2013). *A Companion to Rationalism*. Oxford: Wiley-Blackwell. Markie, P. (2013). Rationalism vs. empiricism. In: E. N. Zalta, ed. *Stanford Encyclopedia of Philosophy*. http://plato.stanford. edu/archives/sum2015/entries/rationalism-empiricism/.

Realism: the belief that reality is mind-independent—often contrasted to idealism. Miller, A. (2014). Realism. In: E. N. Zalta, ed. *Stanford Encyclopedia of Philosophy*. http://plato.stanford.edu/archives/win2014/entries/realism/.

Reductionism: the belief that a complex phenomenon can be investigated and explained in terms of its parts—often contrasted to holism. Ney, A. (2012). Reductionism. In: *Internet Encyclopedia of Philosophy*. http://www.iep.utm. edu/red-ism/. Sachse, C. (2007). *Reductionism in the Philosophy of Science*. Frankfurt: Ontos.

Relativism: the belief that a judgment depends on the context in which it is made—often contrasted to absolutism. Baghramian, M., and Carter, A. (2015). Relativism. In: E. N. Zalta, ed. *Stanford Encyclopedia of Philosophy*. http:// plato.stanford.edu/archives/win2015/entries/relativism/. Kraus, M. (2011). *Dialogues on Relativism, Absolutism, and Beyond: Four Days in India*. Lanham, MD: Roman & Littlefield.

Scientism: the belief that the empirical sciences provide the authoritative understanding of reality—often contrasted to humanism. Sorell, T. (1991). *Scientism: Philosophy and the Infatuation with Science*. New York: Routledge. Williams, R. N., and Robinson, D. N., eds. (2015). *Scientism: The New Orthodoxy*. London: Bloomsbury.

Sex: World Health Organization defines it as "the different biological and physiological characteristics of males and females, such as reproductive organs, chromosomes, hormones, etc." WHO: http://www.who.int/gender-equity-rights/knowledge/glossary/en/. Esplen, E., and Jolly, S. (2006). *Gender and Sex: A Sample of Definitions*. BRODGE: http://www.iwtc.org/ideas/15_def-initions.pdf.

Sickness: the impact of pathology on a person's social role and life. Hahn, R. (1996). *Sickness and Healing: An Anthropological Perspective*. New Haven, CT: Yale University Press. Boyd, K. M. (2000). Disease, illness, sickness, health, healing, and wholeness: Exploring some elusive concepts. *Medical Humanities* 26: 9–17.

Social epistemology: the belief that the production and justification of knowledge, even scientific knowledge, depends on the social context. Fuller, S. (2002). *Social Epistemology*, 2nd edition. Bloomington, IN: Indiana University Press. Haddock, A., Millar, A., and Duncan Pritchard, D. (2010). *Social Epistemology*. New York: Oxford University Press.

Subjectivity: the belief that subjective perspective is critical for decision-making and knowing—often contrasted to objectivity. Hall, D. E. (2004). *Subjectivity*. New York: Routledge. Mandik, P. (2009). The neurophilosophy of subjectivity. In: J. Bickle, ed. *The Oxford Handbook of Philosophy and Neuroscience*, pp. 601–18. New York: Oxford University Press.

Suffering: the existential condition, whether physical or mental, of pain or discomfort. Anderson, R. E. (2013). *Human Suffering and Quality of Life: Conceptualizing Stories and Statistics*. New York: Springer. Langle, A. (2008). Suffering—an existential challenge: Understanding, dealing and coping with suffering from an existential-analytic perspective. *International Journal of Existential Psychology and Psychotherapy* 2(1): http://existentialpsychology.org/journal/index.php?journal=ExPsy&page=article&op=view&path%5B%5D=115&path%5B%5D=58.

Synthesis/Synthetic: a judgment inferred from informal or empirical reasoning—often contrasted to analysis/analytic. Rey, G. (2013). The analytic/synthetic distinction. In: E. N. Zalta, ed. *Stanford Encyclopedia of Philosophy*. http://plato.stanford.edu/archives/win2015/entries/analytic-synthetic/.

Systems medicine: an approach to medical research and practice that incorporates systems science, bioinformatics, and big biology. Hood, L., and Flores, M. (2012). A personal view on systems medicine and the emergence of proactive P4 medicine: Predictive, preventive, personalized and participatory. *New Biotechnology* 29(6): 613–24. Bousquet, J., Jorgensen, C., Dauzat, M., et al. (2014). Systems medicine approaches for the definition of complex phenotypes in chronic diseases and ageing: From concept to implementation and policies. *Current Pharmaceutical Design* 20(38): 5928–44.

Tacit/implicit knowledge: knowledge that is not articulated but rather inferential or prereflective—often contrasted to explicit knowledge. Polanyi, M. (1966). *The Tacit Dimension*. Garden City, NY: Doubleday. Collins,

H. (2010). *Tacit and Explicit Knowledge*. Chicago, IL: University of Chicago Press. Gascoigne, N., and Thornton, T. (2013). *Tacit Knowledge*. Durham, UK: Acumen.

Techné: the epistemic virtue for technical knowing, that is, craft or professional or applied knowledge. Kaplan, D. M., ed. (2009). *Readings in the Philosophy of Technology*, 2nd edition. Lanham, MD: Roman & Littlefield. Parry, R. (2014). Episteme and techne. In: E. N. Zalta, ed. *Stanford Encyclopedia of Philosophy*. http://plato.stanford.edu/archives/fall2014/entries/episteme-techne/. Hofmann, B. (2003). Medicine as techne—a perspective from antiquity. *Journal of Medicine and Philosophy* 28(4): 403–25.

Translational medicine: an approach to medical research and practice that incorporates current laboratory research into the clinical encounter, often defined as "from laboratory bench to patient bedside." Alving, B., Dai, K., and Chan, S. H. H., eds. (2013). *Translational Medicine—What, Why and How: An International Perspective*. Basel: Karger. Shahzad, A., ed. (2016). *Translational Medicine: Tools and Techniques*. London: Academic Press.

Value: the worth or importance of something. McDonald, H. P. (2004). *Radical Axiology: A First Philosophy of Values*. Amsterdam: Rodopi. Hurka, T. (2001). *Virtue, Vice, and Value*. New York: Oxford University Press. Schroeder, M. (2012). Value theory. In: E. N. Zalta, ed. *Stanford Encyclopedia of Philosophy*. http://plato.stanford.edu/archives/sum2012/entries/value-theory/.

Values-based practice: an approach to medical practice that incorporates personal, institutional, and social values. Fulford, K. W. M. (2004). Ten principles of values-based medicine (VBM). In: T. Schramme and J. Thome, eds. *Philosophy and Psychiatry*, pp. 50–80. Berlin: Walter de Gruyter. McCarthy, J., and Rose, P., eds. (2010).*Values-Based Health and Social Care: Beyond Evidence-Based Practice*. London: SAGE.

Vice: a trait that inhibits a person from exhibiting either moral or epistemic excellence—often contrasted to virtue. Hurka, T. (2001). *Virtue, Vice, and Value*. New York: Oxford University Press.

Virtue: a trait that allows a person to exhibit either moral or epistemic excellence—often contrasted to vice. Traditionally there are the four cardinal virtues—justice, prudence, courage, and temperance—and three theological virtues—faith, hope, and charity. Adams, R. M. (2006). *A Theory of Virtue: Excellence in Being for the Good*. New York: Oxford University Press. Hurka, T. (2001). *Virtue, Vice, and Value*. New York: Oxford University Press. Simon, Y. R. (1986). *The Definition of Moral Virtue*. New York: Fordham University Press. Fairweather, A., and Zagzebski, L., eds. (2001).*Virtue Epistemology: Essays in Epistemic Virtue and Responsibility*. New York: Oxford University Press.

Well-being: the physical and psychological state of health and happiness, respectively. Eid, M., and Larsen, R. J., eds. (2008).*The Science of Subjective*

Well-Being. New York: Guilford Press. Walker, P., and John, M., eds. (2012). *From Public Health to Wellbeing: The New Driver for Policy and Action.* New York: Palgrave-Macmillan.

Wholeness: a state of being complete in terms of constitution—often contrasted to fragmentation. Vaught, C. G. (1982). *The Quest for Wholeness.* Albany, NY: SUNY. Bohm, D. (1976). *Fragmentation and Wholeness.* Jerusalem: Van Leer Jerusalem Foundation. Boyd, K. M. (2000). Disease, illness, sickness, health, healing, and wholeness: Exploring some elusive concepts. *Medical Humanities* 26: 9–17.

Research Guide

There are numerous resources, both online and in print, for conducting philosophical investigations into and scholarship on contemporary Western medicine and its practice. In this guide to research sources, several of the salient resources are listed to assist the reader in engaging the literature in contemporary philosophy of medicine.

Dictionaries and Encyclopedia

Boyd, K. M., Higgs, R., and Pinching, A., eds. (1997). *The New Dictionary of Medical Ethics*. London: BMJ Publishing Group.
Duncan, A. S., Dunstan, G. R., and Welborn, R. B., eds. (1981). *Dictionary of Medical Ethics*, revised edition. New York: Crossroad.
Jennings, B., ed. (2014). *Encyclopedia of Bioethics*, 4th edition. New York: Macmillan.

Online Encyclopedia Articles

Arras, J. Theory and bioethics. *The Stanford Encyclopedia of Philosophy* (Summer 2013 Edition), E. N. Zalta (ed.), URL: http://plato.stanford.edu/archives/sum2013/entries/theory-bioethics/.
Donchin, A. Feminist bioethics. *The Stanford Encyclopedia of Philosophy* (Fall 2012 Edition), E. N. Zalta (ed.), URL: http://plato.stanford.edu/archives/fall2012/entries/feminist-bioethics/.
Gannett, L. The Human Genome Project. *The Stanford Encyclopedia of Philosophy* (Winter 2014 Edition), E. N. Zalta (ed.), URL: http://plato.stanford.edu/archives/win2014/entries/human-genome/.
Gordon, J.-S. Bioethics. *The Internet Encyclopedia of Philosophy*: http://www.iep.utm.edu/bioethic/.
Kukla, R., and Wayne, K. Pregnancy, birth, and medicine. *The Stanford Encyclopedia of Philosophy* (Fall 2015 Edition), E. N. Zalta (ed.), URL: http://plato.stanford.edu/archives/fall2015/entries/ethics-pregnancy/.
Marcum, J. A. Philosophy of medicine. *The Internet Encyclopedia of Philosophy*: http://www.iep.utm.edu/medicine/.
Murphy, D. Concepts of disease and health. *The Stanford Encyclopedia of Philosophy* (Spring 2015 Edition), E. N. Zalta (ed.), URL: http://plato.stanford.edu/archives/spr2015/entries/health-disease/.
Murphy, D. Philosophy of psychiatry. *The Stanford Encyclopedia of Philosophy* (Spring 2015 Edition), E. N. Zalta (ed.), URL: http://plato.stanford.edu/archives/spr2015/entries/psychiatry/.

Perring, C. Mental illness. *The Stanford Encyclopedia of Philosophy* (Spring 2010 Edition), E. N. Zalta (ed.), URL: http://plato.stanford.edu/archives/spr2010/entries/mental-illness/.

Ramirez, E. Philosophy of mental illness. *The Internet Encyclopedia of Philosophy*: http://www.iep.utm.edu/mental-i/.

Raphals, L. Chinese philosophy and Chinese medicine. *The Stanford Encyclopedia of Philosophy* (Summer 2015 Edition), E. N. Zalta (ed.), URL: http://plato.stanford.edu/archives/sum2015/entries/chinese-phil-medicine/.

Silvers, A. Feminist perspectives on disability. *The Stanford Encyclopedia of Philosophy* (Spring 2015 Edition), E. N. Zalta (ed.), URL: http://plato.stanford.edu/archives/spr2015/entries/feminism-disability/.

Wasserman, D., Asch, A., Blustein, J., and Putnam, D. Disability: Definitions, models, experience. *The Stanford Encyclopedia of Philosophy* (Winter 2015 Edition), E. N. Zalta (ed.), forthcoming URL: http://plato.stanford.edu/archives/win2015/entries/disability/.

Wendler, D. The ethics of clinical research. *The Stanford Encyclopedia of Philosophy* (Fall 2012 Edition), E. N. Zalta (ed.), URL: http://plato.stanford.edu/archives/fall2012/entries/clinical-research/.

Wikipedia. Philosophy of medicine. https://en.wikipedia.org/wiki/Philosophy_of_medicine.

Introductory Volumes

Bunge, M. (2013). *Medical Philosophy: Conceptual Issues in Medicine*. Singapore: World Scientific Publishing Co.

Culver, C. M., and Gert, B. (1982). *Philosophy in Medicine: Conceptual and Ethical Issues in Medicine and Psychiatry*. Oxford: Oxford University Press.

Johansson, I., and Lynøe, N. (2008). *Medicine & Philosophy: A Twenty-First Century Introduction*. Frankfurt: Ontos.

Lee, K. (2012). *The Philosophical Foundations of Modern Medicine*. New York: Palgrave Macmillan.

Maier, B., and Shibles, W. A. (2011). *The Philosophy and Practice of Medicine and Bioethics: A Naturalistic–Humanistic Approach*. New York: Springer.

Marcum, J. A. (2008). *An Introductory Philosophy of Medicine: Humanizing Modern Medicine*. New York: Springer.

Pellegrino, E. D., and Thomasma, D. C. (1981). *A Philosophical Basis of Medical Practice: Toward a Philosophy and Ethic of the Healing Professions*. New York: Oxford University Press.

Sadegh-Zadeh, K. (2015). *Handbook of Analytic Philosophy of Medicine*, 2nd edition. New York: Springer.

Tauber, A. I. (1999). *Confessions of a Medicine Man: An Essay in Popular Philosophy*. Cambridge, MA: MIT Press.

Van Der Steen, W. J., and Thung, P. J. (1988). *Faces of Medicine: A Philosophical Study*. Dordrecht: Kluwer.

Wulff, H. R., Pedesen, S. A., and Rosenberg, R. (1990). *Philosophy of Medicine: An Introduction*, 2nd edition. Oxford, UK: Blackwell.

Anthologies

Carson, R. A., and Burns, C. R., eds. (1997). *Philosophy of Medicine and Bioethics: A Twenty-Year Retrospective and Critical Appraisal*. Dordrecht: Kluwer.

Engelhardt, Jr, H. T., ed. (2000). *The Philosophy of Medicine: Framing the Field*. New York: Springer.

Evans, M., Louhiala, P., and Puustinen, R., eds. (2004). *Philosophy for Medicine: Applications in a Clinical Context*. Oxford: Radcliffe Publishing.

Gifford, F., ed. (2011). *Philosophy of Medicine*. Oxford: Elsevier.

Huneman, P., Lambert, G., and Silberstein, M., eds. (2015). *Classification, Disease and Evidence: New Essays in the Philosophy of Medicine*. New York: Springer.

Lindemann, N. J., and Lindemann, N. H., eds. (1999). *Meaning in Medicine: A Reader in the Philosophy of Health Care*. London: Routledge.

Schramme, T., and Edwards, S., eds. (2016). *Handbook of the Philosophy of Medicine*. New York: Springer.

Series

Cambridge's *Studies in Philosophy and Health Policy*: http://www.cambridge.org/US/academic/subjects/philosophy/philosophy-social-science/series/studies-philosophy-and-health-policy.

Springer's *Philosophy and Medicine*: http://www.springer.com/series/6414.

The Hastings Center Report: http://www.thehastingscenter.org/Publications/HCR/About.aspx.

Journals

European Journal of Person Centered Healthcare: http://ubplj.org/index.php/ejpch/index.

International Journal of Person Centered Medicine: http://www.ijpcm.org/index.php/IJPCM.

Journal of Evaluation of Clinical Practice: http://onlinelibrary.wiley.com/journal/10.1111/(ISSN)1365–2753.

Journal of Medicine and Philosophy: http://jmp.oxfordjournals.org/.

Journal of Medicine and the Person: http://link.springer.com/journal/12682.

Medicine, Health Care and Philosophy: http://link.springer.com/journal/11019.

Medicine Studies: http://link.springer.com/journal/12376.

Perspectives in Biology and Medicine: https://www.press.jhu.edu/journals/perspectives_in_biology_and_medicine/.

Philosophy, Ethics, and Humanities in Medicine: http://peh-med.biomedcentral.com/.

Social Science and Medicine: http://www.journals.elsevier.com/social-science-and-medicine/?testing=a.

Theoretical Medicine and Bioethics: http://link.springer.com/journal/11017.

Online databases

Goldenberg, M. J. Philosophy of medicine. *PhilPapers*: http://philpapers.org/browse/philosophy-of-medicine/.

Howick, J. Kennedy, A. G., and Mebius, A. Philosophy of evidence-based medicine. *Oxford Bibliographies*: http://www.oxfordbibliographies.com/view/document/obo-9780195396577/obo-9780195396577-0253.xml.

Marcum, J. A. Contemporary philosophy of medicine. *Oxford Bibliographies*: http://www.oxfordbibliographies.com/view/document/obo-9780195396577/obo-9780195396577-0216.xml.

Mendeley. Philosophy of medicine: https://www.mendeley.com/disciplines/philosophy/philosophy-of-medicine/.
Questia. Philosophy of medicine: https://www.questia.com/library/philosophy/branches-of-philosophy/philosophy-of-medicine.
Simon, J. R. Philosophy of medicine. Misc, *PhilPapers*: http://philpapers.org/browse/philosophy-of-medicine-misc.
Tekin, S. Philosophy of psychiatry and psychopathology. *PhilPapers*: http://philpapers.org/browse/philosophy-of-psychiatry-and-psychopathology.

Professional Societies

American Philosophical Society, Newsletter on Philosophy and Medicine: http://www.apaonline.org/?medicine_newsletter.
European Society for Person Centered Healthcare: http://pchealthcare.org.uk/.
European Society for the Philosophy of Medicine and Healthcare: http://www.espmh.org/about.php.
International Philosophy of Medicine Roundtable: https://philosmed.wordpress.com/.

Academic Research Centers

Durham University, Durham, UK, History and Philosophy of Science and Medicine: https://www.dur.ac.uk/philosophy/research/research_centres/hpsmgroup/
Hannover Medical School, Hannover, Germany, Institute for History, Ethics and Philosophy of Medicine: https://www.mh-hannover.de/igepm.html?&L=1.
King's College, London, UK. Philosophy and Medicine: http://www.kcl.ac.uk/artshums/depts/philosophy/research/projects/medicine/index.aspx.
St Catherine's College, Oxford, UK, The Collaborating Centre for Values-Based Practice in Health and Social Care: http://valuesbasedpractice.org/more-about-vbp/research-and-on-going-development-2/the-theory-of-values-based-practice-partner-profiles/.
Ulm University, Ulm, Germany, Institute of the History, Philosophy and Ethics of Medicine: https://www.uni-ulm.de/en/med/institute-of-the-history-philosophy-and-ethics-of-medicine.html.
University of California, Berkeley, CA, USA, Center for Science, Technology, Medicine & Society: http://cstms.berkeley.edu/.
University of Kansas Medical School, Kansas City, KS, USA, Department of History and Philosophy of Medicine: http://www.kumc.edu/school-of-medicine/history-and-philosophy-of-medicine/faculty-development.html.
University of Oxford, Oxford, UK, Centre for Evidence-Based Medicine: http://www.cebm.net/.

Annotated Bibliography

The annotated bibliography lists the salient and relevant literature in the contemporary philosophy of medicine, beginning from the second half of the twentieth century. Although there are several important papers that have had a major impact on the field, only books are listed (those papers are contained in anthologies below). Also, only representative entries from the bioethical and medico-sociological literature are listed. Obviously, the list cannot be exhaustive; but, it does provide a starting point for investigating the various issues in contemporary philosophy of medicine.

Aho, J., and Aho, K. (2008). *Body Matters: A Phenomenology of Sickness, Disease, and Illness*. Lanham, MD: Lexington Books.
The authors explore the phenomenological dimensions of pathology in order to critique common assumptions about its personal and social manifestations and to humanize medical therapies.

Albert, D. A., Munson, R., and Resnik, M. D. (1988). *Reasoning in Medicine: An Introduction to Clinical Inference*. Baltimore, MD: The Johns Hopkins University Press.
The authors initially discuss traditional issues in medical epistemology and then introduce a "cyclical" model of clinical reasoning, which involves an iterative process of diagnosis.

Ars, B., ed. (2001). *The Meaning of Medicine: The Human Person*. The Hague: Kugler.
The contributors to this edited volume examine the impact of the person on the meaning of medicine, with respect to life and death, suffering and illness, and body and mind.

Baer, H. A. (2004). *Toward an Integrative Medicine: Merging Alternative Therapies with Biomedicine*. Oxford: AltaMira Press.
The rise of integrative healthcare and its professionalization are discussed, especially the work of Andrew Weil and Deepak Chopra, along with its potential to transform contemporary medicine.

Barro, S., and Marin, R., eds. (2002). *Fuzzy Logic in Medicine*. New York: Springer.
The edited volume explores the application of fuzzy logic to medicine, ranging from its use in analyzing medical data to diagnosis.

Black, D. (1968). *The Logic of Medicine*. Edinburgh: Oliver & Boyd.
The book explores the role of logic qua intellectual rigor in the practice of medicine, especially in terms of diagnosis and disease management.

Braude, H. D. (2012). *Intuition in Medicine: A Philosophical Defense of Clinical Reasoning*. Chicago: The University of Chicago Press.
The author argues for a central role of intuition in clinical reasoning and decision-making, particularly in connecting medicine's technical and moral mandates.

Broadbent, A. (2013). *Philosophy of Epidemiology*. New York: Palgrave Macmillan.
The author defends epidemiology as a legitimate topic for philosophical reflection and discusses the philosophical notions, such as induction, causation, and prediction, puzzles of attributability, risk relativism, multifactorialism, and legal issues associated with epidemiology.

Brody, H. (2003). *Stories of Sickness*, 2nd edition. New York: Oxford University Press.
The author argues that the stories patients narrate concerning their illness experience are essential for providing optimal care for the individual patient.

Brown, M. M., Brown, G. C., and Sharma, S. (2005). *Evidence-Based to Value-Based Medicine*. Chicago, IL: American Medical Association Press.
The authors argue that value-based medicine, that is, taking into account the patient's values, rounds out evidence-based medicine for optimizing the delivery of quality healthcare.

Bunge, M. (2013). *Medical Philosophy: Conceptual Issues in Medicine*. Singapore: World Scientific Publishing Co.
The author introduces the reader to a variety of topics germane to contemporary philosophy of medicine, including disease and diagnosis, drugs and therapy, iatroethics, and the nature of modern medicine in terms of art or science.

Campaner, R. (2012). *Philosophy of Medicine: Causality, Evidence and Explanation*. Bologna: ArchetipoLibri.
The author discusses a variety of issues facing contemporary philosophy of medicine, including the nature of disease and the notions of causation, explanation, mechanism, and reductionism, as well as the complexities and uncertainties involved in clinical medicine.

Canguilham, G. (1978). *On the Normal and the Pathological*, C. R. Fawcett, trans. Dordrecht: Reidel.
The author demonstrates how traditional notions of health and disease were reshaped not only by science but also by social and political forces.

Caplan, A. L., McCartney, J. J., and Sisti, D. A., eds. (2004). *Health, Disease and Illness: Concepts in Medicine*. Washington, DC: Georgetown University Press.
The book consists of a collection of essays analyzing the concepts of health and disease from a historical perspective, as well as their clinical application in terms of normalcy, enhancement, and genetics.

Carel, H. (2013). *Illness: The Cry of the Flesh*, revised edition. Durham, UK: Acumen.
The author uses her own illness experience to explore philosophical issues concerning the nature of illness with respect to its individual and social dimensions.

Carel, H., and Cooper, R. V., eds. (2012). *Health, Illness and Disease: Philosophical Essays*. Durham, UK: Acumen.
The book is a collection of essays that explore health and disease with respect to organic pathology and to the patient's lived experience and life-world.

Carson, R. A., and Burns, C. R., eds. (1997). *Philosophy of Medicine and Bioethics: A Twenty-Year Retrospective and Critical Appraisal*. Dordrecht: Kluwer.
The book consists of essays that cover the history, theory, and practice of medicine, as well as public policy issues in medicine.

Cassell, E. J. (2004). *The Nature of Suffering and the Goals of Medicine*, 2nd edition. New York: Oxford University Press.
The author provides a convincing argument for the goal of medicine as the relief of suffering through a therapeutic patient–physician relationship.

Cassell, E. J. (2015). *The Nature of Clinical Medicine: The Return of the Clinician*. New York: Oxford University Press.
The author explores the contemporary goals of medicine and how they relate to the practice of clinical medicine, from medical thinking to therapy.

Cassell, E. J., and Siegler, M., eds. (1979). *Changing Values in Medicine*. Frederick, MD: United Publications of America.

In a series of essays, various topics in the practice of medicine related to values are discussed—such as limits of clinical medicine, medical causation, centrality of attending physician, and patient rights.

Charon, R. (2006). *Narrative Medicine. Honoring the Stories of Illness*. New York: Oxford University Press.
The author develops a notion of narrative medicine and explicates the principles involved in its practice, especially with respect to narrative competence.

Childs, B. (1999). *Genetic Medicine: A Logic of Disease*. Baltimore, MD: The Johns Hopkins University Press.
The author's goal is the "geneticization" of medicine, with integration of genetics into medical research and clinical practice.

Clark, W. A. (1997). *The New Healers: The Promise and Problems of Molecular Medicine in the Twenty-First Century*. New York: Oxford University Press.
The author reconstructs the rise of molecular or genetic medicine and discusses the therapeutic and ethical challenges facing it in the twenty-first century.

Culver, C. M., and Bernard G. (1982). *Philosophy in Medicine: Conceptual and Ethical Issues in Medicine and Psychiatry*. Oxford: Oxford University Press.
The authors cover a variety of philosophical issues in medicine and psychiatry, including professional competence, rationality, physical diseases and mental maladies, and definitions of death.

Daly, J. (2005). *Evidence-Based Medicine and the Search for a Science of Clinical Care*. Berkeley: University of California Press.
The author discusses philosophical issues concerning the role of evidence-based medicine in clinical medicine both in terms of its achievements and its limitations.

Dolezal, L. (2015). *The Body and Shame: Phenomenology, Feminism, and the Socially Shaped Body*. Lanham, MD: Lexington Books.
The author explores the philosophical and phenomenological issues surrounding bodily shame and the medical and social efforts to reshape the body.

Dowie, J., and Elstein, A., eds. (1988). *Professional Judgment: A Reader in Clinical Decision Making*. Cambridge: Cambridge University Press.
The collection of essays focuses on uncertainty in clinical decision-making, on the nature of clinical reasoning from psychological, statistical, and process-tracing perspectives, and on the impact of economic, ethical, legal, and professional factors on clinical judgment.

Downie, R. S., Tannahill, C., and Tannahill, A. (1996). *Health Promotion: Models and Values*, 2nd edition. Oxford: Oxford University Press.
The authors examine the health promotion movement initiated in the second half of the twentieth century in terms of the models constructed to promote health and the values underlying the movement.

Drane, J. (1995). *Becoming a Good Doctor: The Place of Virtue and Character in Medical Ethics*, 2nd edition. Kansas City, MO: Sheed & Ward.
The author defines the "good doctor" in terms of virtues for both moral behavior and technical competence.

Engelhardt, Jr, H. T., ed. (2000). *The Philosophy of Medicine: Framing the Field*. New York: Springer.
The papers discuss a variety of philosophical and bioethical issues ranging from the embodied person to the nature of death and euthanasia and even to the role of urbanization and public policy on medical practice.

Engelhardt, Jr, H. T., and Spicker, S. F., eds. (1975). *Evaluation and Explanation in the Biomedical Sciences*. Dortrecht: Reidel.
From epistemological, phenomenological, and ethical perspectives, the essays cover a range of topics concerning the evaluation of medical knowledge and its role in medical explanation.

Engelhardt, Jr, H. T., Spicker, S. F., and Towers, B., eds. (1979). *Clinical Judgment: A Critical Appraisal*. Dordrecht: Reidel.
The papers explore the various elements of clinical judgment, including intuitions, hunches, rules, and the role of logic.

Evans, A. S. (1993). *Causation and Disease: A Chronological Journey*. New York, NY: Plenum Publishing Corporation.
The author traces the historical development of disease causation from germ theory to contemporary chronic diseases.

Evans, M., Louhiala, P., and Puustinen, R., eds. (2004). *Philosophy for Medicine: Applications in a Clinical Context*. Oxford: Radcliffe Publishing.
The essays address the theoretical and practical issues facing medical science, including clinical encounter and uncertainty, clinical aesthetics and morality, and the nature of clinical medicine.

Feinstein, A. R. (1967). *Clinical Judgment*. Huntington, NY: Krieger.
This book is a classic on clinical judgment and has been hailed as revolutionary in its approach.

Foss, L. (2002). *The End of Modern Medicine: Biomedical Science under a Microscope*. New York: SUNY Press.
The author offers a postmodern critique of the standard biomedical model, especially its mind–body dualism, and proposes a "psychobiological" model for disease ontology and etiology.

Frampton, S. B., and Charmel, P. A., eds. (2009). *Putting Patients First: Best Practices in Patient-Centered Care*, 2nd edition. San Francisco: Wiley.
The book is an introduction to the Planetree philosophy of patient-centered healthcare, which stresses proactive healthcare.

Frankel, R. M., Quill, T. E., and McDaniel, S. H., eds. (2003). *The Biopsychosocial Approach: Past, Present, and Future*. Rochester, NY: University Rochester Press.
The essays cover a wide range of topics concerning the biopsychosocial model, from its historical origins and philosophical perspective to its impact on clinical pedagogy and practice.

Fulford, K. W. M., Peile, E., and Carroll, H. (2012). *Essential Values-Based Practice: Clinical Stories Linking Science with People*. New York: Cambridge University Press.
The book is an introductory text to the role of values in clinical practice, with the goal of equipping the clinician with the necessary skills to include values in the clinical encounter.

Gadamer, H.-G. (1996). *The Enigma of Health: The Art of Healing in a Scientific Age*. Stanford, CA: Stanford University Press.
The author argues for a humanistic approach to the practice of medicine in which clinicians engage in hermeneutical interpretation of the patient's illness.

Ghaemi, S. N. (2010). *The Rise and Fall of the Biopsychosocial Model: Reconciling Art and Science in Psychiatry*. Baltimore, MD: The Johns Hopkins University Press.
The author conducts a critical historical and philosophical analysis of the biopsychosocial model, claiming it failed to deliver the promised humanistic care, and he proposes an alternative model to replace it.

Gifford, F., ed. (2011). *Philosophy of Medicine*. Oxford: Elsevier.
A wide range of topics in the philosophy of medicine are presented, from both a theoretical and a practical perspective.

Gluckman, P., Beedle, A., and Hanson, M. (2009). *Principles of Evolutionary Medicine*. New York: Oxford University Press.
The book represents an introduction to the principles of evolutionary medicine and its application to clinical practice.

Golub, E. S. (1997). *The Limits of Medicine: How Science Shapes Our Hope for the Cure*. Chicago, IL: University of Chicago Press.
In terms of the molecular biology revolution in the biomedical sciences, the author explores the limits of medicine and their implications for clinical medicine.

Greenhalgh, T., and Hurwitz, B., eds. (1998). *Narrative Based Medicine: Dialogue and Discourse in Clinical Practice*. London: BMJ Books.
The essays explore the nature of narrative-based medicine and its relevance for clinical practice, as well as for medical education and ethics.

Groopman, J. (2007). *How Doctors Think*. Boston, MA: Houghton Mifflin.
The author discusses the cognitive processes physicians use to make clinical decisions, which he illustrates from his own clinical experience.

Gupta, M. (2014). *Is Evidence-Based Psychiatry Ethical?* Oxford: Oxford University Press.
The author asks an important question about the relationship between evidence-based medicine and psychiatry and provides an insightful analysis of the relationship in terms of the ethics of practice.

Guyatt, G. H., Rennie, D., Meade, M. O., et al., eds. (2008). *Users' Guides to the Medical Literature: A Manual for Evidence-Based Clinical Practice*, 2nd edition. New York: McGraw-Hill.
The book is a practical manual for evidence-based medicine, with an introductory chapter providing a philosophical analysis of its principles.

Halpern, J. (2001). *From Detached Concern to Empathy: Humanizing Medical Practice*. New York: Oxford University Press.
The author argues for the inclusion of empathy in clinical practice, in contrast to the traditional stance of emotionally detached concern.

Higgs, J., and Jones, M. A., eds. (2008). *Clinical Reasoning in the Health Professions*, 3rd edition. Amsterdam: Elsevier.
In close to fifty chapters, almost every topic germane to clinical reasoning is covered, including its nature, the role of clinical expertise, and pedagogical issues.

Howick, J. H. (2011). *The Philosophy of Evidence-Based Medicine*. Hoboken, NJ: Wiley-Blackwell.
The author provides a first-rate philosophical analysis of evidence-based medicine, especially in terms of the nature of "good" evidence and clinical trials, and addresses its critics with respect to clinical expertise and mechanistic reasoning.

Humber, J. M., and Almeder, R. F., eds. (1997). *What Is Disease?* Totowa, NJ: Humana Press.
Focusing on Boorse's naturalistic approach, the contributors address various issues concerning the nature of disease and how to define it.

Huneman, P., Lambert, G., and Silberstein, M., eds. (2015). *Classification, Disease and Evidence: New Essays in the Philosophy of Medicine*. New York: Springer.
The essays canvas recent discussions concerning the nature and classification of disease, from genetic to psychiatric disorders.

Hunter, K. M. (1991). *Doctor's Stories: The Narrative Structure of Medical Knowledge*. Princeton, NJ: Princeton University Press.
The author argues that medicine is an interpretative profession, as well as a science, which depends on the patient's story as reflected in the doctor's story.

Illari, P., and Russo, F. (2014). *Causality: Philosophical Theory Meets Scientific Practice*. Oxford: Oxford University Press.
The authors provide a comprehensive analysis of causation in the natural sciences, especially the biomedical sciences, and propose a "mosaic" model to unify the pluralistic accounts of causation.

Illari, P., Russo, F., and Williamson, J., eds. (2011). *Causality in the Sciences*. New York: Oxford University Press.
The essays explore the notion and models of causality in the natural and social sciences, as well as in the healthcare sciences.

Jensen, U. J., and Mooney, G., eds. (1990). *Changing Values in Medical and Healthcare Decision-Making*. New York: John Wiley & Sons.
The contributors to the edited volume discuss the role of values in clinical decision-making and healthcare policy formation.

Johansson, I., and Lynøe, N. (2008). *Medicine & Philosophy: A Twenty-First Century Introduction*. Frankfurt: Ontos.
The authors provide an introduction to traditional philosophical issues in contemporary philosophy of medicine, especially from a biomedical perspective.

Kleinman, A. (1988). *The Illness Narratives: Suffering, Healing and the Human Condition*. New York: Basic Books.
The author argues for the inclusion of the patient's illness narrative into the treatment and management of chronic diseases.

Kligler, B., and Lee, R., eds. (2004). *Integrative Medicine: Principles for Practice*. New York: McGraw-Hill.
The book represents a comprehensive introduction to the principles of integrative medicine not only for primary care but also for medical specialties.

Larson, J. S. (1991). *The Measurement of Health: Concepts and Indicators*. New York: Greenwood Press.
The author examines the various models of health, as well as the indicators of health and their measurement.

Leder, D. (1990). *The Absent Body*. Chicago, IL: University of Chicago Press.
The author engages in a phenomenological analysis of the body, in terms of the ecstatic, recessive, and dys-appearing body, and then proceeds to discuss the philosophical implications with respect to the immaterial and threatening body.

Leder, D., ed. (1992). *The Body in Medical Thought and Practice*. New York: Springer.
The essays promote the humanization of clinical practice by focusing on the nature of the patient's body, not as object of medical scrutiny but as a person who is worthy of respect.

Lee, K. (2012). *The Philosophical Foundations of Modern Medicine*. New York: Palgrave Macmillan.
The author provides the reader with an introduction to various themes in the philosophy of medicine, especially disease causation, as they relate to contemporary philosophy of science.

Lieberman, D. E. (2013). *The Story of the Human Body: Evolution, Health, and Disease*. New York: Pantheon Books.

The author argues for the inclusion of human evolutionary history into conceptions of health and illness to address modern plagues, such as obesity and type 2 diabetes.

Lindemann Nelson, J., and Lindemann Nelson, H., eds. (1999). *Meaning and Medicine: A Reader in the Philosophy of Health Care*. London: Routledge.
A collection of articles taken from the philosophy of medicine literature that addresses metaphysical, epistemological, and ethical issues—including biomedical research, clinical practice, and healthcare administration and policy—challenging contemporary medicine.

Loughlin, M., ed. (2014). *Debates in Values-Based Practice: Arguments For and Against*. Cambridge: Cambridge University Press.
The essays examine the advantages and disadvantages of values-based medicine from both a philosophical and a practical perspective.

Maier, B., and Shibles, W. A. (2011). *The Philosophy and Practice of Medicine and Bioethics: A Naturalistic–Humanistic Approach*. New York: Springer.
The authors critically investigate the metaphors informing modern medical practices, especially evidence-based medicine, from a humanistic perspective.

Marcum, J. A. (2008). *An Introductory Philosophy of Medicine: Humanizing Modern Medicine*. New York: Springer.
The author examines the metaphysical, ontological, epistemological, and ethical challenges facing the humanization of scientific medicine.

Marcum, J. A. (2012). *The Virtuous Physician: The Role of Virtue in Medicine*. New York: Springer.
The author argues for the role of virtues in the practice of modern medicine to resolve its quality of care and professionalism crises.

McHugh, S., and Vallis, T. M., eds. (1986). *Illness Behavior: A Multidisciplinary Model*. New York: Plenum Press.
The book represents a collection of conference papers that explores illness behavior from multidisciplinary perspectives in order to forge an integrated model.

Meacham, D., ed. (2015). *Medicine and Society: New Perspectives in Continental Philosophy*. New York: Springer.
The essays canvas a wide range of topics within medicine from a continental philosophical framework, including phenomenological, hermeneutical, and poststructuralist perspectives.

Meehl, P. E. (1954). *Clinical versus Statistical Prediction: A Theoretical Analysis and a Review of the Evidence*. Minneapolis, MN: University of Minnesota Press.
The author demonstrates that formal or algorithmic methods are superior to traditional clinical methods for making sound diagnoses and prognoses.

Meza, J. P., and Passerman, D. S. (2011). *Integrating Narrative Medicine and Evidence-Based Medicine: The Everyday Social Practice of Healing*. London: Radcliffe.
The authors explore the social and philosophical issues associated with integrating evidence-based and narrative medicine, beginning with practical problems and culminating in theoretical challenges.

Miettinen, O. S. (2014). *Toward Scientific Medicine*. New York: Springer.
The author contends that contemporary medicine is actually prescientific and then proposes a rational theoretical framework for making it truly scientific, especially in terms of prognosis.

Mol, A. (2002). *The Body Multiple: Ontology in Medical Practice*. Durham, NC: Duke University Press.

Drawing on the medical example of atherosclerosis, the author discusses philosophical issues involved in disease-objectivity and illness-subjectivity distinctions.

Mol, A. (2008). *The Logic of Care: Health and the Problem of Patient Choice*. London: Routledge.
The author argues that quality of healthcare is not a factor of the "logic of choice" on the basis of patient as customer but on the outcome of a "logic of care" from collaborative efforts of those involved in clinical encounters.

Montgomery, K. (2006). *How Doctors Think: Clinical Judgment and the Practice of Medicine*. Oxford, UK: Oxford University Press.
The author contends that clinical judgment should reflect the process of Aristotelian *phronesis* in contrast to the hypothetical–deductive method of positive science.

More, E. S., and Milligan, M. A., eds. (1994). *The Empathic Practitioner: Empathy, Gender, and Medicine*. New Brunswick, NJ: Rutgers University Press.
The collection of essays examines the role of empathy in clinical practice, especially from a gender studies perspective.

Morris, D. B. (1998). *Illness and Culture in the Postmodern Age*. Berkeley, CA: University of California Press.
The author proposes that in the postmodern age the boundary between the concept of disease and the experience of illness has become blurred because of its "biocultural" model of health and disease.

Murphy, E. A. (1997). *The Logic of Medicine*, 2nd edition. Baltimore, MD: The Johns Hopkins University Press.
The author utilizes logic not in terms of formal clinical reasoning but with respect to clarifying ontological issues, such as causation, nature and classification of disease, and diagnostic uncertainty, and to examining epistemological challenges, such as modeling, biases, confounding, and standards in medical knowledge.

National Research Council (US) Committee on a Framework for Developing a New Taxonomy of Disease. (2011). *Toward Precision Medicine: Building a Knowledge Network for Biomedical Research and a New Taxonomy of Disease*. Washington, DC: National Academies Press (US).
The report discusses the efforts of the biomedical research community to define disease at the molecular level and the implications for public health and healthcare delivery.

Nesse, R. M., and Williams, G. C. (1996). *Why We Get Sick: The New Science of Darwinian Medicine*. New York: Vintage Books.
The authors explore the relevance of Darwinian evolution for biomedical research and clinical practice and for answering the question, "Why we get sick?"

Nordenfelt, L. (1995). *On the Nature of Health: An Action-Theory Approach*, 2nd edition. Dordrecht: Kluwer.
The author proposes and defends a holistic theory of health based on action theory in which health reflects the ability of a person to achieve vital goals.

Nordenfelt, L., Ingemar, B., and Lindahl, B., eds. (1984). *Health, Disease, and Causal Explanations in Medicine*. Dordrecht: Kluwer.
The essays cover a range of philosophical topics concerning the nature of health and disease, and medical causation and explanation—especially as they pertain to the practice of medicine.

Nordenfelt, L., and Tengland, P.-A., eds. (1996). *The Goals and Limits of Medicine*. Stockholm: Almqvist & Wiksell International.
The essays address the various goals of modern medicine and the limits that challenge their realization.

Pellegrino, E. D. (1979). *Humanism and the Physician*. Knoxville, TN: University of Tennessee Press.
The author argues for the role of the humanities in medical education and practice, which includes philosophical and ethical issues.

Pellegrino, E. D. (2008). *The Philosophy of Medicine Reborn: A Pellegrino Reader*. Notre Dame, IN: University of Notre Dame Press.
The reader represents a collection of Pellegrino's seminal essays, with an introductory essay discussing their significance for contemporary philosophy of medicine.

Pellegrino, E. D., and Thomasma, D. C. (1981). *A Philosophical Basis of Medical Practice: Toward a Philosophy and Ethic of the Healing Professions*. New York: Oxford University Press.
The authors provide an insightful introduction to the philosophical issues that challenge contemporary medical practice, especially its moral imperative to benefit the patient.

Pellegrino, E. D., and Thomasma, D. C. (1993). *The Virtues in Medical Practice*. New York: Oxford University Press.
The authors explore virtue theory and the role of virtues, such as fidelity, trust, compassion, *phronesis*, justice, fortitude, and temperance in medical education and practice.

Pellegrino, E. D., and Thomasma, D. C. (1996). *The Christian Virtues in Medical Practice*. Washington, DC: Georgetown University Press.
The authors develop a notion of the Christian personalist physician in terms of Christian virtue ethics and the theological virtues of faith, hope, and charity.

Philips, C. I., ed. (1995). *Logic in Medicine*, 2nd edition. London: BMJ Publishing.
The book is a collection of essays, originally published individually in the *British Medical Journal*, which explore the role of logic in clinical reasoning and decision-making.

Rabins, P. V. (2013). *The Why of Things: Causality in Science, Medicine, and Life*. New York: Columbia University Press.
The author discusses the perplexing questions of causality in the natural, biomedical, and social sciences, and introduces a "three-facet" model of causality to address them.

Rakel, D., ed. (2012). *Integrative Medicine*, 3rd edition. Philadelphia: Elsevier.
The textbook chapters inform the reader about a variety of practical topics for practicing integrative medicine, including an introductory chapter on its philosophical issues.

Reznek, L. (1987). *The Nature of Disease*. London: Routledge & Kegan Paul.
The author contends that disease is not a natural kind as a mind-independent object but rather a value-dependent concept.

Rothman, K. J., ed. (1988). *Causal Inference*. Chestnut Hill, MA: Epidemiology Resources.
The essays examine the conceptual and methodological issues surrounding the notion of causal inference in epidemiology, especially from a Popperian perspective.

Sadegh-Zadeh, K. (2015). *Handbook of Analytic Philosophy of Medicine*, 2nd edition. New York: Springer.
The author's intention is to bring clarity to philosophical issues for the metaphysical, methodological, epistemological, logical, and ethical foundations of medicine in order to improve the clinical encounter.

Schaffner, K. F., ed. (1985). *Logic of Discovery and Diagnosis in Medicine*. Berkeley, CA: University of California Press.
The essays discuss a number of topics related to diagnosis, discovery, clinical evaluation, and nosology, as well as the role of computers in clinical diagnosis.

Schaffner, K. F. (1993). *Discovery and Explanation in Biology and Medicine*. Chicago, IL: University of Chicago Press.

The author argues for logical pragmatism in analyzing discovery, natural laws, empirical testing, causation, historical and teleological explanations, and reductionism in the biomedical sciences.

Seifert, J. (2004). *The Philosophical Diseases of Medicine and Their Cure. Philosophy and Ethics of Medicine, Vol. 1: Foundations*. New York: Springer.
The author discusses the philosophical "diseases" or crises facing modern medicine, especially with its emphasis on the scientific and technological, and explores a possible "cure" or resolution.

Seising, R., and Tabacchi, M. E., eds. (2013). *Fuzziness and Medicine: Philosophical Reflections and Application Systems in Health Care*. New York: Springer.
The essays serve as a companion to Sadegh-Zadeh's *Handbook of Analytic Philosophy of Medicine*, by exploring the intersection between fuzziness and medicine.

Shelp, E. E., ed. (1985). *Virtue and Medicine: Explorations in the Character of Medicine*. Dordrecht: Reidel.
The essays represent one of the first contemporary explorations for the role of virtues in medical practice.

Slatman, J. (2014). *Our Strange Body: Philosophical Reflections on Identity and Medical Interventions*. Amsterdam: Amsterdam University Press.
The author argues that the conception of the body entails a "strangeness," which allows the body to be reshaped through medical technology—without compromising its individual identity.

Smart, B. (2016). *Concepts and Causes in the Philosophy of Disease*. New York: Palgrave Macmillan.
The author explores the debate over the nature of disease, especially in terms of what it means for the practicing clinician.

Solomon, M. (2015). *Making Medical Knowledge*. New York: Oxford University Press.
The author proposes a pluralistic account to address the epistemological issues associated with the production of medical knowledge in terms of consensus conferences, evidence-based medicine, translational medicine, and narrative medicine.

Spiro, H., McCrea Curnen, M. G., Peschel, E., et al., eds. (1992). *Empathy and the Practice of Medicine: Beyond Pills and the Scalpel*. New Haven, CT: Yale University Press.
In the collection of essays, the contributors discuss the nature of empathy and its role in clinical practice and medical education.

Stearns, S. C., and Koella, J. C., eds. (2008). *Evolution in Health and Disease*, 2nd edition. Oxford: Oxford University Press.
The essays address a variety of topics concerning medical theory and practice from an evolutionary perspective.

Stempsey, W. E. (2000). *Disease and Diagnosis: Value-Dependent Realism*. Dordrecht: Kluwer.
The author proposes "value-dependent realism" to account for the role of values in clinical diagnoses and practice.

Stewart, M., Brown, J. B., Weston, W. W., et al. (2003). *Patient-Centered Medicine: Transforming the Clinical Method*, 2nd edition. Abington, UK: Radcliffe Medical Press.
The authors introduce the fundamental principles of patient-centered medicine and discuss the six components comprising the patient-centered clinical method.

Svenaeus, F. (2000). *The Hermeneutics of Medicine and the Phenomenology of Health: Steps towards a Philosophy of Medical Practice*. Dordrecht: Kluwer.
The author applies phenomenological hermeneutics to examine the nature of health and illness, and the practice of clinical medicine—especially in terms of the patient–physician relationship.

Tauber, A. I. (1999). *Confessions of a Medicine Man: An Essay in Popular Philosophy.* Cambridge, MA: MIT Press.
Although partly autobiographical, the book is deeply philosophical in that the author engages substantive metaphysical, epistemological, and ethical issues that face clinicians daily.

Tauber, A. I. (2005). *Patient Autonomy and the Ethics of Responsibility.* Cambridge, MA: MIT Press.
The author argues that the principle of patient autonomy unfortunately has crippled the clinician in terms of fulfilling his or her fiduciary responsibility to the patient and proposes an ethic of care to revive the delivery of quality care.

Tavris, D. R. (1997). *Philosophy in Epidemiology and Public Health.* Commack, NY: Nova Science.
The author examines the philosophical issues emerging in both epidemiology and public health, such as causation, animal experimentation, infectious diseases, health and disease, and confidentiality and malpractice.

Ten Have, H. A. M. J., Kimsma, G. K., and Spicker, S. F., eds. (1990). *The Growth of Medical Knowledge.* Dordrecht: Kluwer.
The essays focus on the question of whether progress in the biomedical sciences is comparable to progress in the natural sciences; and if so, how the former is similar or different from the latter.

Thagard, P. (1999). *How Scientists Explain Disease.* Princeton, NJ: Princeton University Press.
The author explores the philosophical issues with how biomedical scientists explain the cause of disease through their discoveries of pathophysiological mechanisms.

Toombs, S. K. (1993). *The Meaning of Illness: A Phenomenological Account of the Different Perspectives of Physician and Patient.* Dordrecht: Kluwer.
The author enlists phenomenology to discuss various perspectives of the patient–physician relationship with respect to the meaning of the illness experience and for forming a healing relationship.

Toombs, S. K., ed. (2001). *Handbook of Phenomenology and Medicine.* New York: Springer.
The essays begin with an introduction to the role of phenomenology in medicine and then proceed to topics such as the body in illness and the patient's lived experience, as well as practical issues in clinical practice and research.

Toon, P. D. (1999). *Towards a Philosophy of General Practice: A Study of the Virtuous Practitioner.* London: Royal College of General Practitioners.
The author provides an introduction to the role of virtues in the practice of general or family medicine to benefit both patient and physician.

Trevathan, W., Smith, E. O., and McKenna, J. J., eds. (2008). *Evolutionary Medicine and Health: New Perspectives.* New York: Oxford University Press.
The essays explore various research topics in evolutionary medicine, particularly from an anthropological perspective, such as nutrition and diet, sex and reproduction, and the evolutionary role of environment and ecology in health and disease.

Tutton, R. (2014). *Genomics and the Reimagining of Personalized Medicine.* Farnham, UK: Ashgate.
The author explores the role of genomics in grounding personalized medicine and discusses its limits.

Twaddle, A., and Nordenfelt, L. (1994). *Disease, Illness and Sickness: Three Central Concepts in Theory of Health.* Linköping, Sweden: Linköping University, Department of Health and Society.

The book is a record of a dialogue between Twaddle and Nordenfelt over their conceptions of disease, illness, and sickness.

Van Der Steen, W. J., and Thung, P. J. (1988). *Faces of Medicine: A Philosophical Study*. Dordrecht: Kluwer.
The authors discuss the philosophical themes emerging from medicine's theoretical basis, such as health and disease, and medical cure, as well as from its practice, including psychosomatic, biopsychosocial, and alternative medicine.

Weil, A. (2004). *Health and Healing: The Philosophy of Integrative Medicine and Optimum Health*, revised edition. New York: Houghton Mifflin.
The author provides a popular approach to the integration of complementary medicine and traditional Western medicine and covers a wide range of topics, such as the nature of health, curing and healing, the mind–body relationship, and allopathic and homeopathic therapies.

West, B. J. (2006). *Where Medicine Went Wrong: Rediscovering the Path to Complexity*. Hackensack, NJ: World Scientific Publishing Co.
The author argues for a reorientation of the biomedical science in terms of complexity science and fractal physiology in order to account for health and disease.

White, M., and Epston, D. (1990). *Narrative Means to Therapeutic Ends*. New York: Norton & Co.
The authors discuss the importance of patient's illness narrative in the therapy process and provide stories illustrating narrative's therapeutic power.

Wulff, H. R., Pedesen, S. A., and Rosenberg, R. (1990). *Philosophy of Medicine: An Introduction*, 2nd edition. Oxford, UK: Blackwell.
The authors provide an introductory philosophical analysis of issues challenging clinical practice, including the nature of medicine and disease, empiricism and realism, causality, the mind–body problem, psychiatric naturalism, and medical sociology and ethics.

Zaner, R. M. (1981). *The Context of Self: A Phenomenological Inquiry Using Medicine as a Clue*. Athens, OH: Ohio University Press.
The author develops a phenomenological notion of self and embodiment for a robust practice of medicine.

Zaner, R. M. (2004). *Conversations on the Edge: Narratives of Ethics and Illness*. Washington, DC: Georgetown University Press.
The author explores a variety of narratives concerning death and dying and the philosophical lessons learned from them.

Zeiler, K., and Käll, L., eds. (2014). *Feminist Phenomenology and Medicine*. New York: SUNY Press.
The essays explore the multiple dimensions involved in the intersection between medical practices and feminist phenomenology, from both conceptual and methodological perspectives.

Index

abnormal 7, 78, 81, 85–6, 135, 221, 236–8, 242, 244, 263, 285
absolutism 14, 371, 383
adaptation 50, 150, 153, 157, 280, 356
allocation bias 8, 120–1, 123–5
alternative medicine 3, 20, 379, 402
analytical 3, 14, 34, 207, 210, 329, 371
Arendt, H. 11, 193, 195, 206
Aristotle 33, 176, 210, 219, 230, 281–2, 317, 335–9
art of medicine 5, 10, 13, 24, 325
autonomy 13, 189, 192, 237, 250–3, 267, 269, 290, 330, 371

Beauvoir, S. de 228, 231, 235, 244
being-in-the-world 11–12, 193, 196, 200, 208, 210–17, 220, 263
Beneficence 371
Bernard, C. 136–7, 175, 317
bioethics 209, 214, 260–1, 270, 343
biomarker 7, 73–6, 78–82, 87, 371
biomedical/medical ethics 33, 172, 206–7, 259, 275
biomedical/medical research 7, 13, 18, 20, 46–7, 49–51, 54, 66, 68, 70, 72, 74–5, 82–7, 186, 188–9, 238, 241, 287, 343, 345–7, 349, 358–63, 384–5, 393, 397–8
biopsychosocial model 4, 19, 21, 24, 252
Boorse, C. 15, 155, 227, 276–9, 284–5, 395

Canguilhem, G. 75–6, 78, 88
caring 158, 173, 235, 250, 265–7
cascade model of disease 7, 74, 76–7, 79, 82–3, 87
Cassell, E. 14, 214, 252, 254, 262, 325, 336
causal inference 8, 97, 102–5, 108–9, 310, 344, 399
causal interpretation problem 8, 97, 101–3
causal mosaic metaphor 15–17, 299–302, 316–9, 396
causal pie 8, 98, 315–16
causal reasoning 30, 260, 300, 307, 310–11
causality/causation 4, 7–8, 15–17, 29–31, 34, 39, 47–8, 52, 71, 96–7, 99, 101, 104–5,

108–10, 128, 131, 176, 297–319, 337, 344, 372–3, 391–4, 396, 398–402
clinical care 7, 18, 38, 183, 251, 347
clinical decision-making 15, 17, 22, 30, 38–9, 42–4, 48, 58, 129, 250, 264–5, 302, 324, 327–9, 331–4, 336, 391, 393, 399
clinical expertise 8–9, 39, 119, 134, 324, 372, 395–5
clinical judging/judgment 17, 34, 117, 253, 325–30, 339, 372, 393–4, 398
clinical knowing/knowledge 17, 20, 200, 255, 323–38
clinical outcome 19, 21–2, 46, 52, 73, 254–6, 371
clinical reasoning 4, 17, 33–4, 36, 58, 323–39, 391, 393, 395, 398–9
cognition 17, 164–6, 227, 255, 264, 324, 327–34, 336–8, 357–8, 372–3, 377–8, 395
cognitive bias 328–9, 337, 372
cohort study 8, 105, 121, 301, 372, 374, 383
comparative clinical study 116–17, 119–20, 129–31
compassion 11, 18, 23, 36–7, 184–5, 189, 201, 219, 250, 256, 266–7
complexity 6, 16–18, 53, 82–5, 167, 185, 303, 312, 338, 358, 360
consciousness 173, 198, 214, 260, 264, 324, 334, 338, 372, 382
contingency 84–6, 196, 201, 315
counterfactual 8, 16, 105, 107, 316–17, 372
critical reasoning/thinking 328, 372, 382
cure 11–12, 23, 38–40, 45, 68, 113, 120, 136, 138, 148, 150, 190, 193, 206, 220, 256, 262, 286, 317, 359, 372–3

Darwin/Darwinian evolution 147–8, 150–7, 169–70, 175–6, 375, 398
Dasein 175, 193–6
death 11–12, 118, 120, 128, 130, 148, 153, 157, 183–5, 188, 191–200, 215, 222–3, 231–2, 283, 287, 313–15, 391, 393, 401
decision analysis 17, 326–7, 333
deficiency disease 16, 307, 314
demedicalization 16, 290–1

403